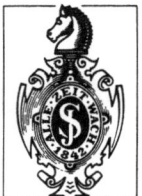

Margot Shiner

Ultrastructure of the Small Intestinal Mucosa

Normal and disease-related appearances

Foreword by Sir Francis Avery Jones

With 165 Figures

Springer-Verlag
Berlin Heidelberg New York 1983

Margot Shiner FRCP, FRCPath, DCH

Member, Scientific Staff, Medical Research Council,
Clinical Research Centre, Harrow, Middlesex
Hon. Consultant in Gastroenterology,
Central Middlesex Hospital, Park Royal, London
and Northwick Park Hospital, Harrow, Middlesex, UK

ISBN-13: 978-1-4471-1340-9   e-ISBN-13:978-1-4471-1338-6
DOI: 10.1007/978-1-4471-1338-6

Library of Congress Cataloging in Publication Data
Shiner, Margot, 1923– Ultrastructure of the Small Intestinal Mucosa
Bibliography: p. Includes index. 1. Intestine, Small – Diseases. 2. Ultrastructure (Biology).
3. Diagnosis, Electron microscopic. I. Title. [DNLM: 1. Intestinal mucosa – Ultrastructure.
2. Intestine, Small – Ultrastructure. 3. Microscopy, Electron. WI 500 S556s] RC802.9.S48 1982
616.3′4 82-10333

2128/3916 543210

To my mother,
husband and children,
and in memory of my father

Foreword

This book represents the culmination of the major aspect of Dr. Margot Shiner's professional career. It was she who devised the technique of jejunal biopsy which opened up whole new fields of small intestinal research, including microbiology, immunology, histochemistry and histopathology, thus greatly expanding our knowledge of fundamental aspects of absorptive pathophysiology. Later the application of electron microscopy demonstrated the individual cell with its mechanisms both for absorption and for the production of so many chemicals such as mucus, enzymes and hormones. Like the vision from the peak in Darian, it opened up new worlds. The contribution to our understanding of cell structure and function has been greater than the direct elucidation of specific diseases but nevertheless, there are pointers to different mechanisms which could have wide applications.

It is a book which serves a double function: On the one hand it is highly technical and a publication for the super expert, recording new landmarks of knowledge and interpretation. On the other hand, it is a book which can indeed fire the imagination of the rising generation of gastroenterologists, paediatricians, pathologists and medical scientists.

Having seen the emergence of the art and science of present-day gastroenterology within my professional lifetime and having been able to provide the facilities for her work in the very early days, it is with particular pleasure and pride that I write this foreword.

London, October 1982

Sir Francis Avery Jones,
CBE, MD(London), FRCP(London)
Consulting Gastroenterologist
Central Middlesex Hospital

Acknowledgements

It is with intense gratitude that I acknowledge all the physicians who kindly referred their patients to me for study and all scientific and nursing staff whose help has made it possible to carry out this work.

To my former teachers, Sir Francis Avery Jones, Professor Dame Sheila Sherlock, Dr. E. N. Rowlands and Dr. P. D. Kellock, I owe a debt which words are inadequate to express. Without their generous support and encouragement over the years of gastroenterological investigation and research, this work would not have been possible. I can only hope that this book will justify their trust in me.

I also gratefully and specifically acknowledge the help of my associates, Mrs. E. E. Cox, Mrs. J. Ballard and Mr. R. Sapsford, in the technical execution of this study.

Lastly my thanks go to my husband Alex, who for 35 years of 'coexistence' with my professional activities has patiently borne my eccentricities, which go inevitably with the medical profession and research. His help and encouragement in writing this book have been invaluable.

Preface

No comprehensive book on the electron microscopy of the human jejunal mucosa in disease has been published to date. This atlas of normal and pathological ultrastructure is aimed at extending present knowledge in this field [5], though it is recognised that the gastrointestinal diseases studied are necessarily limited.

With the development of peroral small bowel biopsy [1–4], the human jejunal mucosa became the subject of intense biological and morphological interest. Though the technique is recognised today as an important tool in the diagnosis of gastrointestinal disease and much is known about the histopathological changes affecting the mucosa, less attention has been paid by clinicians and pathologists to advance that knowledge to the field of the electron microscope (EM). This book therefore aims to correlate a brief clinical and histological presentation of diseases such as coeliac disease (adults and children), cow's milk protein intolerance in infants, protein-energy malnutrition in childhood and a variety of other gastrointestinal diseases with the representative ultrastructural illustrations, and thereby hopes to provide an insight into the organisation of specialised cells of the mucosa essential for an appreciation of the derangement in functions which results when cells undergo pathological changes.

The EM should be used first and foremost to complement and extend the field of light microscopy, for only at higher magnification can the intricate structure of the enterocyte (villous columnar epithelium) and its microvilli, forming the histologist's brush border, be appreciated. These microvilli vastly increase the surface area of each enterocyte and the numerous digestive enzymes located in or on their membranes facilitate the transport of luminal substances through the cell itself. The fine structure of the organelles of the enterocyte allows an appreciation of its function as a 'factory' where organised information is passed from the nucleus to the endoplasmic reticulum and the mitochondria by ribosomes and from there to the Golgi complex, which elaborates material necessary for the protection and function of the cell. A very different picture is seen when the function and ultrastructure of normal enterocytes is altered, as in coeliac disease. The EM clearly shows the loss as well as the structural deformity of the microvilli which undoubtedly results in defects in their digestive-absorptive function. It further demonstrates the cellular immaturity and lack of organisation of its organelles. We cannot be certain that these are specific for coeliac disease, for excessive extrusion of enterocytes, lesser changes in their microvilli, increase in lysosomes and abnormalities in mitochondrial structure are also observed in other diseases affecting the mucosa. The identification and heterogeneity of the fine structure of the interepithelial cells (theliolymphocytes) so clearly seen with the light microscope offer an excellent chance for study with the EM. This also applies to the structure of cells supported by the connective tissue of the lamina propria, their relation to each other and to the enterocytes themselves and their fine structural alteration in the diseased mucosa. The importance of further study of the lamina propria cells cannot be over-estimated, and their role in the pathogenesis of gastrointestinal diseases affecting the jejunal mucosa may await more specialised techniques than conventional EM.

Lastly the EM allows the identification of specific disease-associated abnormalities denied to light microscopy. A foremost example of this is Whipple's disease, characterised by the fine structural identification of intact bacterial forms in the cells and connective tissue of the jejunal mucosa. In acrodermatitis enteropathica, specific (? lysosomal) abnormalities with Paneth cells have been identified with this disease. The intimate association of bacteria, viruses and parasites with mucosal cells in certain diseases can usefully be studied only with the EM. The recognition of early malignant changes in the fine structure of mucosal cells deserves special attention. No doubt this list of indications for ultrastructural investigation in specific gastrointestinal diseases will be greatly extended in the future.

This collection of EM material represents the personal and subjective study of a clinician whose overriding interest for the past 25 years has been the morphology of the human jejunal mucosa and its diagnostic significance. It has been a natural follow-up of the author's development of the peroral jejunal biopsy tube, which has opened new horizons in gastroenterology—including EM. The book is intended to arouse the interest and enthusiasm of gastroenterologists, paediatricians, pathologists and the medical student.

Harrow, Middlesex, 1982   Margot Shiner

References

1. Crosby WH, Kugler HW (1957 Intraluminal biopsy of the small intestine. The intestinal biopsy capsule. Am J Dig Dis 2:236–241
2. Royer M, Croxatto O, Biempica L, Ballazer-Morrison AJ (1955) Biopsia duodenal por aspiracion bajo control radioscopico. Prensa Med Argentina 42:2515–2519
3. Shiner M (1956) Duodenal biopsy. Lancet i: 17–19
4. Shiner M (1956) Jejunal biopsy tube. Lancet i:85
5. Toner, PG, Carr KE, Al Yassin TM (1980) Small intestine. In: Johannessen JV (ed) Electron microscopy in human medicine, vol 7. Digestive system. McGraw-Hill, London, pp 132–168

Contents

Introduction

Clinical material

Jejunal mucosal biopsies were obtained from more than 250 patients:

Chapter 1. Adults and children suspected of having gastrointestinal disease but not proven after extensive investigation. Their biopsies were histologically normal (Fig. 1) and therefore the EM was regarded as a *control.*

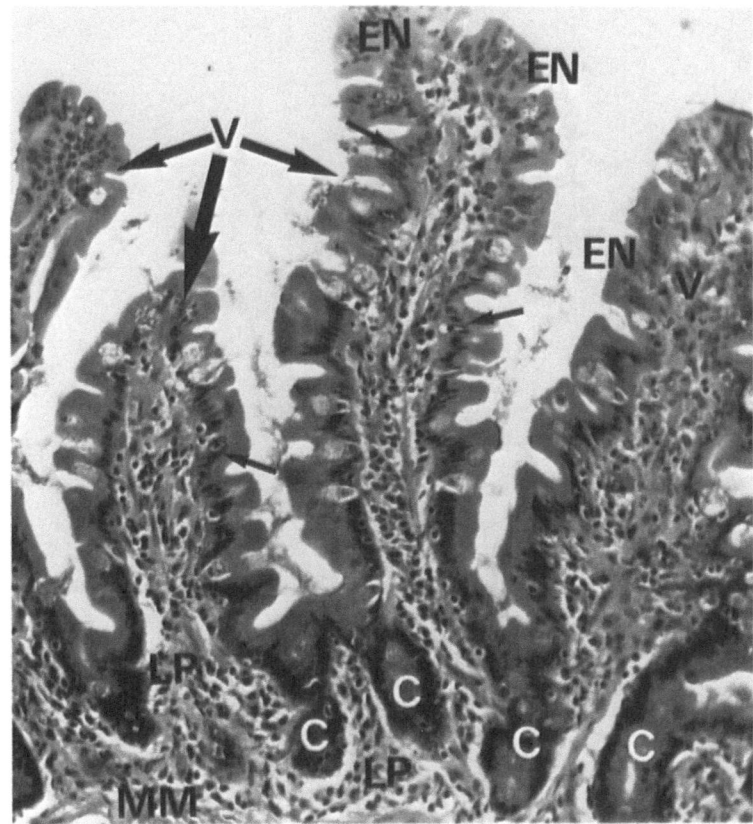

Fig. 1. Histology of normal jejunal mucosa. The villi are tall and covered by columnar epithelium enterocytes with basally situated nuclei (*arrows*). The crypts of Lieberkühn are short and straight and extend from the crypt–villus junction to the muscularis mucosae. The lamina propria contains many different types of cell nuclei. *V*, villi, *EN*, columnar epithelium or enterocyte; *C*, crypts; *MM*, muscularis mucosae; *LP*, lamina propria. (H & E ×200)

Chapter 2. Adults and children clinically diagnosed as having *coeliac disease*, a diagnosis confirmed by the histological mucosal appearance of a subtotal villous atrophy (Fig. 2a). The EM of these patients was regarded as an example of untreated coeliac disease and contrasted with that obtained after a period of gluten-free diet in which the histology had reverted to normal or near normal. Diagnostic challenge studies with gluten were carried out in a number of these patients at various time-intervals after gluten ingestion and, following repeat biopsy, the material was studied both histologically and ultrastructurally.

Chapter 3. Children clinically diagnosed as having an *allergy to cow's milk proteins*. The jejunal mucosa of these patients showed, in most instances, the third type of histological abnormality—a partial villous atrophy (Fig. 2b). The patients were also subjected to repeat biopsies after a period of milk elimination diet and subsequent milk challenge. All mucosal biopsies (as well as those in Chaps. 4 and 5) were studied histologically and ultrastructurally.

Chapter 4. Kwashiorkor and marasmus in children.

Chapter 5. Miscellaneous. This heading includes adults with malignancies affecting the small intestinal tract, mainly lymphomas and immunoprolifera-

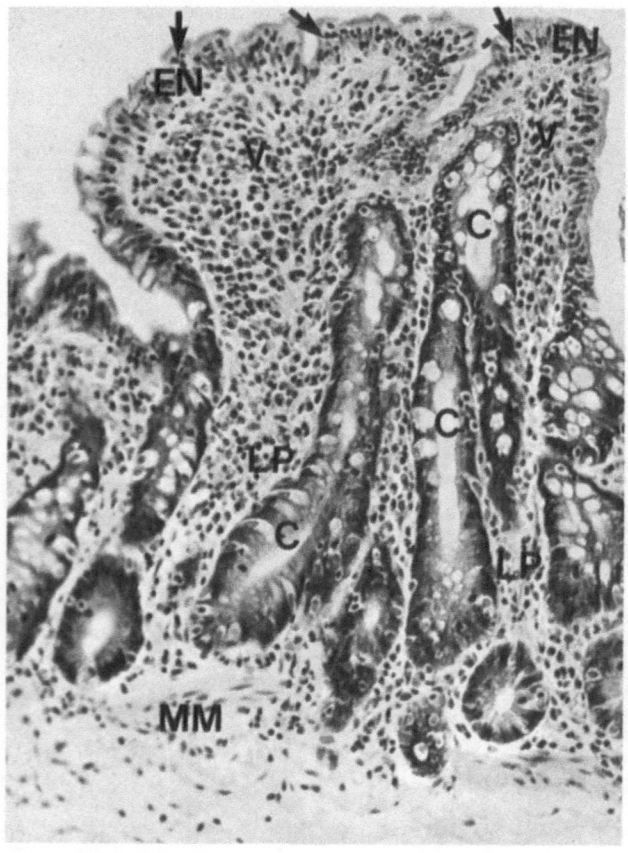

Fig. 2a Histology of jejunal mucosa in subtotal villous atrophy. The villi (*V*) are very short and broad and are covered by cuboidal epithelium (*EN*). Numerous theliolymphocyte nuclei (*arrows*) are seen in the epithelial layer. The crypts (*C*) are elongated and the villi and lamina propria (*LP*) contain increased numbers of inflammatory cells. *MM*, muscularis mucosae. (H & E ×200)

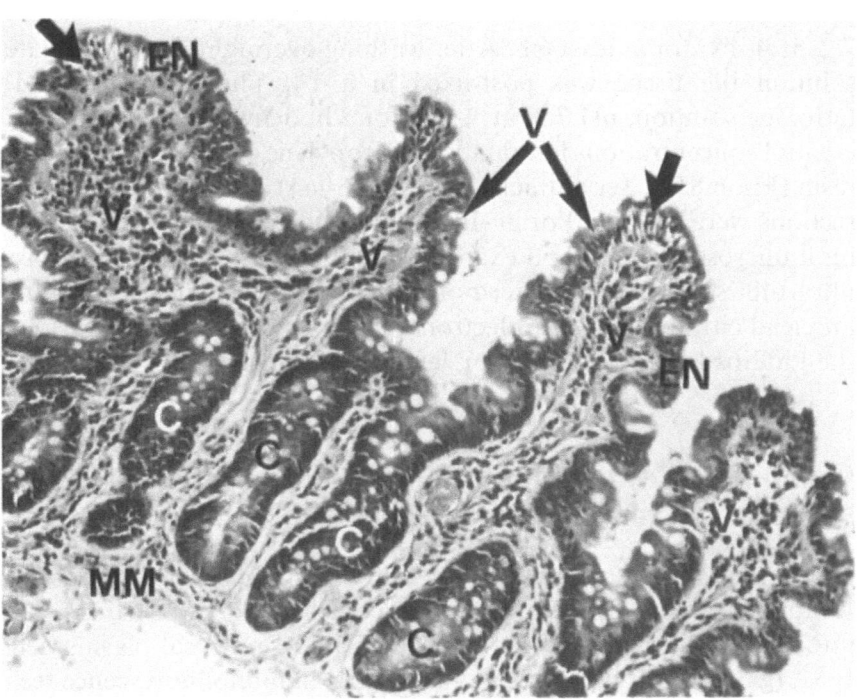

Fig. 2b Histology of jejunal mucosa in partial villous atrophy. The villi (*V*) are shorter than normal and often broader. The villous epithelium (*EN*) is usually normal but may be reduced in height. Theliolymphocytes (*arrows*) are increased. The crypts (*C*) are invariably lengthened and the inflammatory infiltrate is greater than normal. *MM*, muscularis mucosae. (H & E × 180)

tive small intestinal disease, identification of parasites, cysts or ova and their relation to the underlying mucosa, Whipple's disease, acrodermatitis enteropathica, multiple sclerosis and inflammatory bowel disease.

Technique of peroral jejunal biopsy

The great majority of mucosal biopsies were obtained with the Shiner jejunal biopsy capsule or the Crosby capsule (or a modification of the latter) [1]. The capsule was guided to the first part of the jejunum under fluoroscopic control. The adult capsule has a biopsy port of up to 3.5 mm diameter and the children's capsule may have a 1.0- to 2.5-mm diameter port, using a one or two port hole capsule [4]. Thus either single or multiple biopsies were obtained. These biopsies were apportioned into various fixatives for histology and electron microscopy, great care being taken to avoid delay between severing and fixing the mucosal samples.

Technique for electron microscopy

The portion of mucosa destined for electron microscopy was cut into 1- to 2-mm cubes and routinely fixed in a 3 % glutaraldehyde–cacodylate solution, pH

7.2, at +4°C for at least 6 h. After washing overnight in a cacodylate–sucrose solution the tissue was post-fixed in a 1% phosphate buffered osmium tetroxide solution, pH 7.3, at +4°C for 2 h, dehydrated in a graded series of ethanol concentrations terminating in propylene oxide and embedded in epoxy resin (Epon 812). Serial thick (0.25- to 0.5-μm) and ultra-thin (500- to 800-A) sections were cut on a Porter–Blum ultramicrotome. The former were placed on a microscope slide and examined with a phase contrast microscope. The ultra-thin sections were placed on EM grids and stained with uranyl acetate and lead citrate solutions. Electron microscopic viewing was carried out with the Phillips EM 300, AEI 6B or Jem 7A instruments.

Comparison of histology, thick and thin ultramicrotome sections and immunofluorescence

The jejunal mucosa from each patient was studied with routine histological techniques and compared with phase contrast and EM sections. In addition, information on the quantity and specificity of mucosal plasma cells of IgA, IgM, IgG and IgE type was obtained by an immunofluorescence technique [2, 5].

Challenge studies

Challenge with the appropriate antigen (gluten or cow's milk) was carried out by the oral route [3,5,6] and was given to patients (children) after weeks or months of antigen-free diets so as to allow the jejunal mucosa to recover. Jejunal biopsies were performed before the challenge and repeated between 2 and 96 h after challenge. In the case of gluten, the antigen was given in briefly cooked form as a single dose. Milk was given either as a single dose of whole cow's milk or in repeated small doses for a period of 8–10 h. All patients were fasted at least 8 h before each biopsy.

References

1. McCarthy CF, Gough KR, Rodrigues M, Read AE (1964) Peroral intestinal mucosal biopsy with a small Crosby capsule. Br Med J i:1620
2. Maffei HVL, Kingston D, Hill ID, Shiner M (1979) Histological changes and the immune response within the jejunal mucosa in children under and over 2 years. Pediatr Res 13:733–736
3. Schmerling DH, Shiner M (1970) The response of the intestinal mucosa to the intraduodenal instillation of gluten in patients with coeliac disease. In: Booth CC, Dowling RH (eds) Coeliac disease. Churchill Livingstone, Edinburgh, pp 64–75
4. Sebus J, Fernandes J, Bult JA (1968) A new twin hole capsule for peroral intestinal biopsy in children. Digestion 1:193–199
5. Shiner M, Ballard J (1972) Antigen-antibody reactions in jejunal mucosa in childhood coeliac disease after gluten challenge. Lancet i:1202–1205
6. Shiner M, Ballard J, Smith ME (1975) The small intestinal mucosa in cow's milk allergy. Lancet i:136–140

Chapter 1

Cells of the Normal Mucosa

The enterocyte (see schematic representation Fig. 1.1)

Enterocytes are the epithelial cells covering the villi of the small intestinal mucosa (Fig. 1.2). They are highly specialised cells, the function of which is to absorb food products and other material from the lumen of the bowel. These cells mature as they move towards the tip of the villus [15] where eventually cell death occurs (Fig. 1.3). Cell maturation and degeneration appear to be regulated by an as yet unknown mechanism.

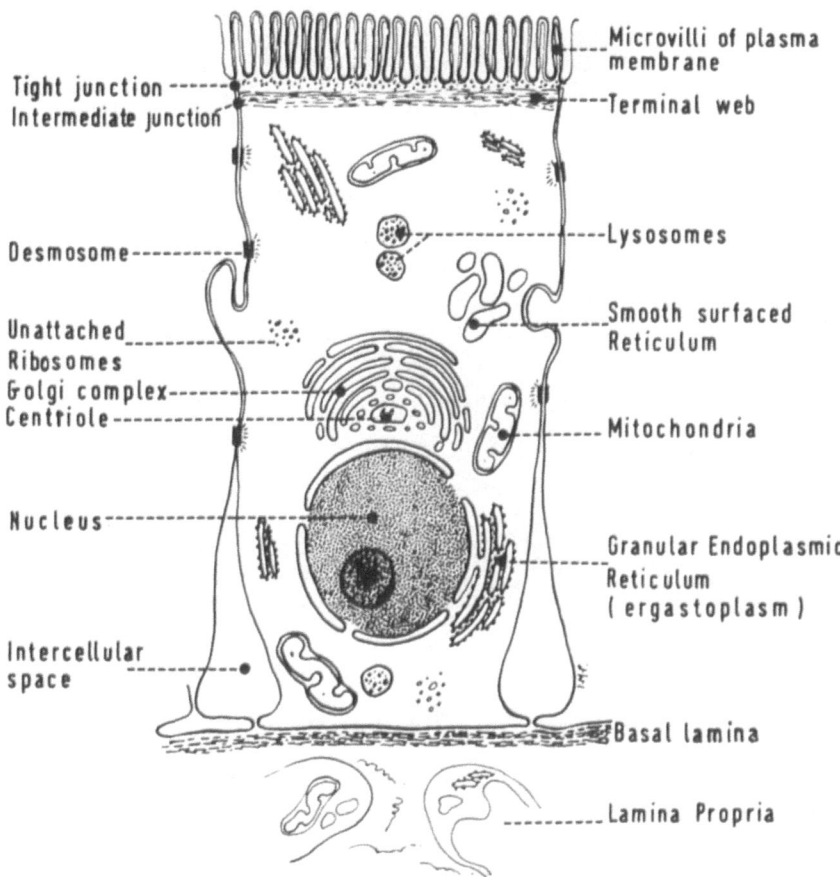

Fig. 1.1. Schematic drawing of enterocyte.

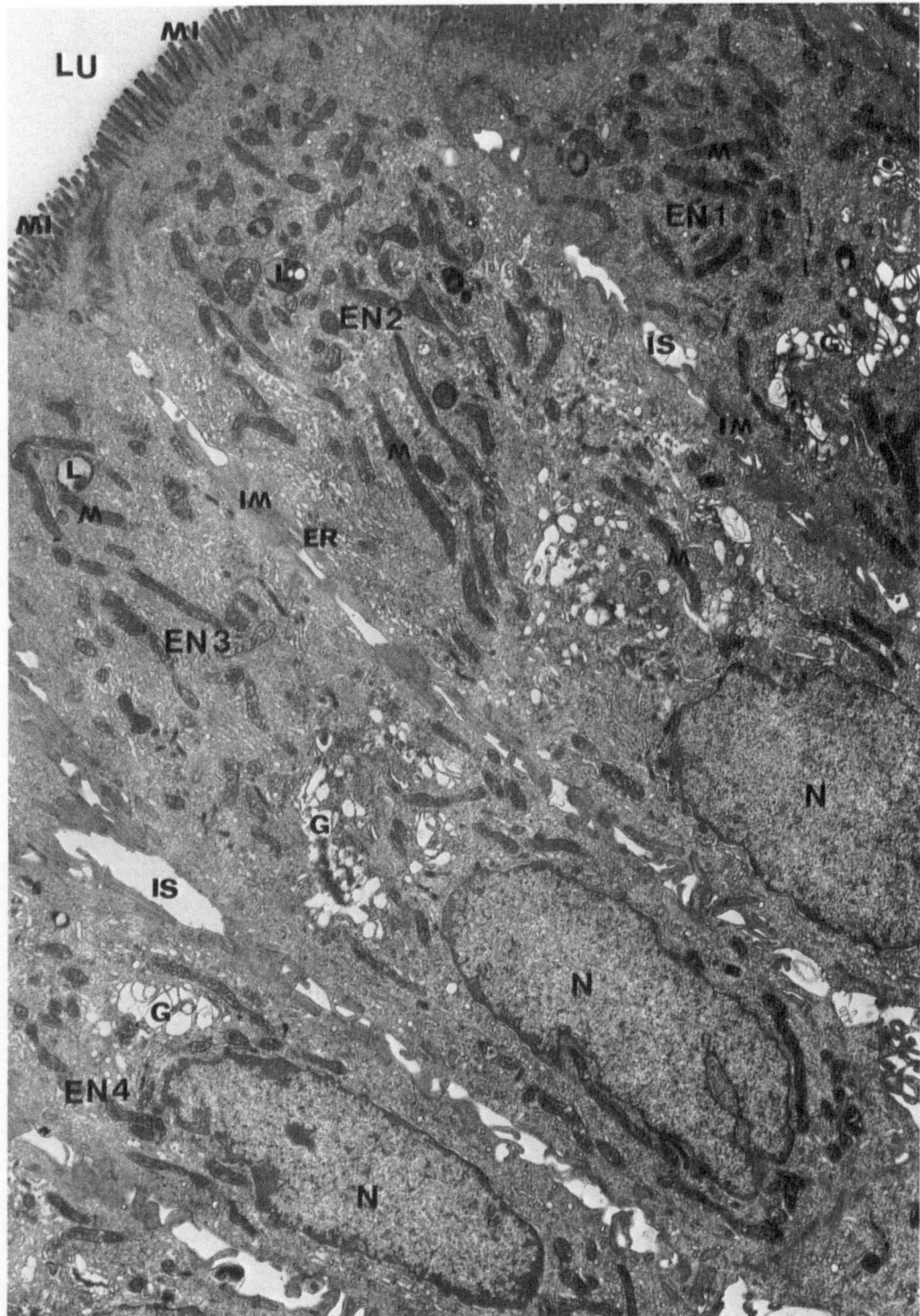

Fig. 1.2. EM. Four enterocytes (*EN 1–4*) from the upper half of a normal villus. The cells are tall columnar with basally situated nuclei (*N*). The microvilli (*MI*) face the lumen (*LU*) of the bowel. The cytoplasm contains mitochondria (*M*), lysosomes (*L*), membrane-bound vacuoles lined by smooth and rough endoplasmic reticulum (*ER*) and those of the Golgi complex (*G*) and free-lying ribosomes. The cells are bound laterally by membranes (*IM*) which allow separation and formation of intercellular spaces (*IS*). (× 6100)

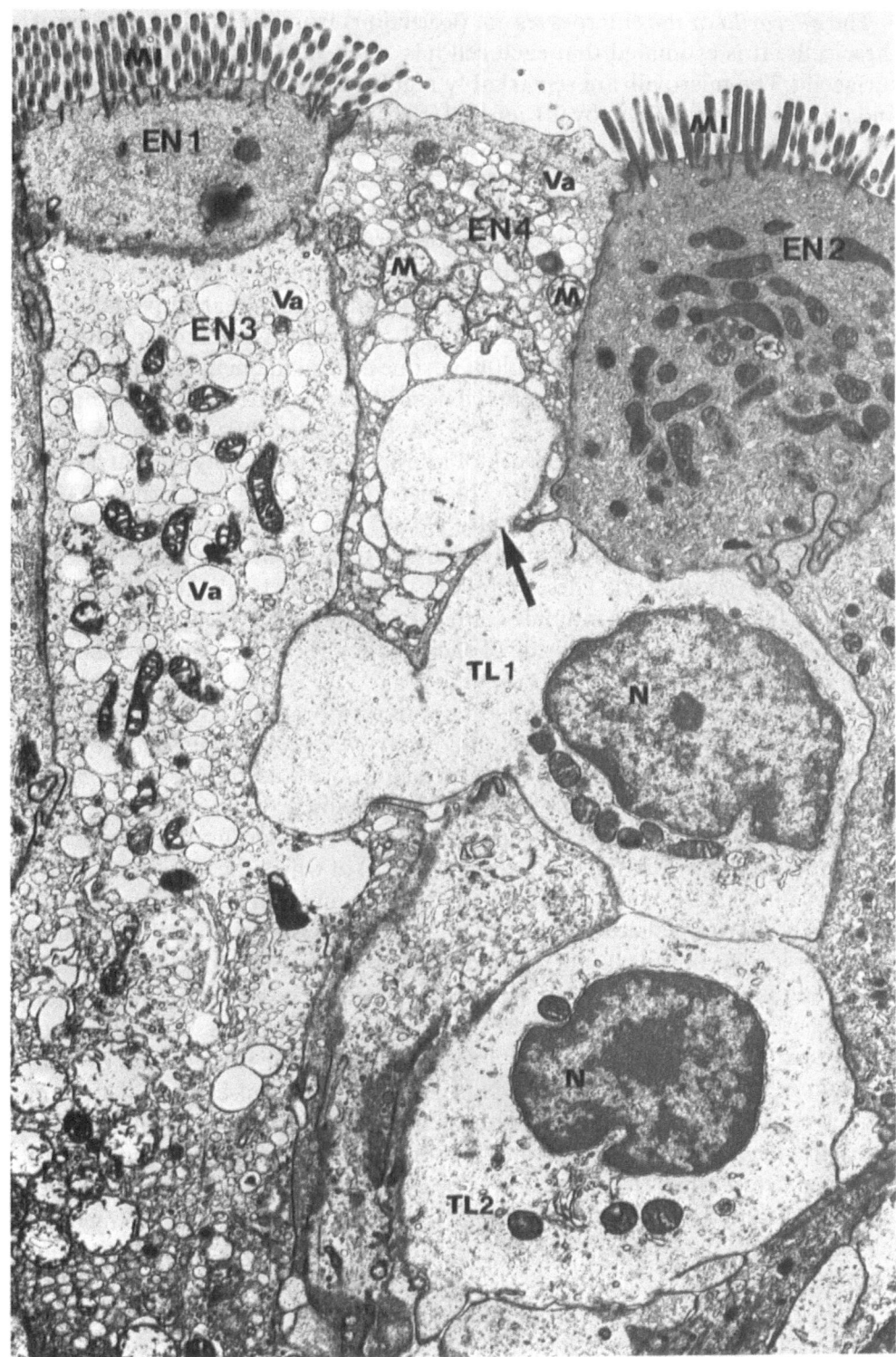

Fig. 1.3. Enterocytes near the tip of a normal villus, showing two viable cells (*EN 1* and *2*) and two disintegrating cells (*EN 3* and *4*) as well as two theliolymphocytes (*TL 1* and *2*). The cytoplasm of the disintegrating cells is vacuolated (*Va*) and contains swollen mitochondria (*M*). The microvilli (*MI*) are absent from cell EN 4. A cytoplasmic process of TL 1 (*arrow*) extends into cell EN 4. *N*, nuclei of TL 1 and 2. (× 10 000)

The *microvilli* of the enterocytes are projections from the luminal surface of these cells. It is estimated that each cell has 1000–4000 such processes on its surface[9]. The microvilli are remarkably regular in height, width and spacing and measure about 1.0 μm by 0.1 μm [17] (Figs. 1.4, 1.5). As they approach the tip of the villi they become somewhat shorter and more irregular. Each microvillus is surrounded by unit membrane consisting of two layers of dense lines separated by a light intermediate zone—the so-called trilaminar structure. These membranes are continuous with the surface and lateral membranes of the enterocyte. Various disaccharidases [3] and proteases [6] are bound in intimate contact with the microvillous membranes, of great importance in absorption. The core of the microvilli (Fig. 1.5) consists of actin filaments [10] which are arranged in an axial fashion, i.e. one central filament surrounded by a concentric ring of other filaments. These filaments extend into the apical cytoplasm of the enterocyte (Figs. 1.4, 1.6–1.8) where they join those from neighbouring microvilli in a network of interlacing fibres (? myosin) arranged parallel to the surface of the cell. This network is called the terminal web (Fig. 1.6). Fine filaments (Fig. 1.7) also extend from the sides and tips of the free surface of the microvillous membrane into the lumen of the bowel to form part of the glycocalyx [7]. These fibres are thus attached only at one end, the other end lying free and in intimate contact with a material of enterocyte origin composed of mucopolysaccharide. Together they form part of the unstirred layer of the physiologist.

The trilaminar structure of the microvillous membranes is continuous with a similar structure composing the *lateral or inter-cell membranes* of the enterocyte (Fig. 1.1) and these are in turn continuous with the *basal membrane* of the cell. Each is composed of lipids and proteins through which there are aqueous channels. The lateral (unit) membranes of adjacent enterocytes are held together by various junctions (Figs. 1.8, 1.9) of which the only structurally (but not functionally) inseparable one is the *tight* junction (zonula occludens). This is situated immediately below the microvilli and is formed by the fusion of the outer leaflets of the plasma membrane, thus sealing the intercellular spaces from the outer environment, i.e. the luminal space. The *intermediate* junction (zonula adherens) lies just below the tight junction and appears as an electron-dense small linear area separated by a small gap and surrounded by fuzz extending into the adjacent cytoplasm. The third, most prominent and numerous, lateral cell junctions are the *desmosomes* (macula adherens). These are dense plaques composed of four membrane leaflets and a gap, surrounded by dense cytoplasmic fuzz (Fig. 1.9). The desmosomes are found in the upper and lower parts of the lateral cell membranes and they, like the intermediate junctions, bind the two adjacent cells loosely together. Below the desmosomes

Fig. 1.4. Longitudinal section of several microvilli (*MI*) projecting from the apical portion of the enterocyte cytoplasm (*EN*) into the lumen of the bowel. Each microvillus is bound by unit membranes (*arrows*) which are continuous with the surface membranes of the enterocyte (*EN*) and also with those of adjacent microvilli. Note filamentous core (*F*) of microvilli. (× 50 184)   ▷

Fig. 1.5. Microvilli in cross section, showing unit membranes (*arrow*) and filamentous core (*F*). (× 73 500)   ▷

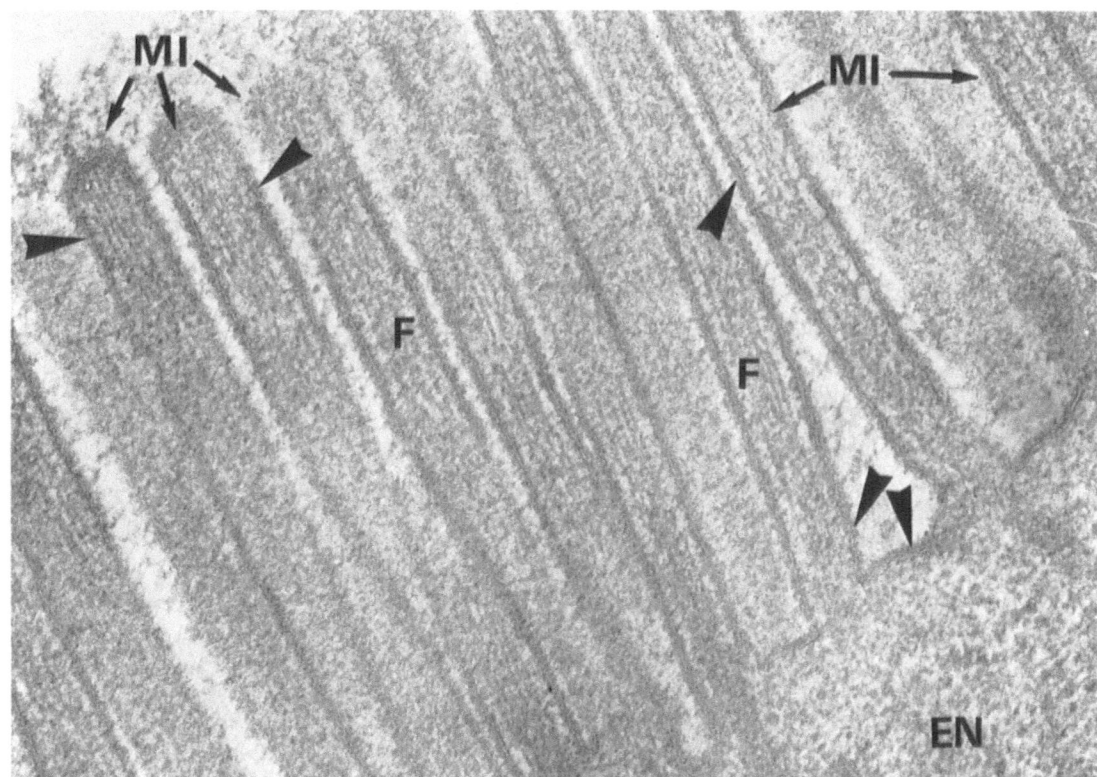

Fig. 1.4. △   Fig. 1.5. ▽

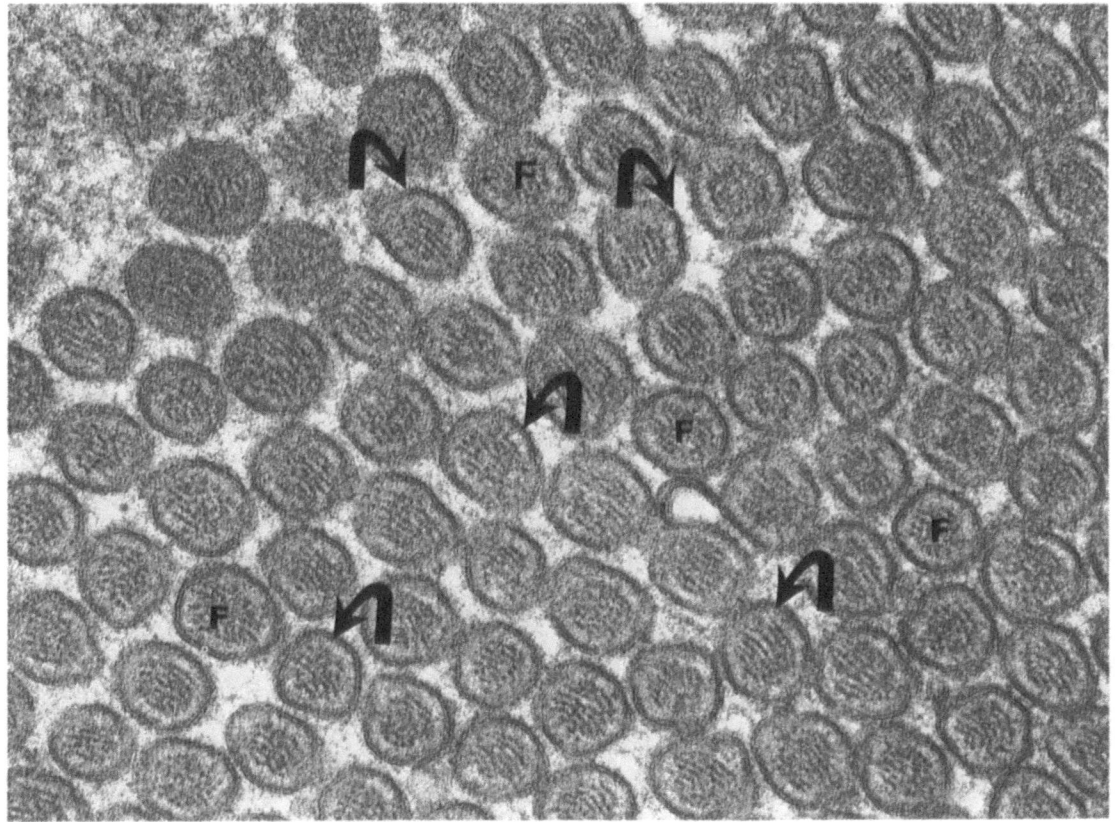

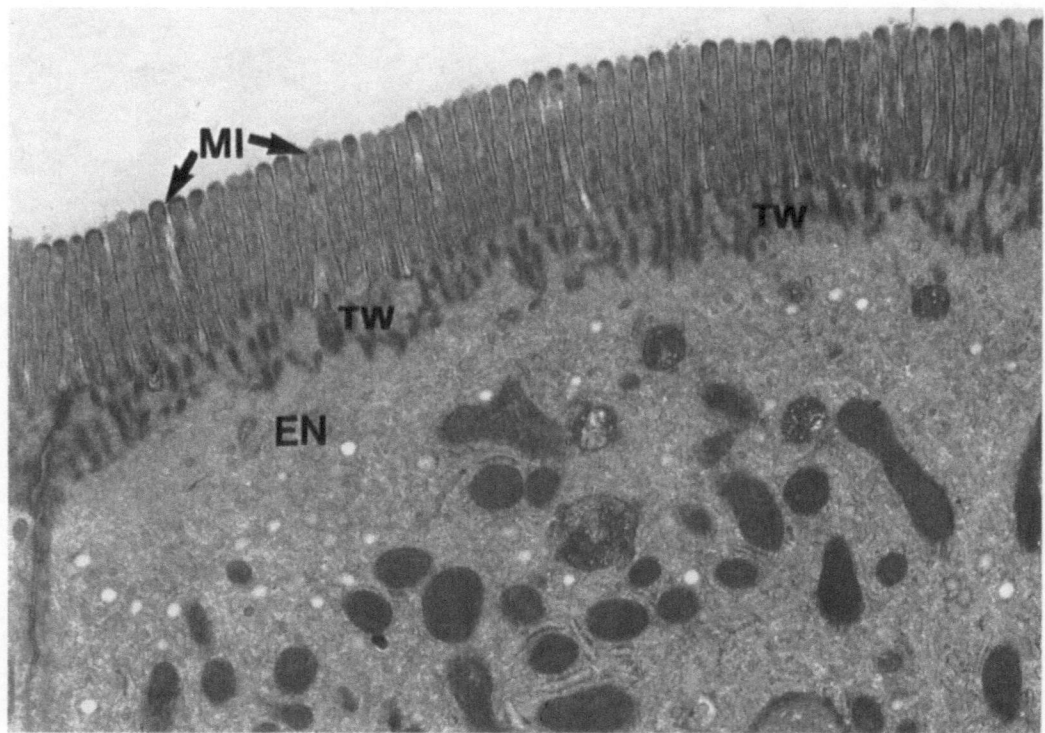

Fig. 1.6. Apical portion of enterocyte (*EN*) showing extension of filaments of microvillous core into the cytoplasm below to form the network of fibrils known as the terminal web (*TW*). MI, microvilli (× 20 592)

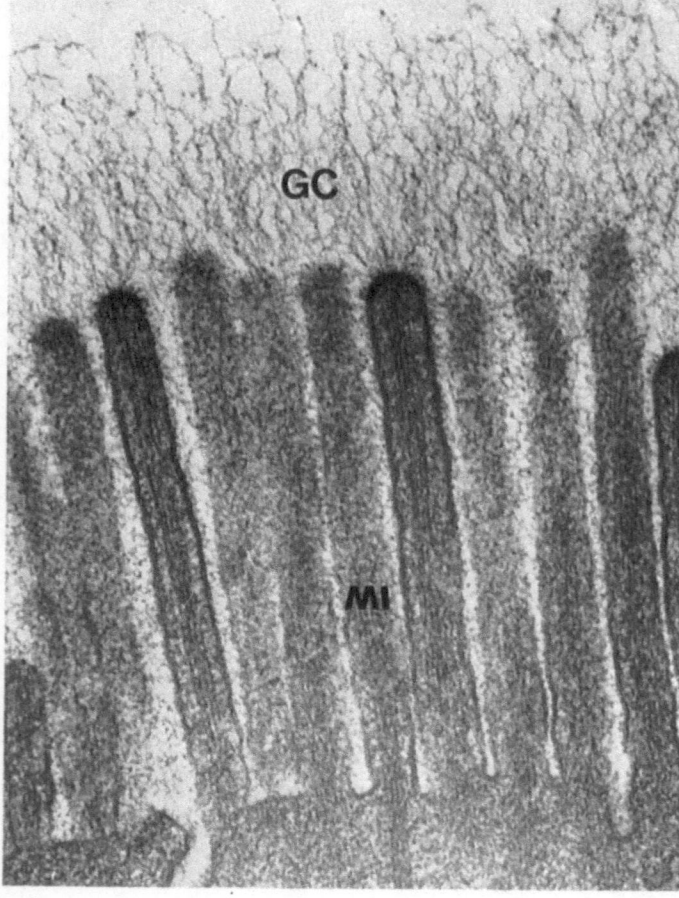

Fig. 1.7. Filaments of the glycocalyx (*GC*) arising from the tips of the microvilli (*MI*). They form the basal structure supporting the mucopolysaccharide layer that surrounds the outer surface of the microvilli (× 40 400)

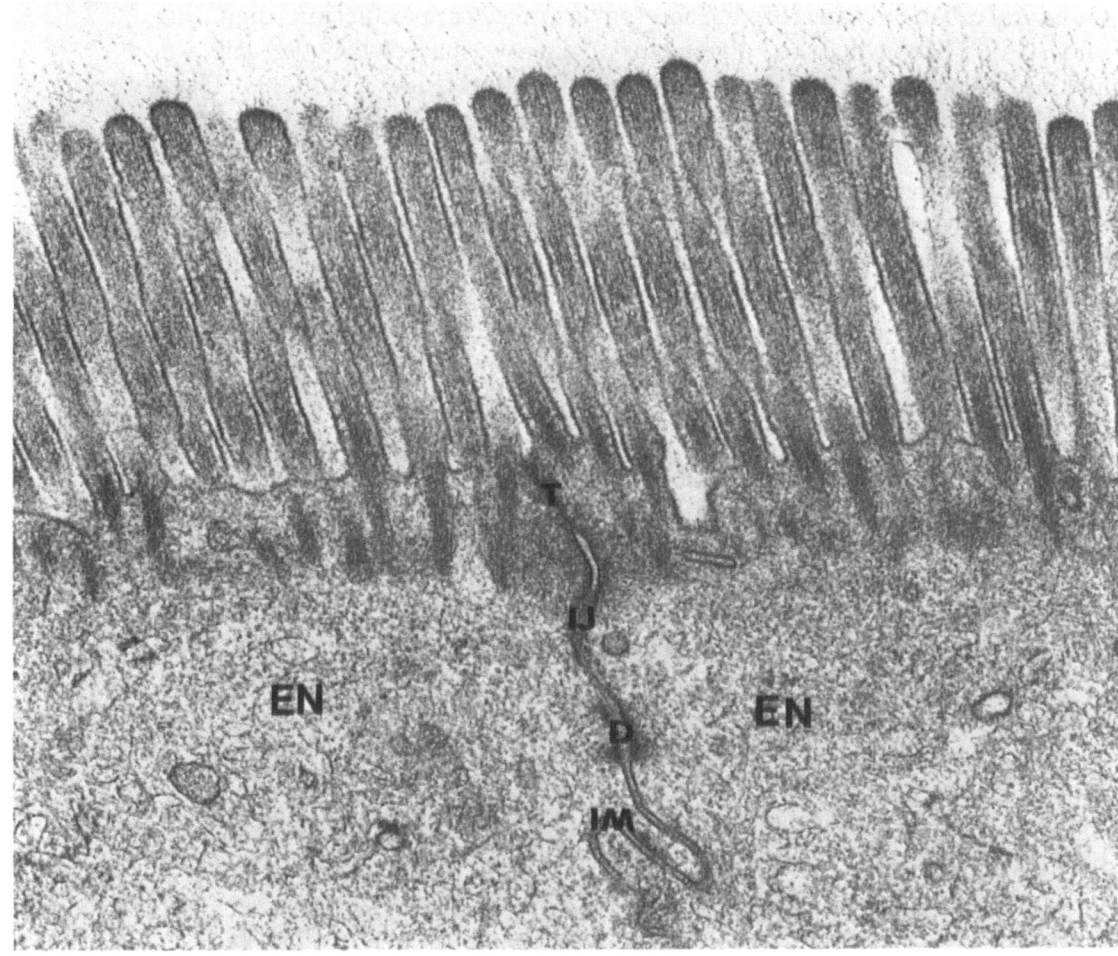

Fig. 1.8. Apical portion of two enterocytes (*EN*) showing the lateral or intercellular membranes (*IM*) and the three types of junctions seen as plaques of increased densities. *T*, tight junction: *IJ*, intermediate junction; *D*, desmosome. (× 31 500)

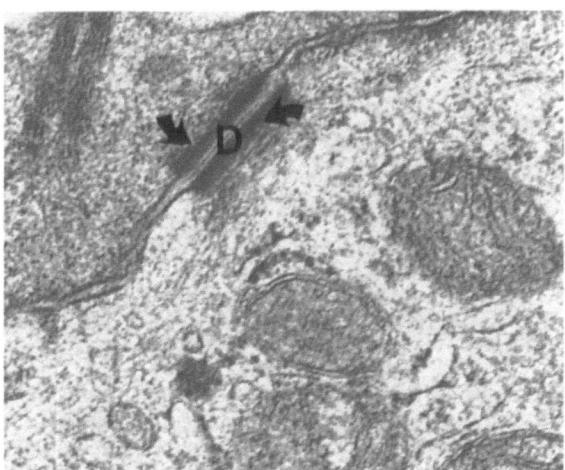

Fig. 1.9. The desmosome (*D*) at higher magnification, showing a central clear space which is bisected by a thin intermediate line and short fibrils extending laterally into the enterocyte cytoplasm (*arrow*). (× 53 880)

the lateral cell membranes of each enterocyte are seen as parallel interdigitating folds (Fig. 1.10) which are divided by a narrow space when the cells are 'fasting' but open into wide spaces during digestion (Figs. 1.10, 1.11). These intercellular spaces are important areas which allow the transport of material from within the absorbing cells to reach the extracellular tissue below. The basal cell membranes separate the basal cytoplasm of the enterocyte from the connective tissue and the various structures lying in it (Fig. 1.12). It is in turn separated by a clear space from the basal *lamina*, a structure composed of a fine filamentous material running parallel to the basal membranes (Fig. 1.12). Like the glycocalyx, it contains polysaccharide-rich material but it is not certain whether the basal lamina is part of the cell membrane or the matrix below.

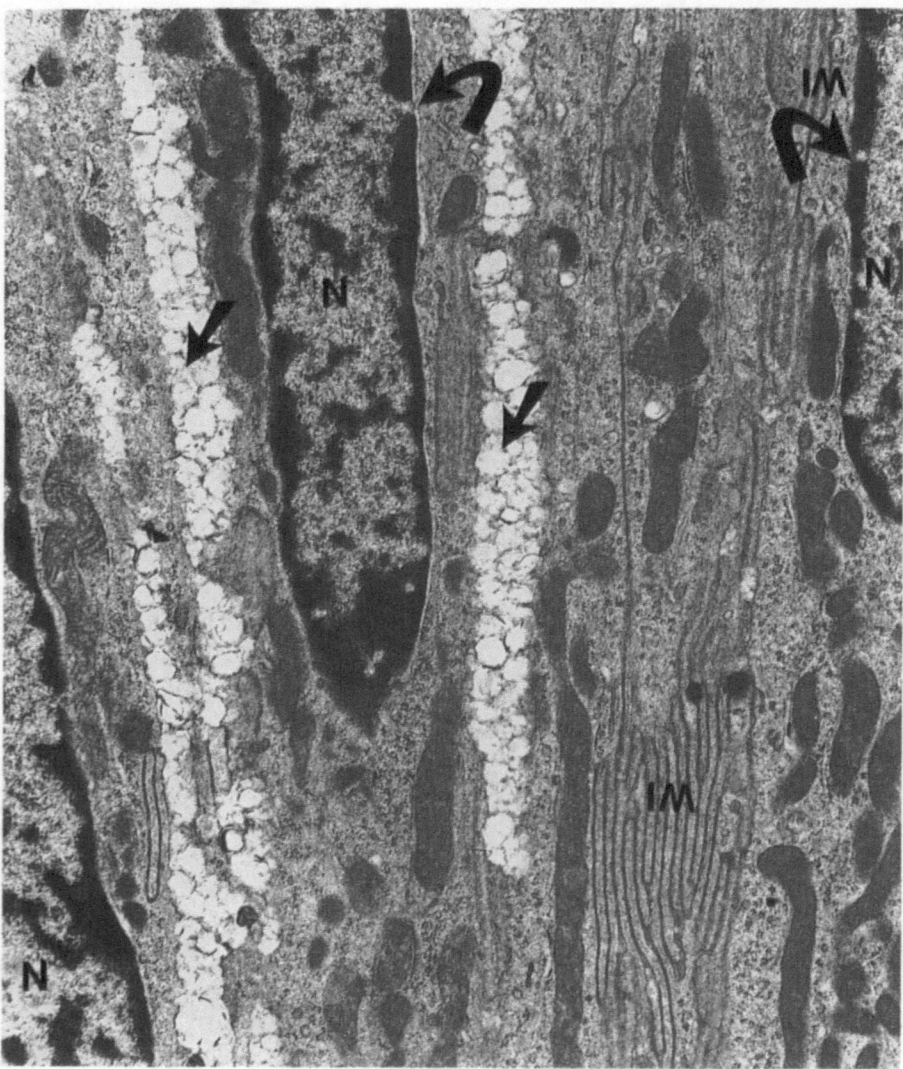

Fig. 1.10. Lower portions of enterocytes showing interdigitating folds of the lateral membranes (*IM*) which separate during digestion to form spaces (*arrows*). The spaces are filled with electron-translucent globular material. Also shown are several enterocyte nuclei (*N*) with nuclear pores (*curved arrows*) in their outer membranes. (× 12 100)

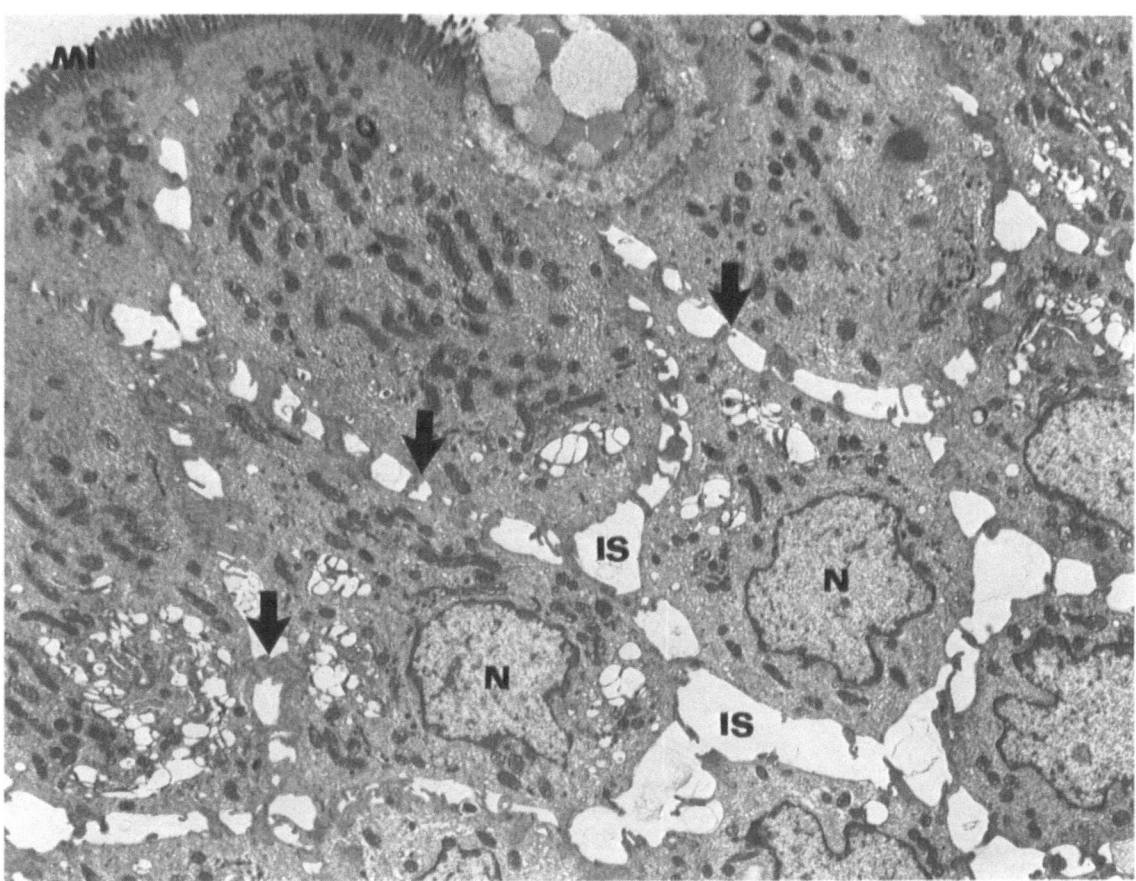

Fig. 1.11. Oblique section across several enterocytes at apical and nuclear levels after water ingestion. The lateral membranes (*arrows*) are partly or wholly separated to form clear spaces (*IS*) between the enterocytes. *N*, nucleus; *MI*, microvilli. (× 5048)

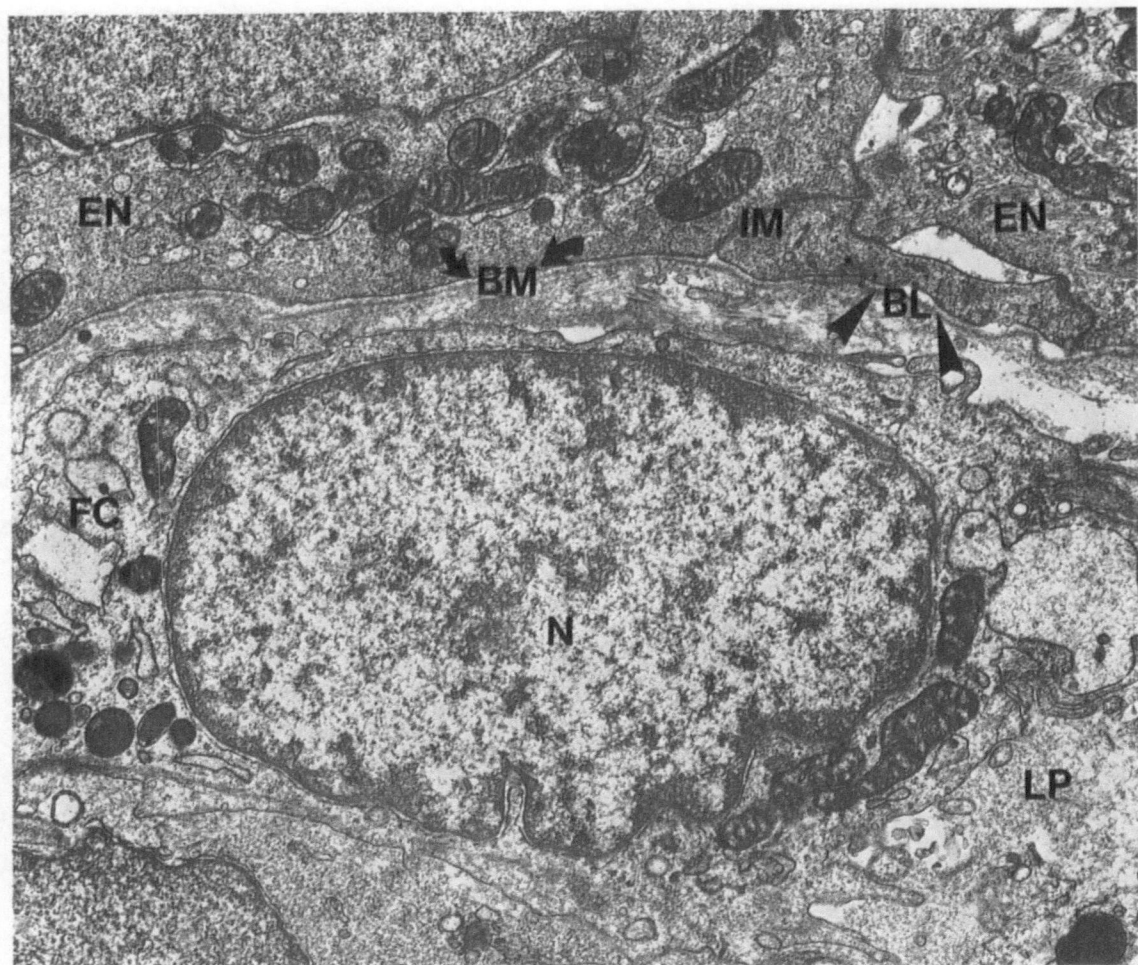

Fig. 1.12. Lower portion of two enterocytes (*EN*) showing the basal cell membranes (*BM + arrow*) as a continuation of the lateral membranes (*IM*). A clear space separates the basal membranes from the basal lamina (*BL + arrows*), a fine fibrillar linear structure running parallel to it. A 'palisading' fibrocyte (*FC*) with its nucleus (*N*) is seen immediately below the basal lamina in the connective tissue of the lamina propria (*LP*). (× 16400)

The *cytoplasmic organelles* of the enterocyte (Fig. 1.13) are typical of absorbing epithelium and rich in *endoplasmic reticulum* of both smooth (ER) and rough (RER) type. The ER and RER is a membranous reticulum of interlacing tubules, vacuoles and vesicles, whose function is the transport, metabolism, secretion and excretion of exogenous and endogenous substances. The mature enterocyte contains relatively few free-lying *ribosomes* and *polysomes* since these are mostly attached to the endoplasmic reticulum

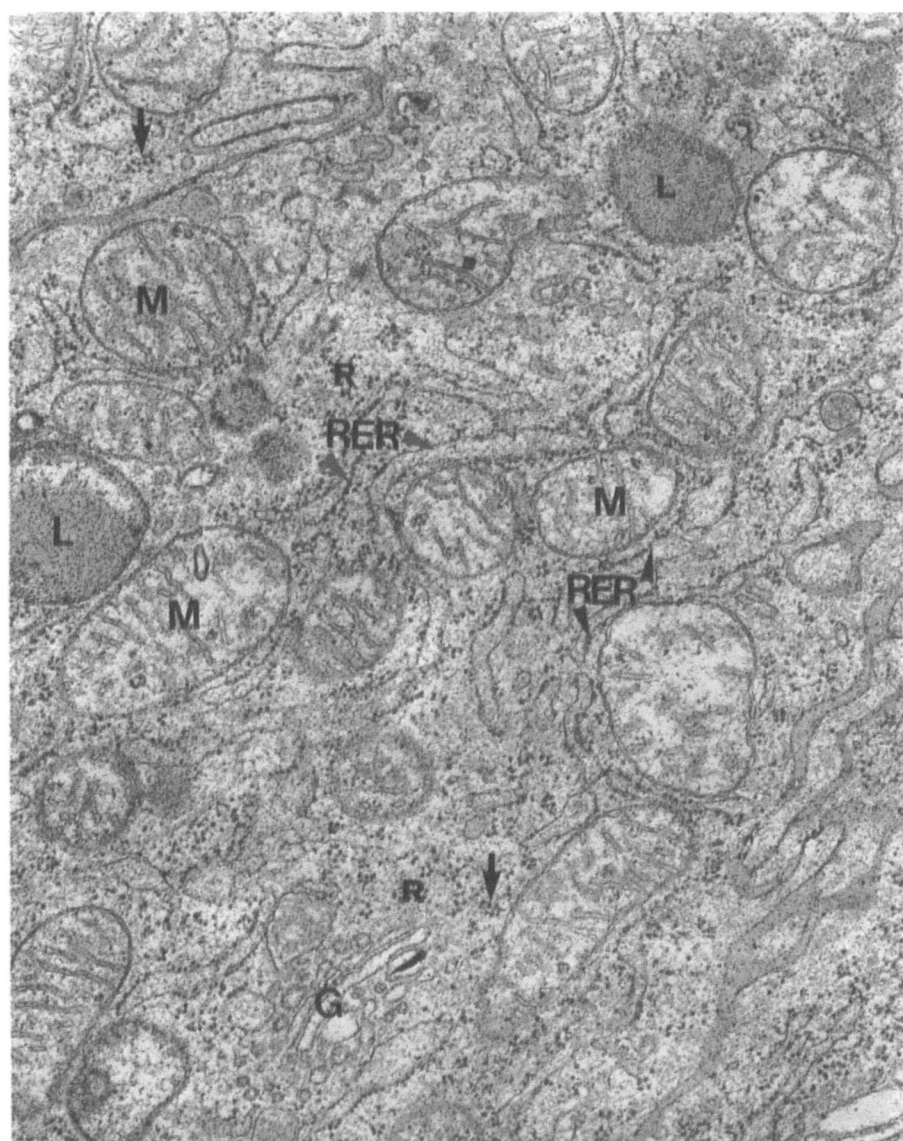

Fig. 1.13. Cytoplasmic organelles of the supranuclear portion of an enterocyte. Note the endoplasmic reticulum, mainly *RER*, in intimate relation to the mitochondria (*M*), and the ribosomes (*R*) lying free as single ribosomes or in clusters as polysomes (*arrow*). *L*, lysosomes; *G*, Golgi complex. (× 30 750)

(RER). Both types of endoplasmic reticulum are intimately related to the *Golgi complex* as well as to the *perinuclear membrane* (Fig. 1.14) and the outer cell membranes, and also participate in endocytotic and exocytotic packaging of materials taken in or out of the enterocyte. The Golgi complex is a pleomorphic, smooth-membraned organelle typically situated in the supranuclear cytoplasm. In the resting cell it presents as a series of stacked, flattened sacs or cisternae (Fig. 1.14) arranged in a curved fashion and a large number of small

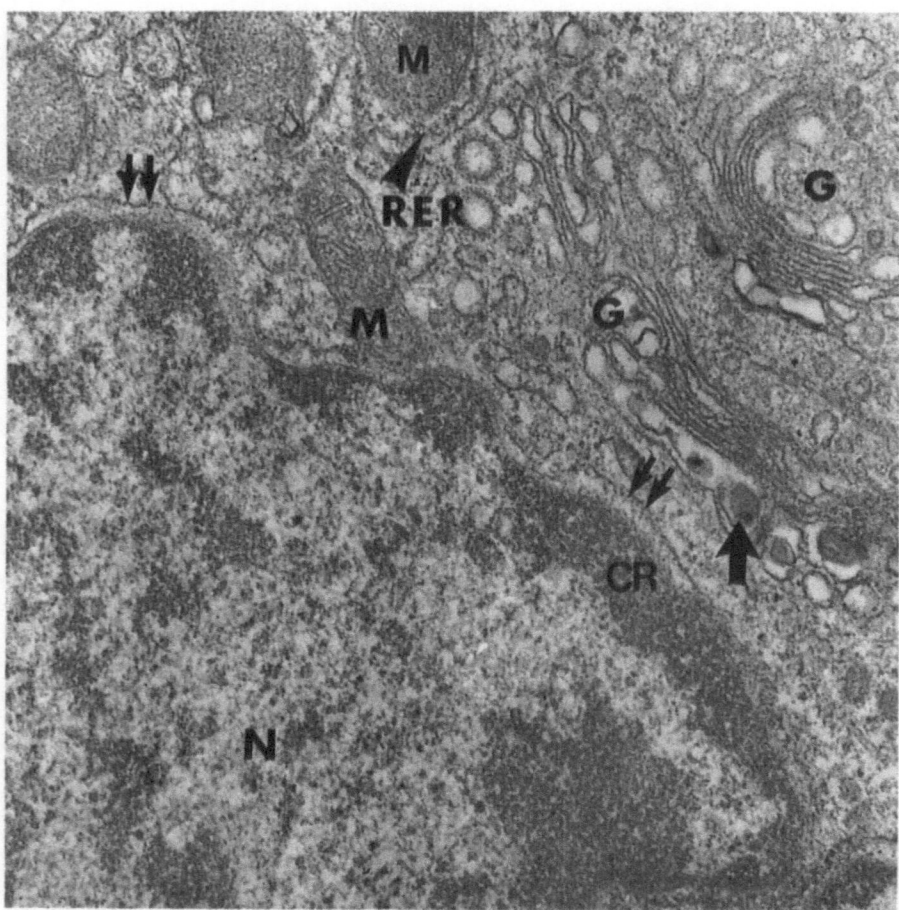

Fig. 1.14. Nuclear and supranuclear portion of an enterocyte showing the Golgi complexes (*G*) in which some of the vesicles or cisternae are dilated and contain globular, electron-dense material (*thick arrow*). Note the intimate relation of the Golgi complex to the mitochondria (*M*), the *RER*, and part of the nucleus (*N*) with its perinuclear membrane (*double arrows*). *CR*, nuclear chromatin. (×31 800)

smooth-membraned vesicles lying on their concave and convex side. The sacs and vesicles dilate during digestion (Fig. 1.15) and are involved in the transport and secretion of material within the cell. The *mitochondria* (Figs. 1.13, 1.16) are longitudinal structures bound by two layers of membrane and containing a matrix in which the mitochondrial cristae, and often dense small bodies, are found. In the enterocyte the mitochondria are found in intimate relation to the rough endoplasmic reticulum (Fig. 1.13), evidently concerned with the supply of energy for protein synthesis. The numerous mitochondrial enzymes have different locations within the outer and inner membranes or the matrical components of this organelle. Cytochrome *c* reductase is situated on the outer membrane, respiratory chain enzymes and ATPase on the inner membrane and most of the enzymes of the Krebs cycle within the matrix. During digestion the mitochondria appear to migrate from their resting position around the nucleus towards the apical portion of the enterocyte.

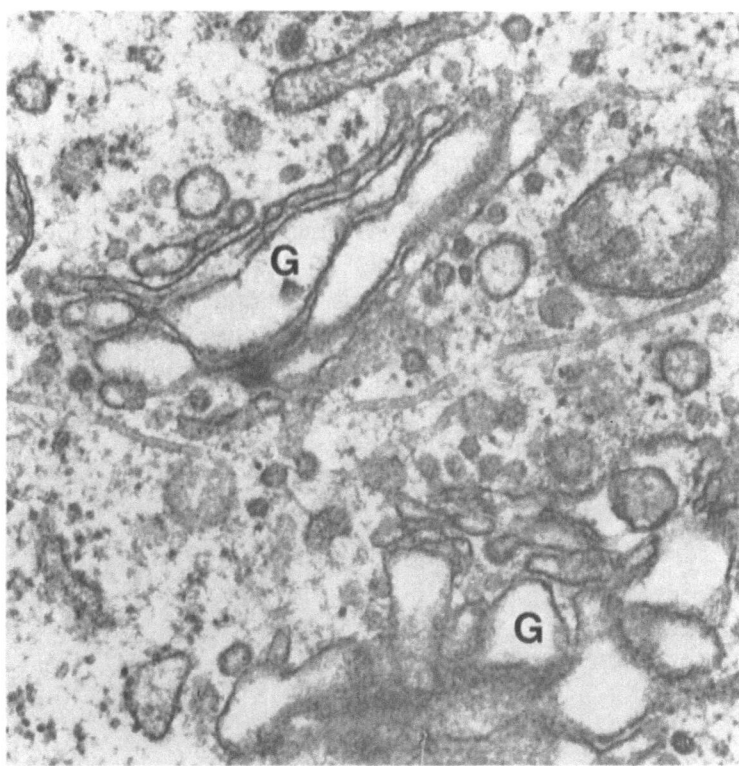

Fig. 1.15. Supranuclear portion of enterocyte cytoplasm showing dilated vesicles of the Golgi complex (*G*). (× 54 500)

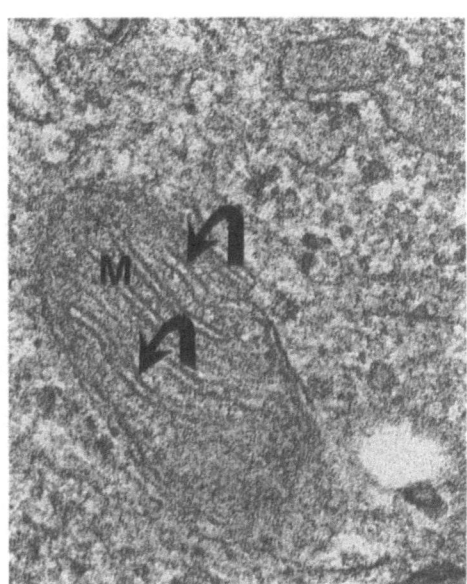

Fig. 1.16. A mitochondrion (*M*) bound by two layers of membrane which are continuous with those of the mitochondrial cristae (*arrows*). The cristae extend into the interior of the mitochondria. The mitochondrial matrix is more electron dense than the surrounding cytoplasm. (× 84 000)

The enterocyte normally contains a number of *lysosomes*, usually not more than five. These are situated in the apical cytoplasm of the cell (Fig. 1.17) and consist of heterogeneous round or oval bodies bound by smooth membrane containing material which is usually denser than that of the surrounding cytoplasm. On a functional basis they have been divided into primary lysosomes, which elaborate a number of acid hydrolases such as acid phosphate, and secondary lysosomes, which act on exogenous or endogenous substrates and are then called phagolysosomes (heterolysosomes) and cytolysosomes (autolysosomes). Residual bodies are another example of secondary lysosomes in which digestion of material has already been completed. Another type of lysosome found in the enterocyte is the

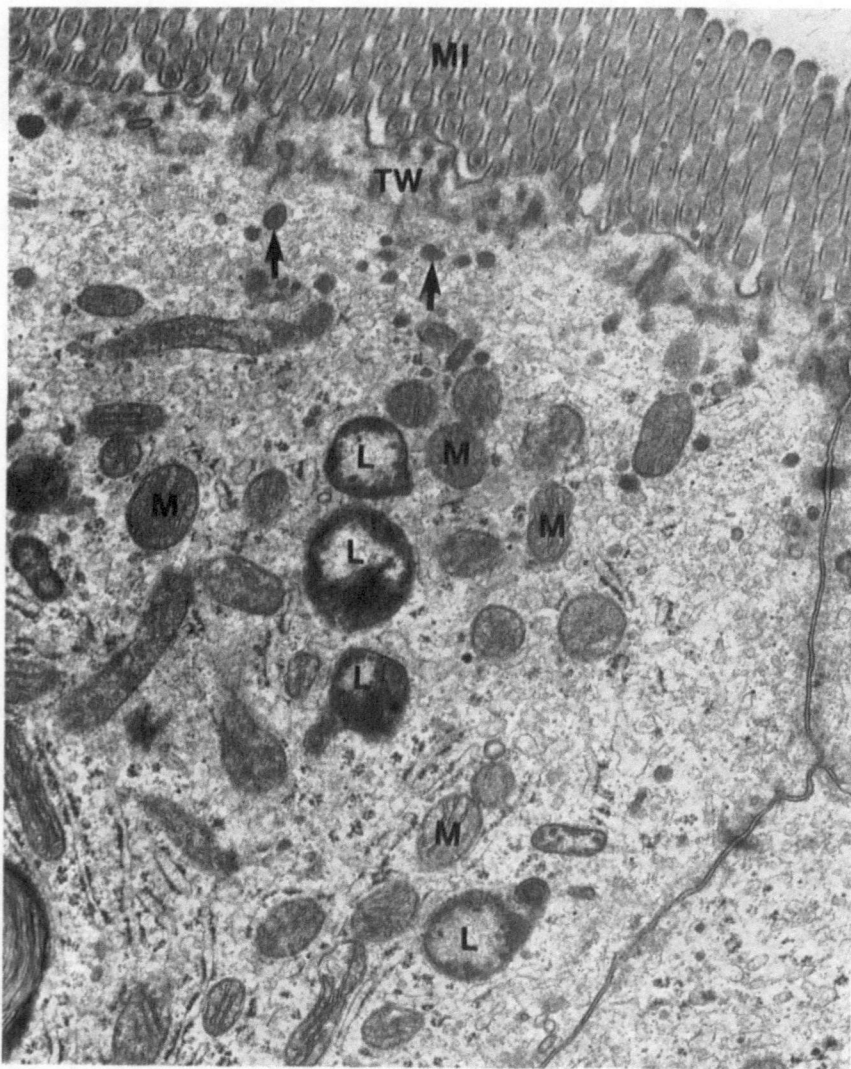

Fig. 1.17. Apical portion of enterocyte showing lysosomes (*L*) in close proximity to the mitochondria (*M*). In addition numerous smaller round vesicles (?lysosomes) filled with electron-dense material (*arrows*) may be seen in the cytoplasm close to the terminal web (*TW*). *MI*, microvilli. (×20 433)

multivesicular body (Fig. 1.18). These bodies are easily identified as round membrane-bound structures containing a number of small vesicles. These vesicles may be replaced by electron-dense whorls of membranes and are then identified as *myelin or myelinoid bodies* (Fig. 1.19). The multivesicular and myelinoid bodies also contain acid phosphatase. It is not clear whether their presence in the enterocyte cytoplasm should be regarded as normal or abnormal and whether they constitute primary or secondary lysosomes. Occasionally *microbodies or peroxisomes* are seen within the cytoplasm and are identified by their round, oval or elongated structure surrounded by a single membrane and containing dense granular material. They contain oxidases and catalases but their function is poorly understood. The *microtubules or microfilaments* are cytoplasmic organelles whose visualisation may be difficult (Figs. 1.20, 1.21). They may be arranged in bundles (Fig. 1.21) or may be loosely distributed. They are often associated with the *centrioles* (Figs. 1.20, 1.22a, b, c). These are in pairs at right angles to each other situated in a juxtanuclear position (Figs. 1.20, 1.22c) and are partly surrounded by the Golgi complex. They occupy a central position within the cell and replicate in

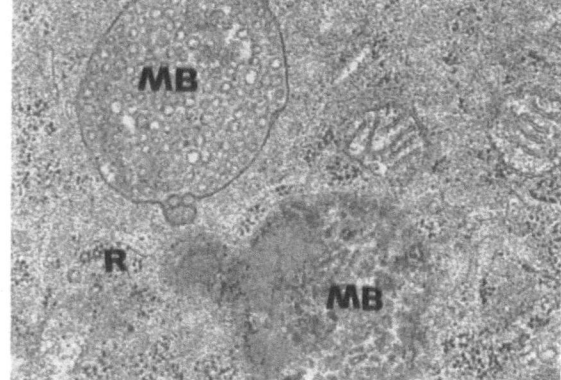

Fig. 1.18. Two multivesicular bodies (*MB*) in the apical cytoplasm of the enterocyte. These bodies are bound by smooth membrane and contain a number of small vacuoles (?vesicles ?tubules). *R*, ribosome. (× 27 000)

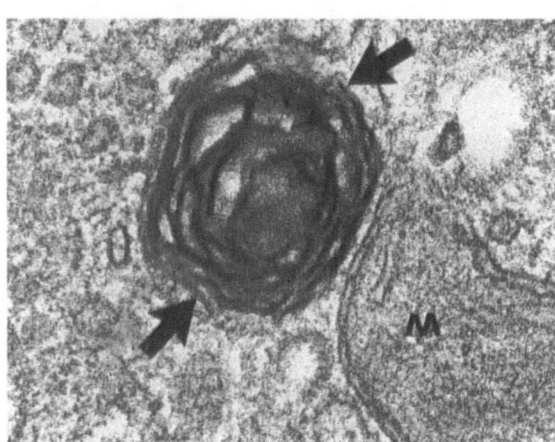

Fig. 1.19. Myelin body (*arrows*) in cytoplasm of enterocyte showing dense, whorl-like appearance. *M*, mitochondrion. (× 101 200)

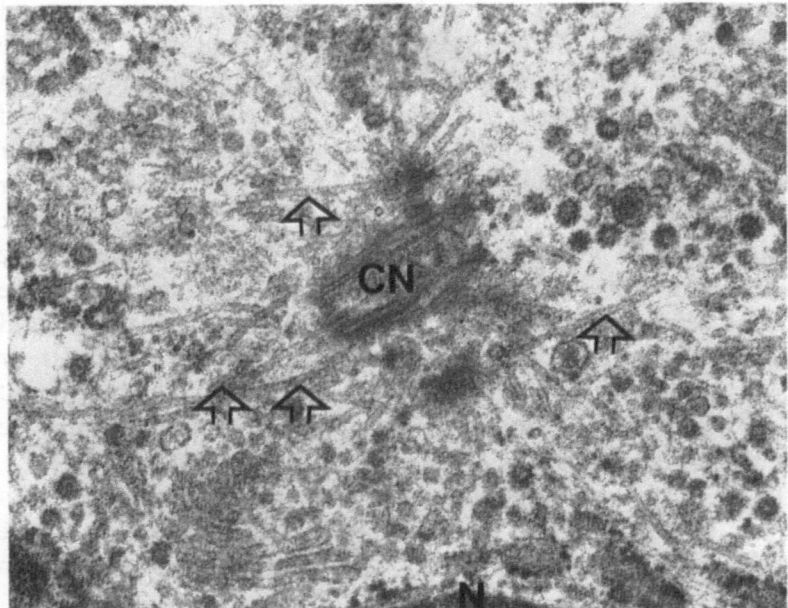

Fig. 1.20. Supranuclear portion of the enterocyte showing cytoplasmic microtubules (*arrows*) surrounding a centriole (*CN*). Note the position of the centriole in relation to the apical portion of the nucleus (*N*). (× 73 350)

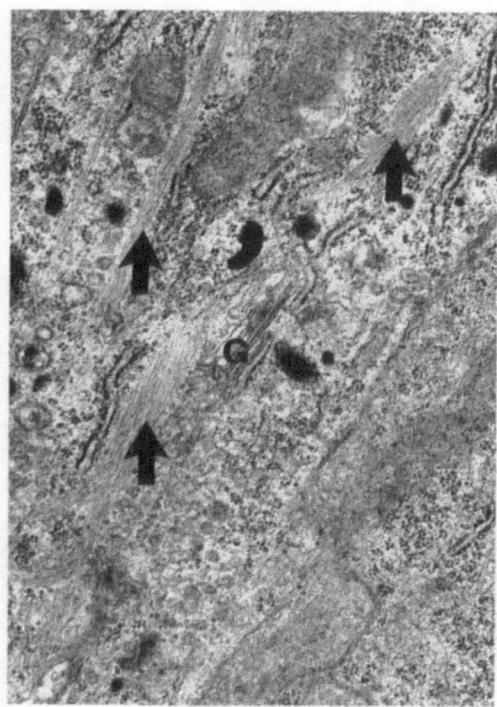

Fig. 1.21. Microfilaments (*arrows*) in the apical portion of the enterocyte cytoplasm. These are arranged in bundles. *G*, Golgi complex. (× 40 350)

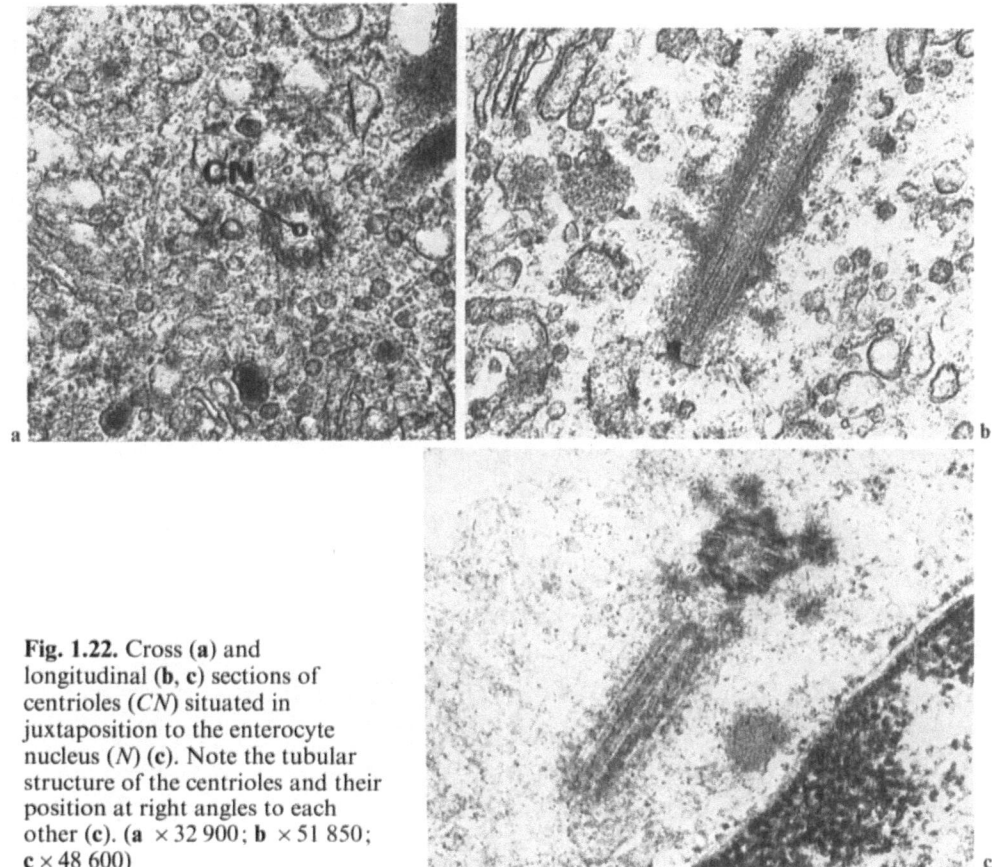

Fig. 1.22. Cross (**a**) and longitudinal (**b, c**) sections of centrioles (*CN*) situated in juxtaposition to the enterocyte nucleus (*N*) (**c**). Note the tubular structure of the centrioles and their position at right angles to each other (**c**). (**a** ×32 900; **b** ×51 850; **c** ×48 600)

relation to mitosis of the nucleus. The centrioles are composed of a series of hollow tubules arranged concentrically (Figs. 1.20, 1.22b) and are easily recognised in cross-section (Figs. 1.22a, c) as a series of nine triplets in rotational symmetry. The function of the centrioles is not established, but it is thought that they are associated with nuclear division and possibly with the formation of the microtubules of the mitotic spindle.

The *nucleus* of the enterocyte is normally situated within the basal region of the cell cytoplasm (Figs. 1.1, 1.2). It has an oval, smooth-contoured structure and is surrounded by the two nuclear membranes (Fig. 1.14). The chromatin within the nucleoplasm contains DNA and consists of aggregates of electron-dense, granular material (Figs. 1.14, 1.23). In the interchromatin areas the nuclear matrix appears as a clear material, containing fibrils and granular material, rich in both DNA and RNA. This granular material may be thought of as the nuclear ribosomes. The enterocyte nuclei possess only occasional nucleoli (Fig. 1.23) which are recognised as dense, granular and fibrillar aggregates, usually near the centre of the nuclear matrix. The nucleoli are rich in RNA but also contain DNA and other proteins, and it is the nucleolar RNA which may synthesise the ribosomal and polysomal RNA of the cell cytoplasm.

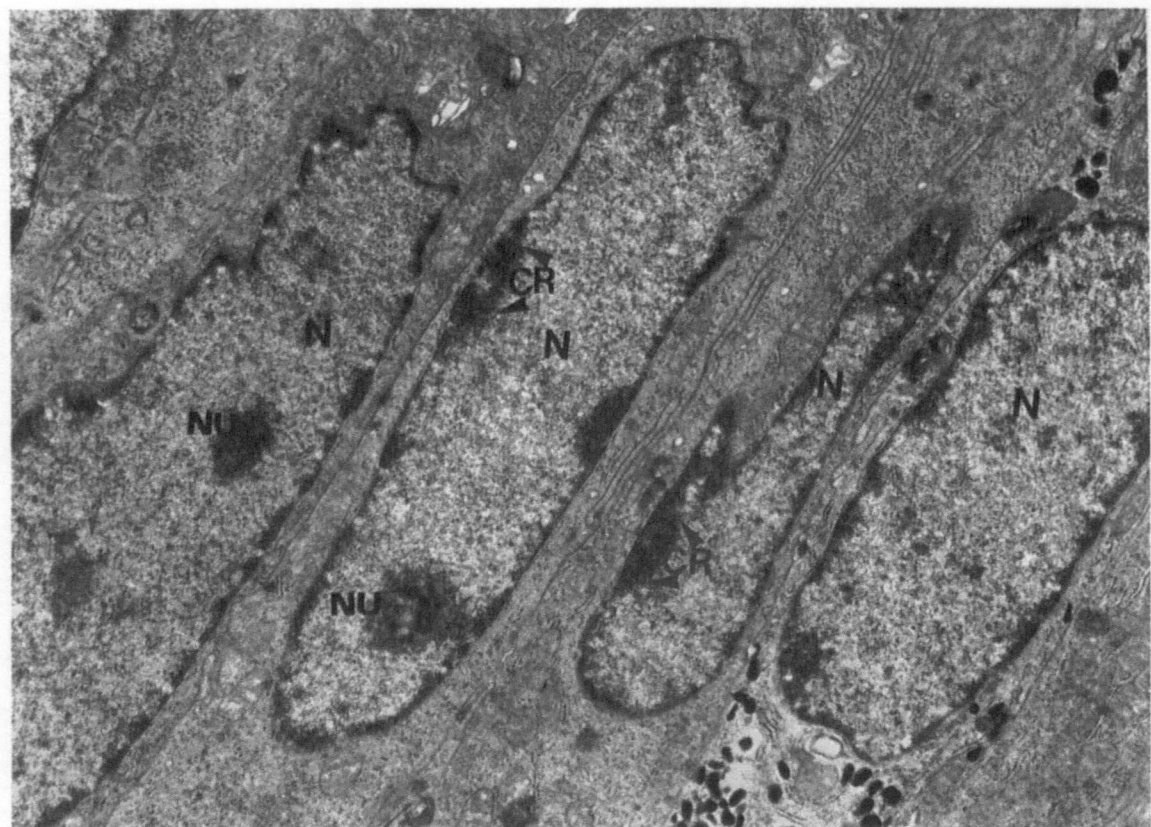

Fig. 1.23. Several nuclei (*N*) of enterocytes, two of which contain a nucleolus (*NU*). *CR*, nuclear chromatin. (× 12 500)

The nuclear membranes are separated by a clear space and are interrupted by a number of nuclear pores or fenestrations (Fig. 1.10). These present either as a discontinuity of the two nuclear membranes or as a single diaphragm between them. They thus facilitate exchanges of protein material from nucleus to cytoplasm. The outer membrane of the nucleus may have ribosomes on its outer surface (Figs. 1.14, 1.2c) and is often seen in intimate relation to the cytoplasmic RER. Towards the tip of the small-intestinal villi, where enterocytes are often seen in a degenerative state (Fig. 1.24), the nuclei may show disintegration or necrobiosis with swelling and loss of chromatin material. Towards the base of the villi occasional epithelial cells may be seen in mitosis (Fig. 1.25).

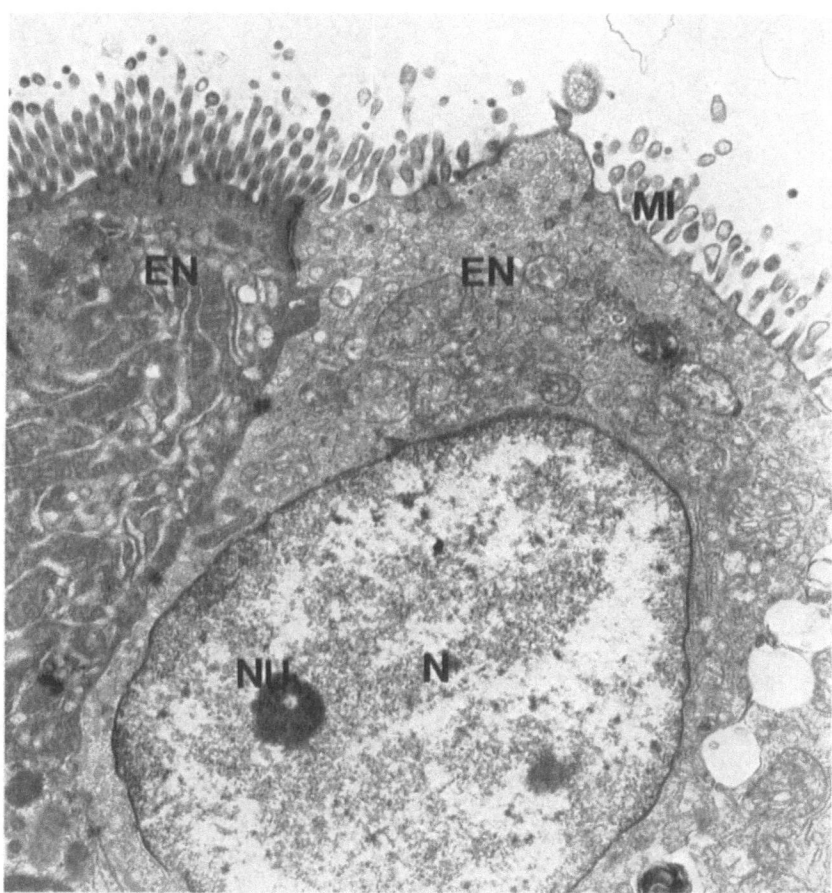

Fig. 1.24. Two enterocytes (*EN*), one of which shows certain features of necrobiosis such as a large nucleus (*N*) with loss of matrix density and chromatin material. The microvilli of this cell (*MI*) appear bulbous compared with the normal microvilli of the adjacent cell. *NU*, nucleolus. (× 10 900)

Crypt cells (Fig. 1, p. 1)

The crypt cell epithelium (Fig. 1.26) contains a variety of different cell types:

1) the precursor cells of the enterocyte
2) the goblet cells, which may mature in the crypt regions or may not differentiate until they reach the villi
3) the Paneth cells, which are entirely confined to the basal regions of the crypts
4) the APUD (amine precursor uptake and decarboxylation) cells, which belong to the neuro-endocrine system of the gut and are mainly found in the crypts though some, like the argentaffin cells, also ascend the villi.

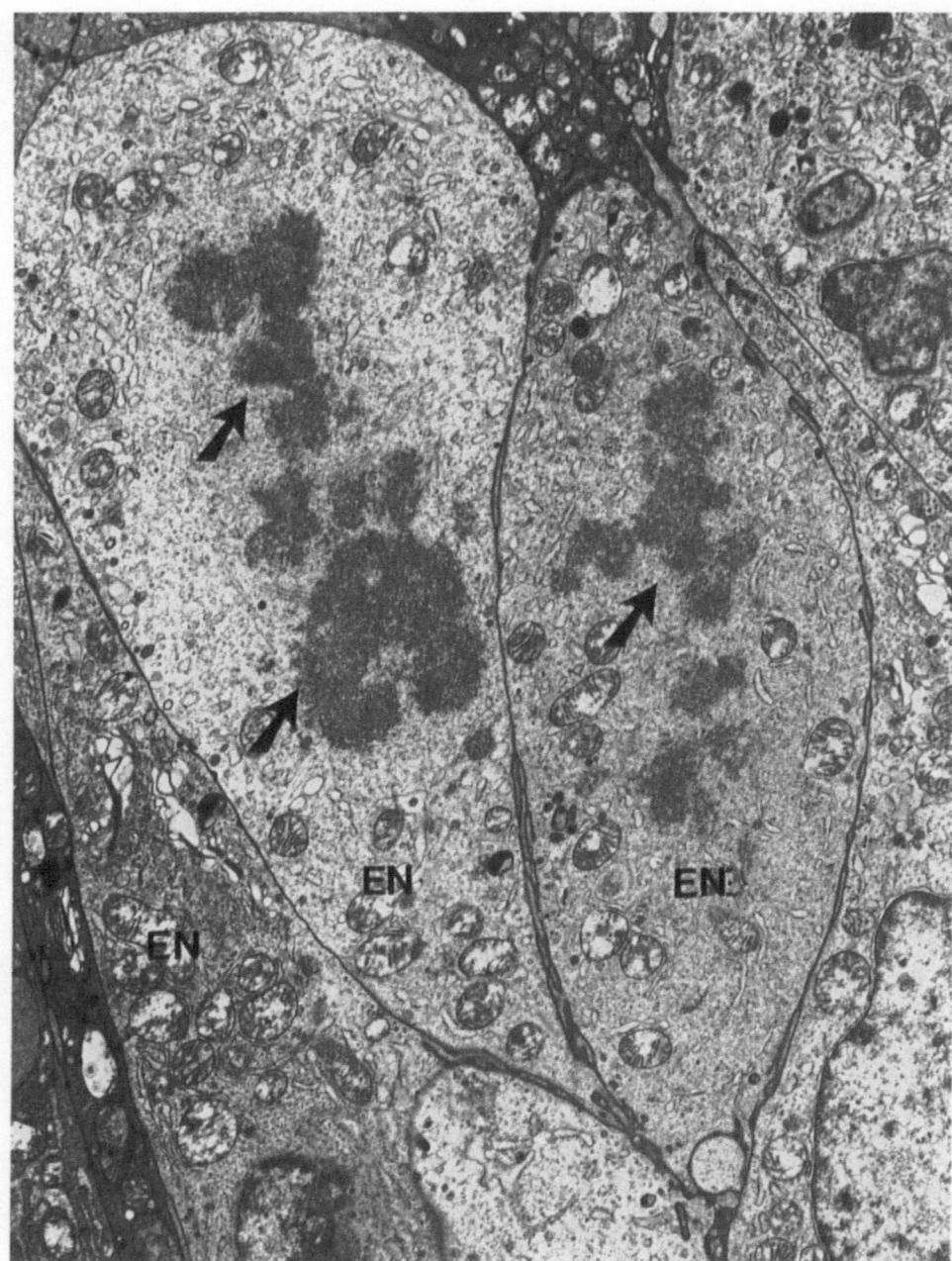

Fig. 1.25. Several enterocytes (*EN*) near the crypt–villous junction. Mitosis may be seen in two of the cells (*arrows*). (× 7716)

Fig. 1.26. Low magnification of crypt epithelium showing various types of cells. Note the short, sparse microvilli (*MI*) of all the cells facing the lumen (*LU*) of the crypt. *GO*, goblet cell; *PR*, precursor cell; *PA*, Paneth cell; *UD*, undifferentiated cell. (× 2507)   ▷

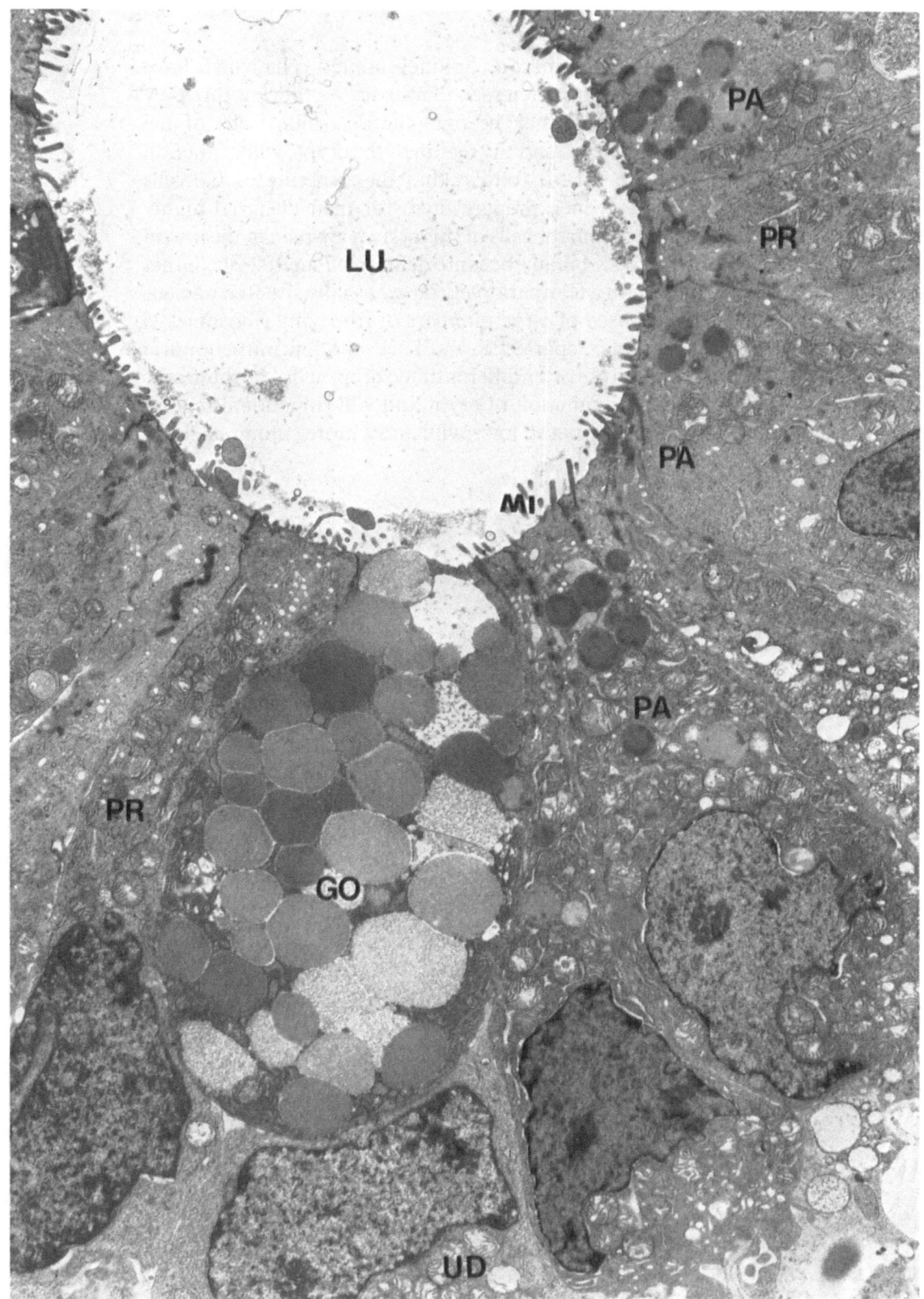

Fig. 1.26.

Precursor cells of the enterocytes

The base of the crypts contains numerous undifferentiated cells which have poorly developed microvilli and are often seen in mitosis. As they mature they move up towards the villi, where they become the absorbing cells of the enterocytes. Maturity is attained around the region of the crypt–villus junction and in the lower third of the villi. It follows that the structure of the cells undergoes important changes which prepare them for their eventual highly specialised function. Certain precursor cells of this system are seen in the lowest parts of the crypts (Fig. 1.26) and many become definitive Paneth cells. Other cells have a cuboidal shape with a comparatively large, basally situated nucleus and their cytoplasm is composed of large numbers of free-lying ribosomes, a poorly developed Golgi complex, sparse ER and RER and few mitochondria (Fig. 1.27). They are the immature or undifferentiated crypt cells. As these cells move up the crypt towards the junction of crypt and villi (junctional region) they acquire taller, more densely spaced microvilli and a more columnar shape

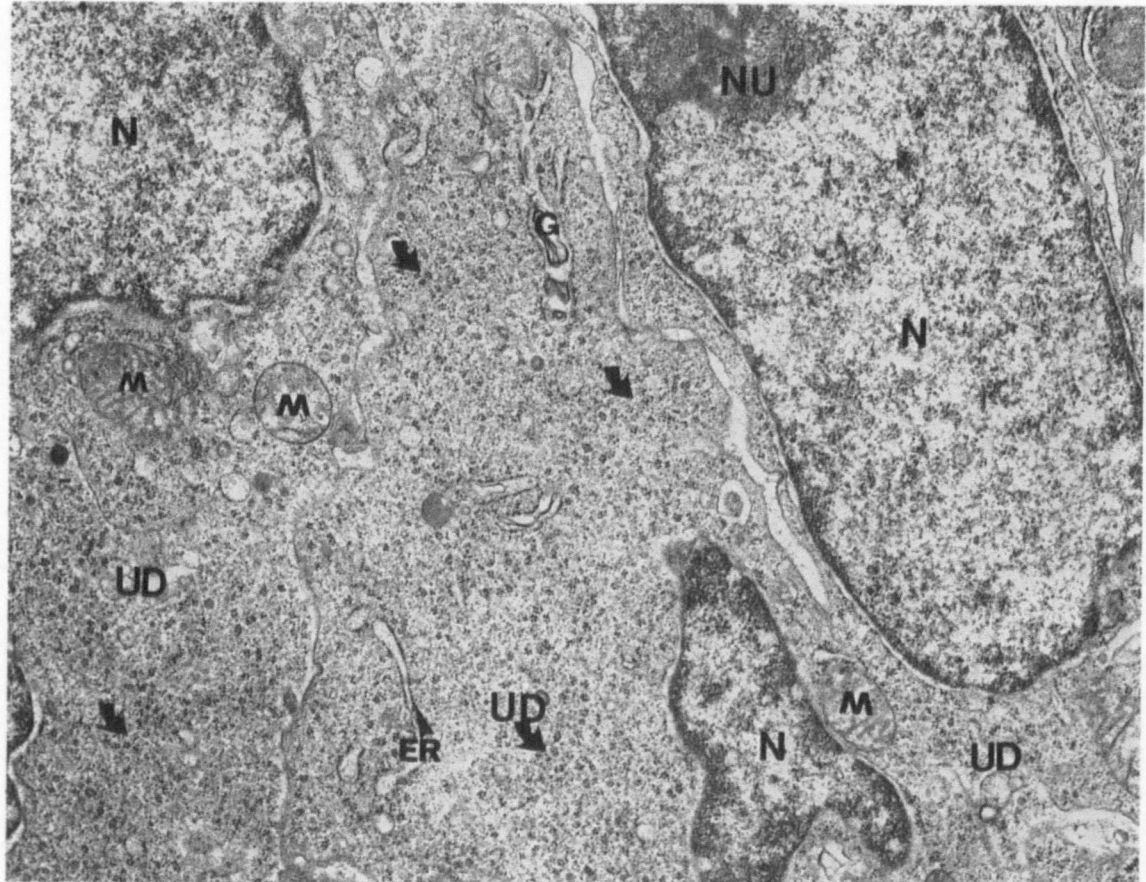

Fig. 1.27. Part of several immature or undifferentiated crypt cells (*UD*) at the nuclear level. The nuclei (*N*) are broad or oval, deficient in chromatin material and may contain a nucleolus (*NU*). The cytoplasm is relatively electron translucent and contains large numbers of free ribosomes (*arrow*), few mitochondria (*M*), little endoplasmic reticulum (*ER*) and a poorly developed Golgi complex(*G*). (×22 390)

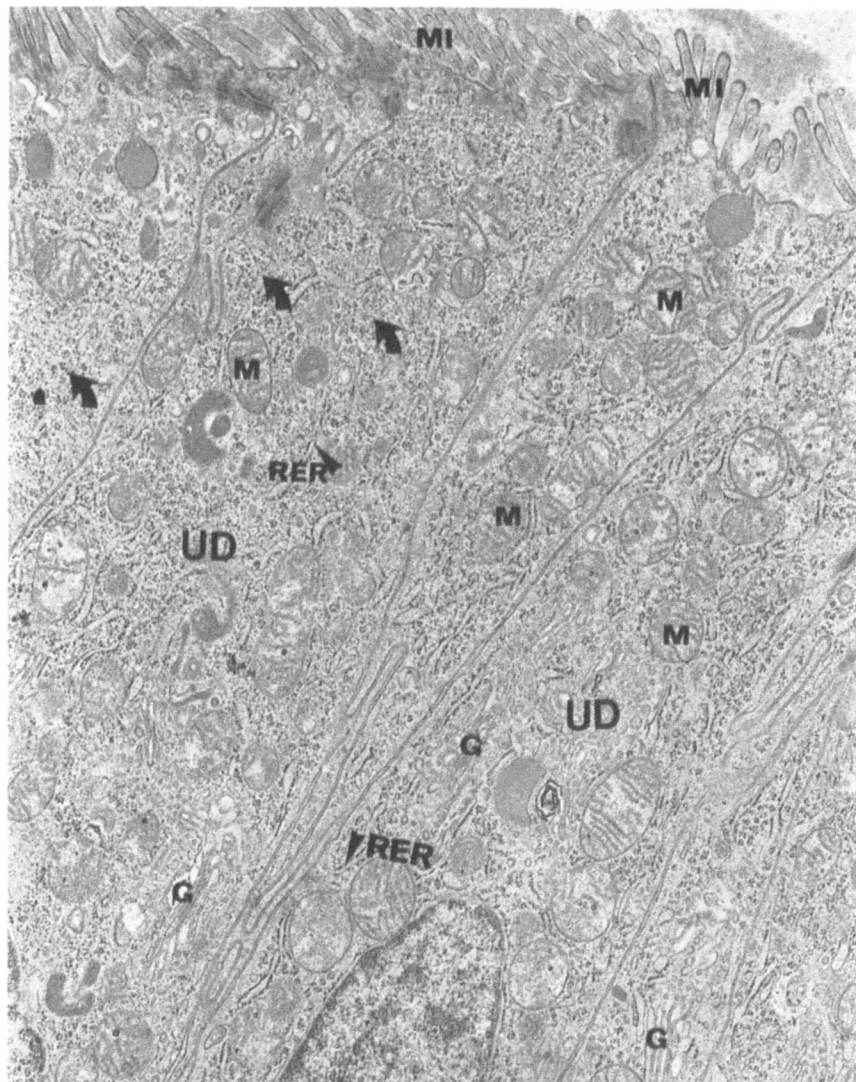

Fig. 1.28. Apical portion of undifferentiated crypt epithelium (*UD*) at a later stage of maturity. Short though densely spaced microvilli (*MI*) are seen. Mitochondria (*M*) and *RER* become more numerous. Several poorly developed Golgi complexes (*G*) are present. Most ribosomes (*arrow*) are still free-lying. (× 19 930)

(Fig. 1.28). Differentiating cells acquire intracytoplasmic organelles which are more numerous and densely packed so that the cell appears more electron dense (Fig. 1.29). The ER and RER systems occupy most of the space within the cytoplasmic matrix. The Golgi complex becomes well developed with numerous vesicles. Lysosomes are few (Fig. 1.29). As these cells mature further, the cytoplasmic organelles become organised to take up their distinctive position, in which the ribosomes attach themselves to ER, usually related to the mitochondria, and the Golgi complex is positioned in relation to the nucleus. The cytoplasmic matrix acquires a relatively light background typical of the mature enterocyte (Fig. 1.13).

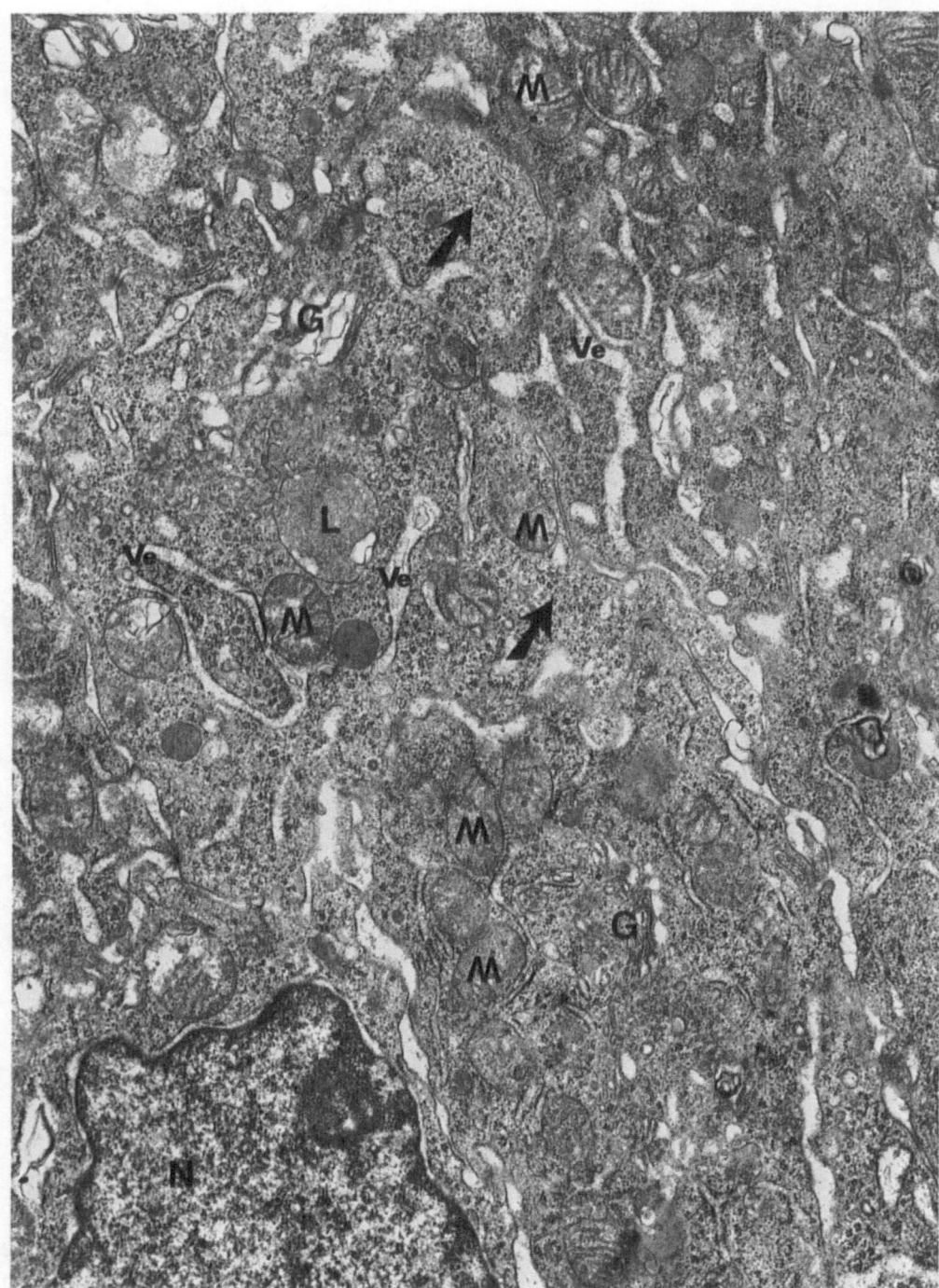

Fig. 1.29. Several differentiating crypt cells at the supranuclear level, showing dense cytoplasmic packing by numerous organelles which include ribosomes and polysomes (*arrow*), dilated elongated vesicles (*Ve*) usually lined by RER, large numbers of mitochondria (*M*) and developing Golgi complexes (*G*). *N*, nucleus; *L*, lysosomes. (× 21 500)

Goblet cells

It is not clear whether the precursor cell of the goblet cell is distinct from the precursor cell of the definitive enterocyte or whether these arise from a common stem cell. In its developmental stages the definitive goblet cell synthesises protein-rich material in the RER. This is passed on to the Golgi complex in which the smooth-membraned sacs proliferate and vesicles dilate around, but mainly above, the nucleus (Fig. 1.30). Carbohydrates are added and form part of the mucopolysaccharide material of the secretory granules which eventually becomes concentrated in round, smooth-membraned

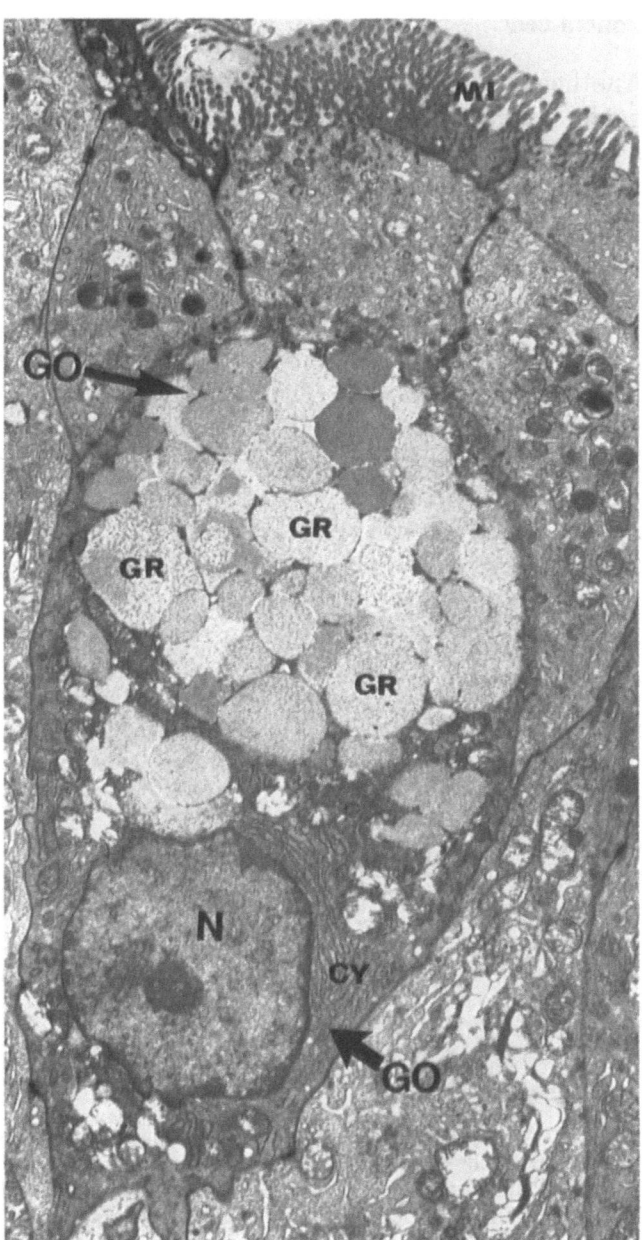

Fig. 1.30. A maturing goblet cell (*GO*) at the crypt-villous junction surrounded by several differentiating cells. The goblet cell shows a basally situated nucleus (*N*), concentrically arranged cisternae (*CY*) and large numbers of secretory granules (*GR*) lined by smooth membrane and containing light-coloured granular material. *MI*, microvilli of differentiating cells. (See also Fig. 1.26 showing a goblet cell with microvilli). (×7500)

droplets. These droplets occupy the proximal part of the cell and push the nucleus into a basal position. The mature goblet cell (Figs. 1.26, 1.30) has a microvillous surface and secretory granules which are enclosed laterally and basally by a limiting membrane that walls them off from the rest of the cytoplasm. The secretory material is homogeneous, light coloured and granular. As the granular material is ready for discharge the microvilli at the surface of the cell separate and the material in the form of masses of mucous droplets escapes into the lumen. The remainder of the cell appears to retain its viability. Goblet cells are most numerous in the crypts and form the second most numerous cell type of the villi.

Paneth cells

Another type of secretory cells are the Paneth cells (Fig. 1.31), but unlike the goblet cells they are entirely confined to the crypts where they take up a position at the base of the crypts. In their early developmental stages the Paneth cells appear indistinguishable from the goblet cells in that they show the same increase in Golgi vesicles and in RER. As the secretory granules form they also become enveloped in smooth membrane. There are however two distinguishing features in Paneth cells: 1) The secretory granules are denser than the goblet material and often show a lighter ring on the outside (halo) with a darker core (inset); and 2) the granules remain discrete and are not walled off from the rest of the cell. The round secretory granules very in size and are somewhat smaller than the goblet secretory granules. They also contain homogeneous, finely granular material which is intensely eosinophilic on light microscopy. The mature granules are discharged into the crypt lumen by an apocrine and merocrine secretory process. The granular material contains mucoproteins and carbohydrates as well as lysozyme [4] and zinc [1]. Their function is poorly understood.

APUD cells

These peptide hormones (*A*mine *P*recursors *U*ptake and *D*ecarboxylation) are found in cells of neural crest ectoderm origin belonging to the gut endocrine system [14]. The cells are widely distributed in the mucosa of the stomach, pancreas and small and large intestine, and contain electron-dense, round granules from which the peptide hormones are discharged directly into the blood. Numerous peptide hormones which have important physiological functions have been characterised as a result of endocrine tumours in which an

---

Fig. 1.31. A Paneth cell (*PA*) amongst several undifferentiated crypt epithelial cells (*UD*). The Paneth cell has a ▷ luminal microvillous border (*MI*) (see also Fig. 1.26) and a basally situated nucleus (*N*). The cytoplasm is rich in RER-bound cisternae (*arrow*) and in Golgi complexes (*G*). The supranuclear cytoplasm is filled with round, densely staining homogeneous or finely granular secretory granules (*GR*) varying in size. Inset shows secretory granules (*GR*) with 'halo' (*arrow*). G, Golgi complex. (× 10 330)

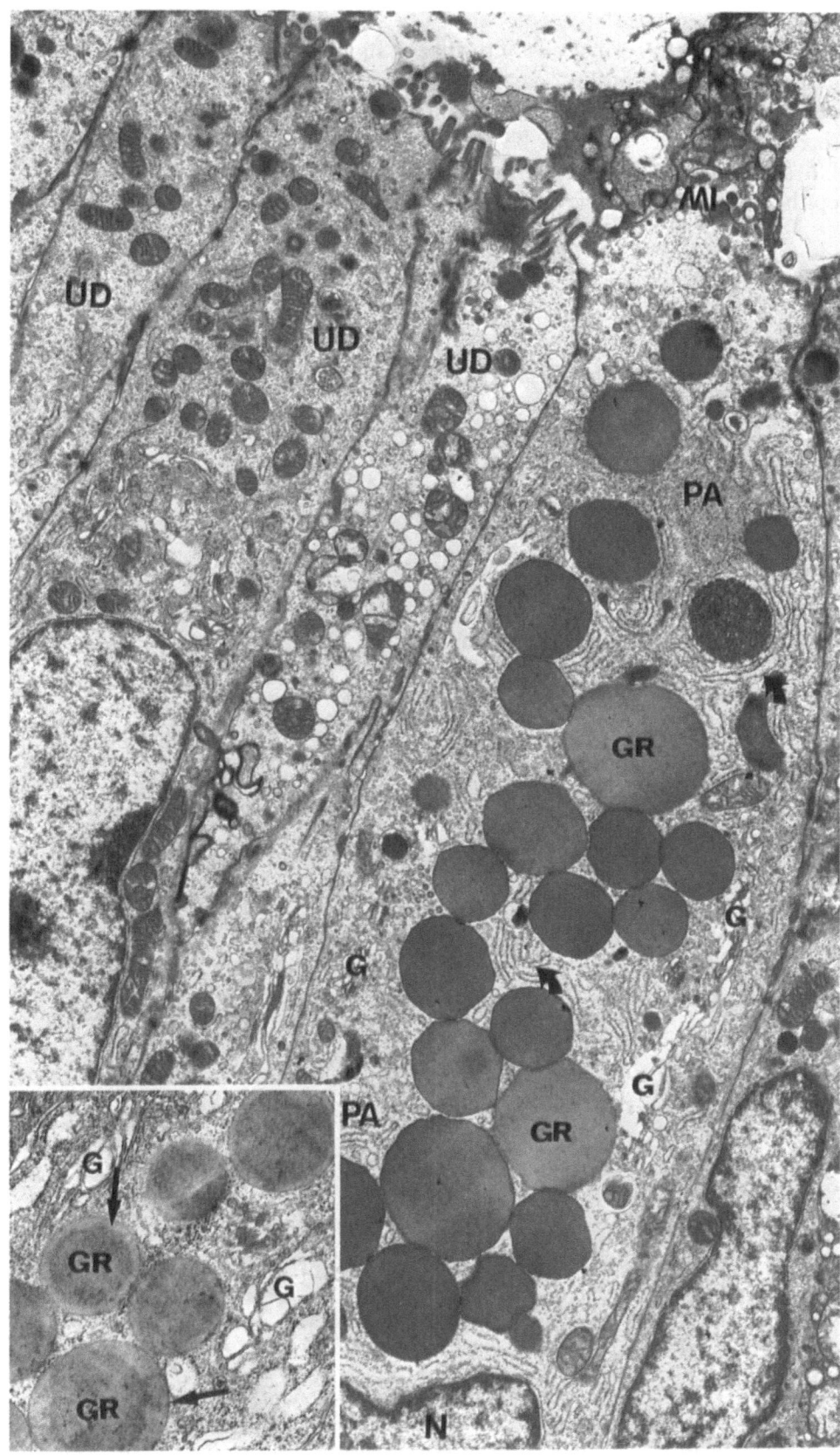

Fig. 1.31.

excess of any particular hormone may be secreted. Of the hormones hitherto described, the endocrine cells of the upper small intestine secrete only secretin, cholecystokinin, motilin, gastric inhibitory peptide, vasoactive intestinal peptide, pancreatic peptide and enteroglucagon. These are stored in the secretory granules and can be studied by immunocytochemical techniques. Ultrastructurally these endocrine cells are mainly found amongst the crypt cell epithelium but also in the villous cells. Various types of cells can be recognised

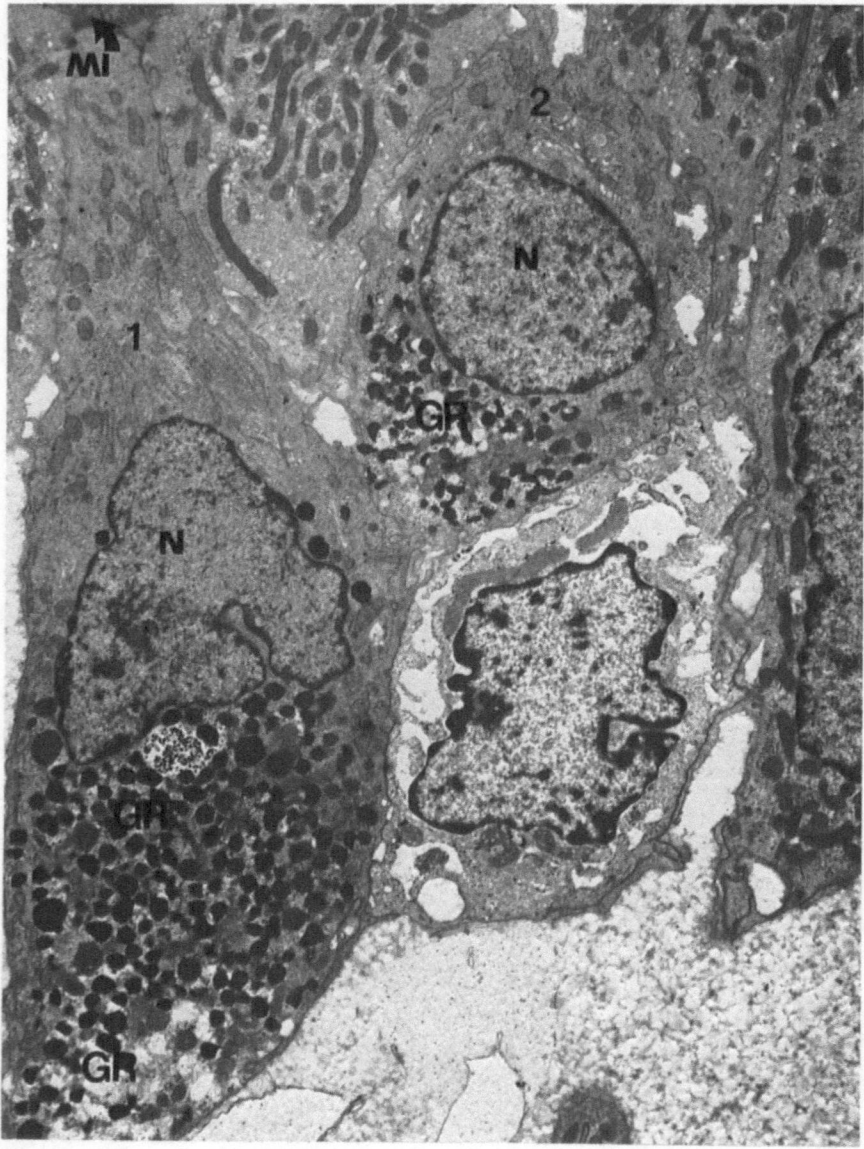

Fig. 1.32a. Two APUD cells (*1* and *2*) with dense secretory granules (*GR*) in the cytoplasm and round or indented nuclie (*N*) situated above the granules in relation to the crypt lumen. Cell 1 extends to the lumen and has microvilli (*MI*). (× 9060)

becauseof their dense secretion granules, which vary from about 100 to 500 μm in size. Some are small triangular-shaped cells situated near the basal end of the epithelial line (Figs. 1.32a, b) and do not appear to extend to the crypt or bowel lumen. Others are longer and narrower cells which share a common brush border with the rest of the epithelium and contain secretory granules on either side of the more centrally placed nucleus (Fig. 1.32a). Either type may discharge its granules through the basal lamina (Fig. 1.33).

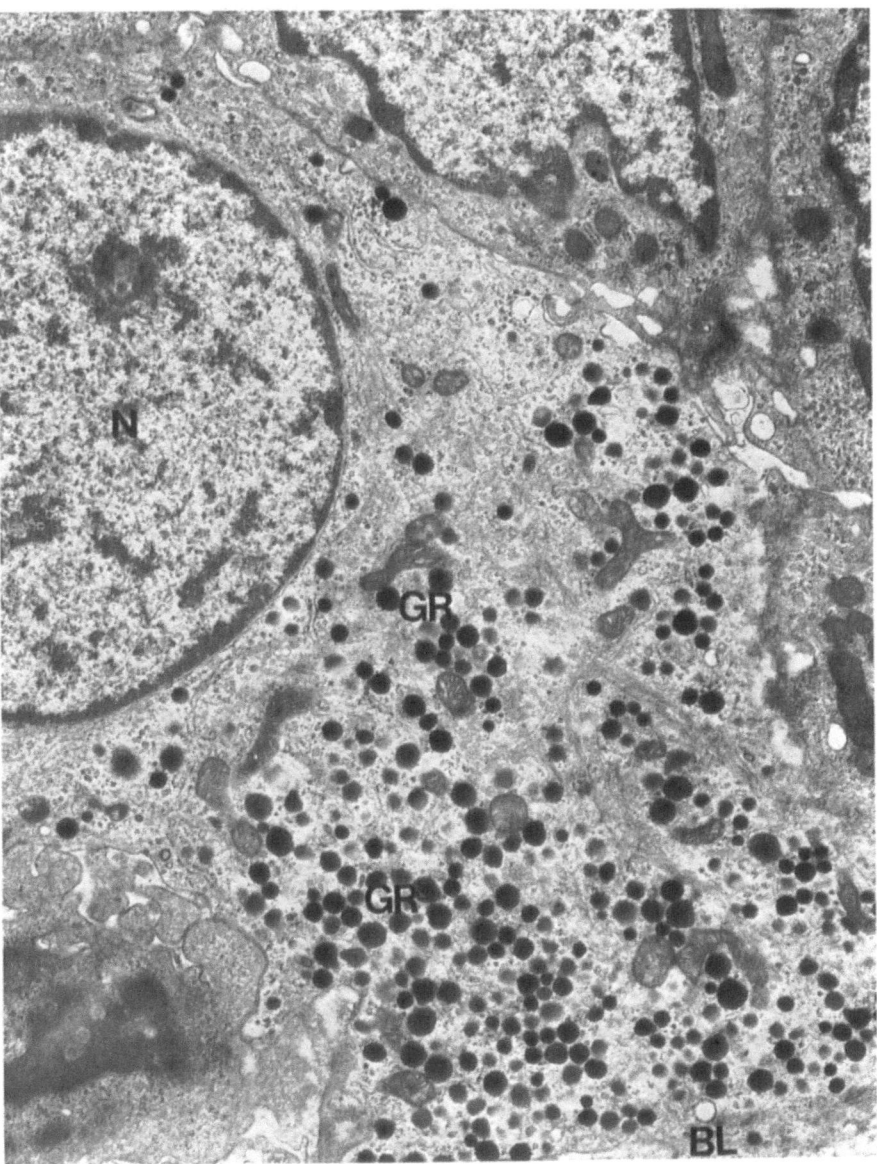

Fig. 1.32b. Lower portion of an APUD cell, showing dense small cytoplasmic granules (*GR*) in relation to the basal lamina (*BL*). Nearly all the granules are found below the nucleus (*N*). (× 11 340)

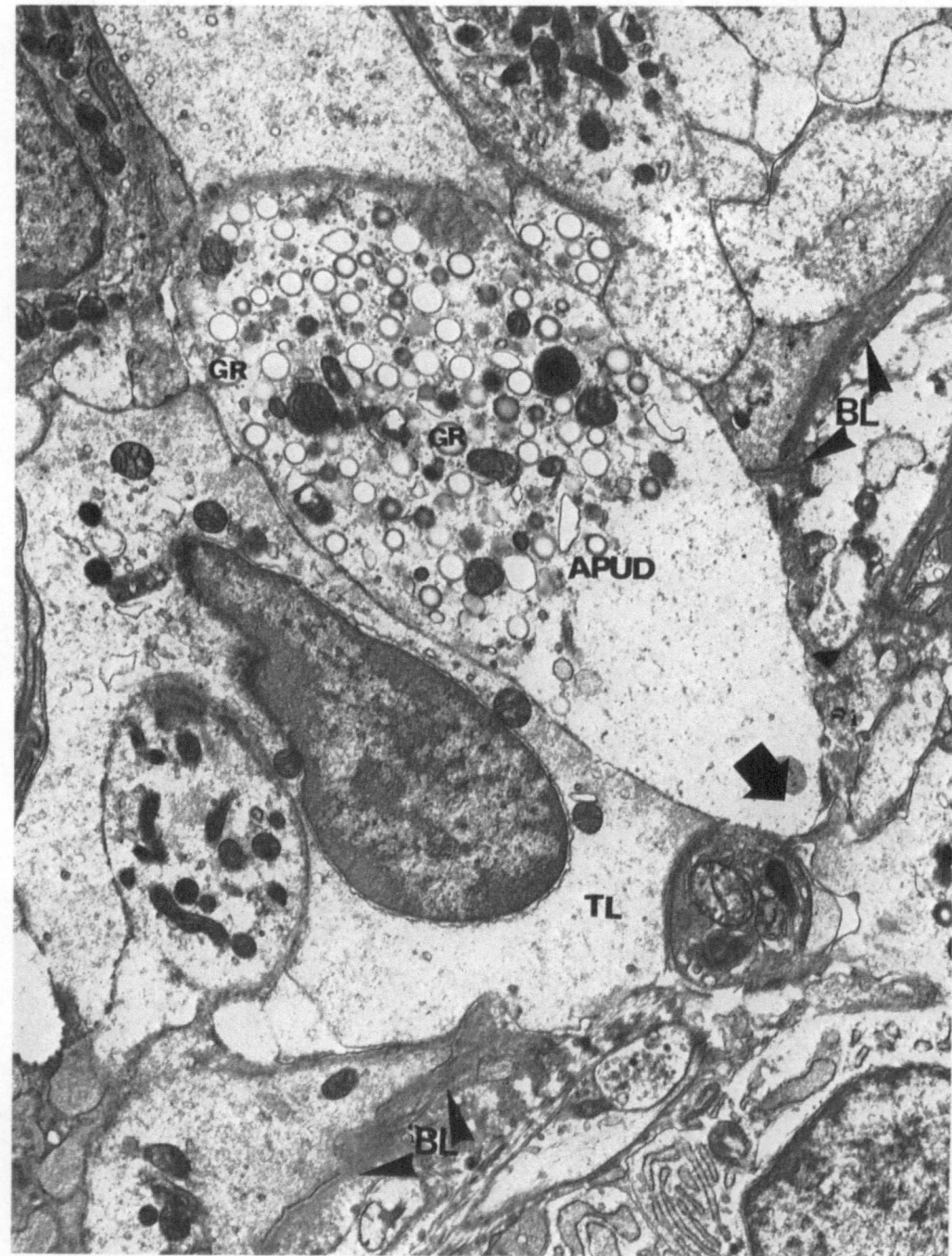

Fig. 1.33. A partly degranulated *APUD* cell with cytoplasmic projection (*arrow*) through the basal lamina (*BL*) of the crypt epithelium. The secretion granules (*GR*) are mostly empty vacuoles. *TL*, theliolymphocyte. (× 7500)

Theliolymphocytes

Amongst the epithelium of villi and crypts another cell type can be identified which has aroused great interest in recent years. These are small cells with a clear cytoplasm containing relatively few organelles and a more or less central nucleus (Figs. 1.3, 1.33). They are found to occupy the spaces between adjacent epithelial cells and are therefore also called inter- (or intra-) epithelial [18] lymphocytes, although they were first described by Fichtelius as theliolymphocytes [5]. Morphologically they resemble the small and large lymphocytes of the lamina propria, and indeed appear to arise from that region since they may be seen to occupy a position just above or between the basal laminae of the epithelial layer (Fig. 1.34). Their cytoplasm is relatively rich in ribosomes and contains a variable amount of ER and RER. Some cells resemble blast cells [8]

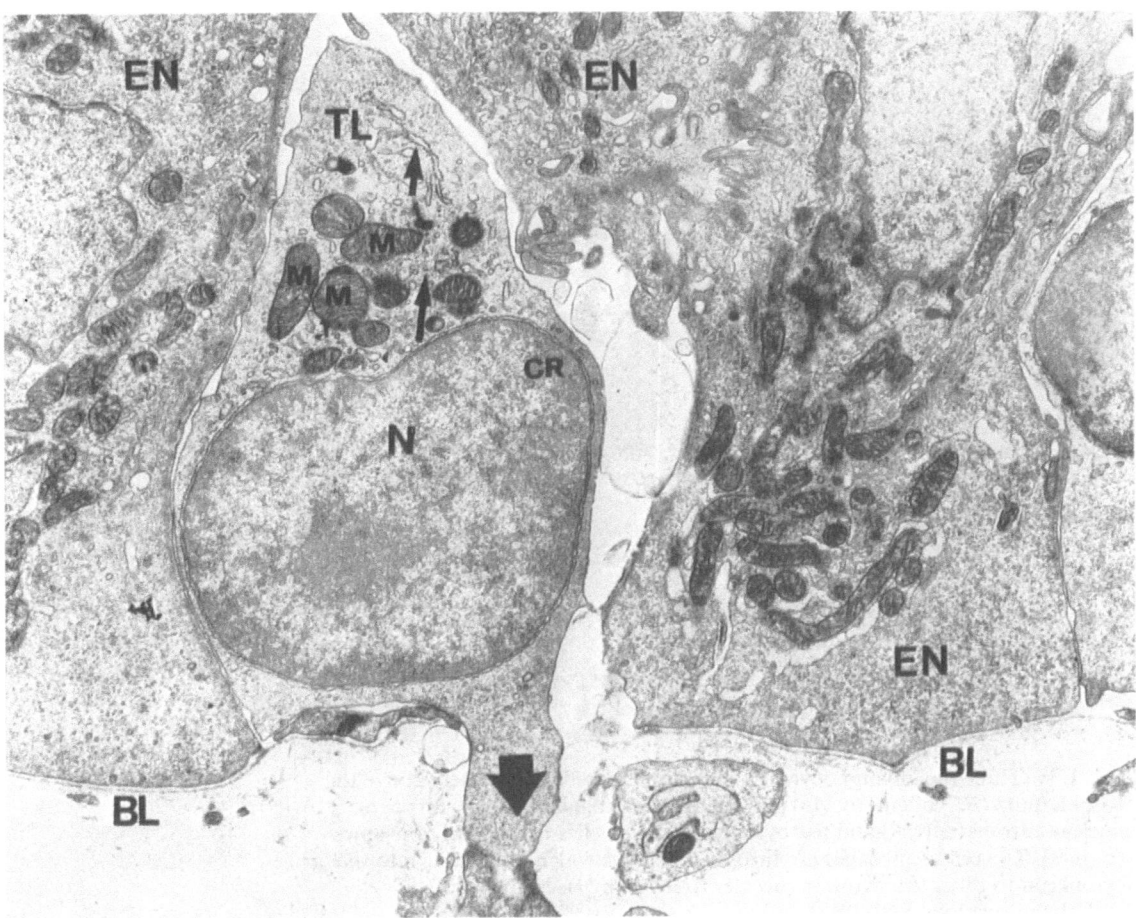

Fig. 1.34. Theliolymphocytes (*TL*) between enterocytes (*EN*) situated immediately above the basal lamina (*BL*). The large nucleus (*N*) and peripherally arranged chromatin (*CR*), as well as the relatively large numbers of cytoplasmic mitochondria (*M*) and endoplasmic reticulum (*arrow*), suggest that the cell is of large lymphocyte type. Below the nucleus a cytoplasmic process (*thick arrow*) extends into the lamina propria, dividing the basal lamina. (×9705)

(Fig. 1.35) with sparse nuclear chromatin and cytoplasmic organelles consisting almost entirely of ribosomes. Other cells resemble macrophages (Fig. 1.36a) with large indented nuclei and numerous cytoplasmic organelles including mitochondria, ER, RER, Golgi and a few dense granules [2]. It is important to appreciate that theliolymphocytes are normal components of villi and crypt cells, though they may greatly increase in number under pathological conditions. Their movement is not properly understood but although they may originate from the lamina propria and return to that position eventually, a few

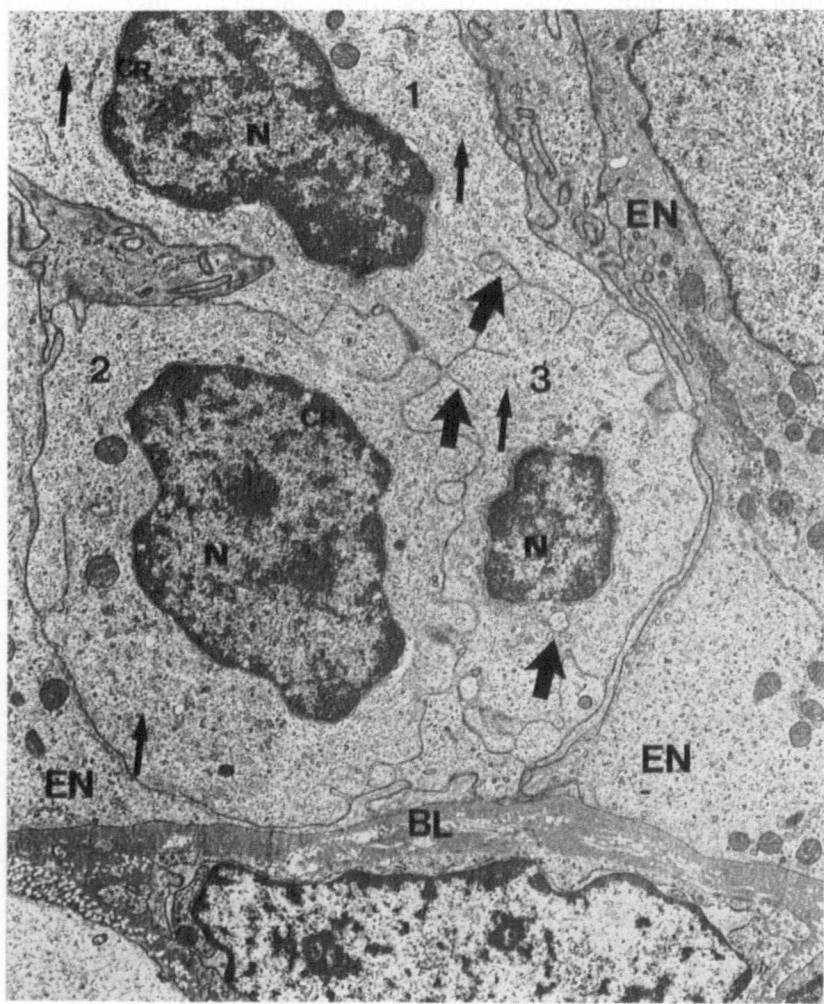

Fig. 1.35. Three theliolymphocytes (*1*, *2* and *3*) situated immediately above the basal lamina (*BL*) of enterocytes (*EN*). They resemble blast cells with sparse nuclear chromatin (*CR*) and few cytoplasmic organelles other than ribosomes (*arrows*). The cell membranes are thrown into folds which invaginate into the cytoplasm to form pinocytotic processes (*thick arrows*). *N*, nuclei of theliolymphocytes. (× 8140)

Fig. 1.36a. Interepithelial cell located between enterocytes (*EN*) showing a large indented nucleus (*N*) and cytoplasm rich in ribosomes (*R*) and polysomes, mitochondria (*M*), *ER* and *RER*, a well-developed Golgi complex (*G*) and a few granules containing dense homogeneous material (*arrows*). (× 25 300)   ▷

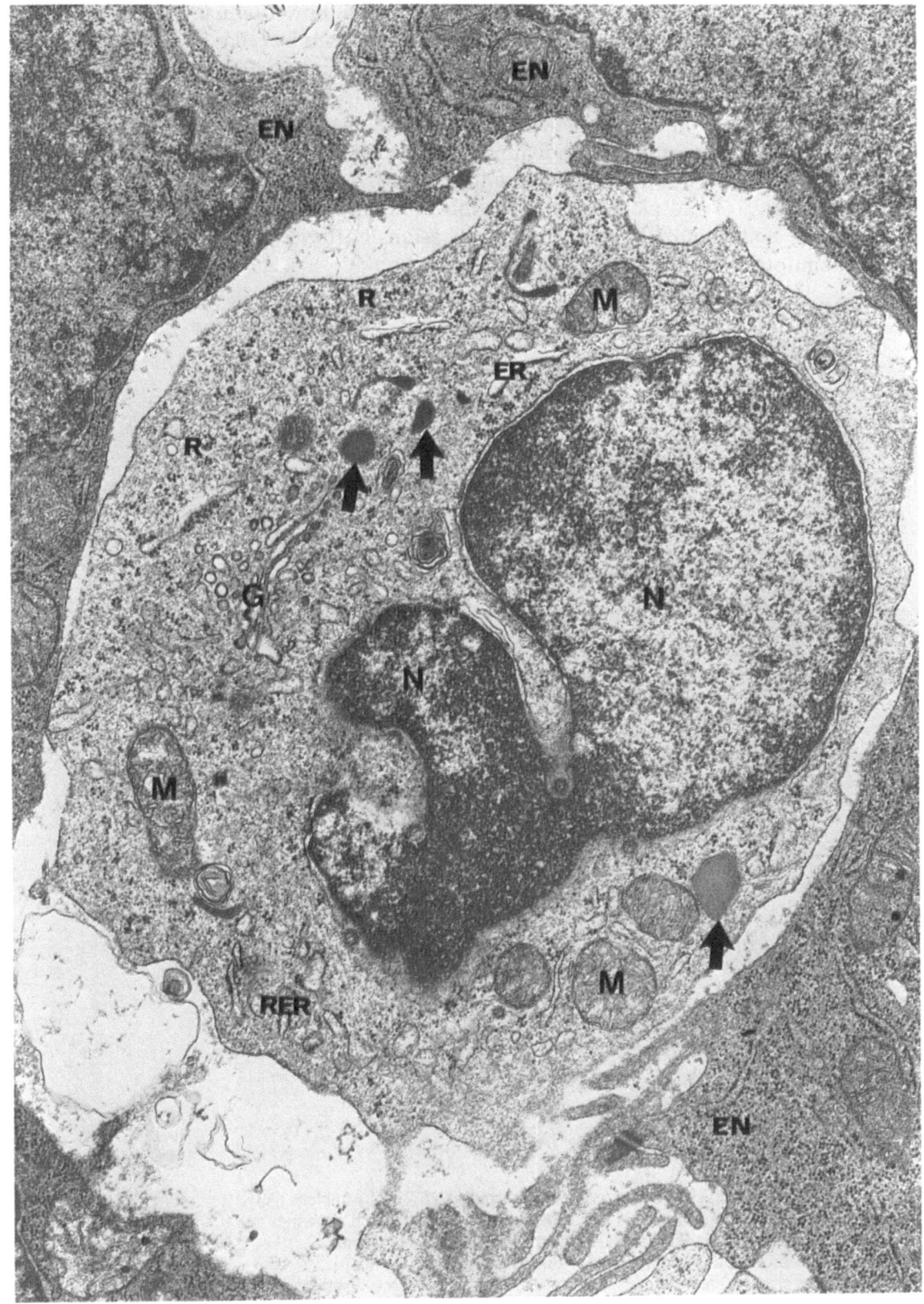

Fig. 1.36a.

of the theliolymphocytes can occasionally be seen in the bowel lumen. It is possible that they escape to the lumen through spaces created by cell lysis and cell death.

The theliolymphocytes are thought, but by no means proven, to possess specialised functions different from the lymphocytes of the lamina propria. The surface membrane of human theliolymphocytes reacts with antisera to T-lymphocyte antigens but not to IA-like antigens. It is possible that they are effector T-cells [16] and pick up antigenic information during their passage between the epithelium (Fig. 1.36b). Very occasionally they can be seen to undergo mitotic division.

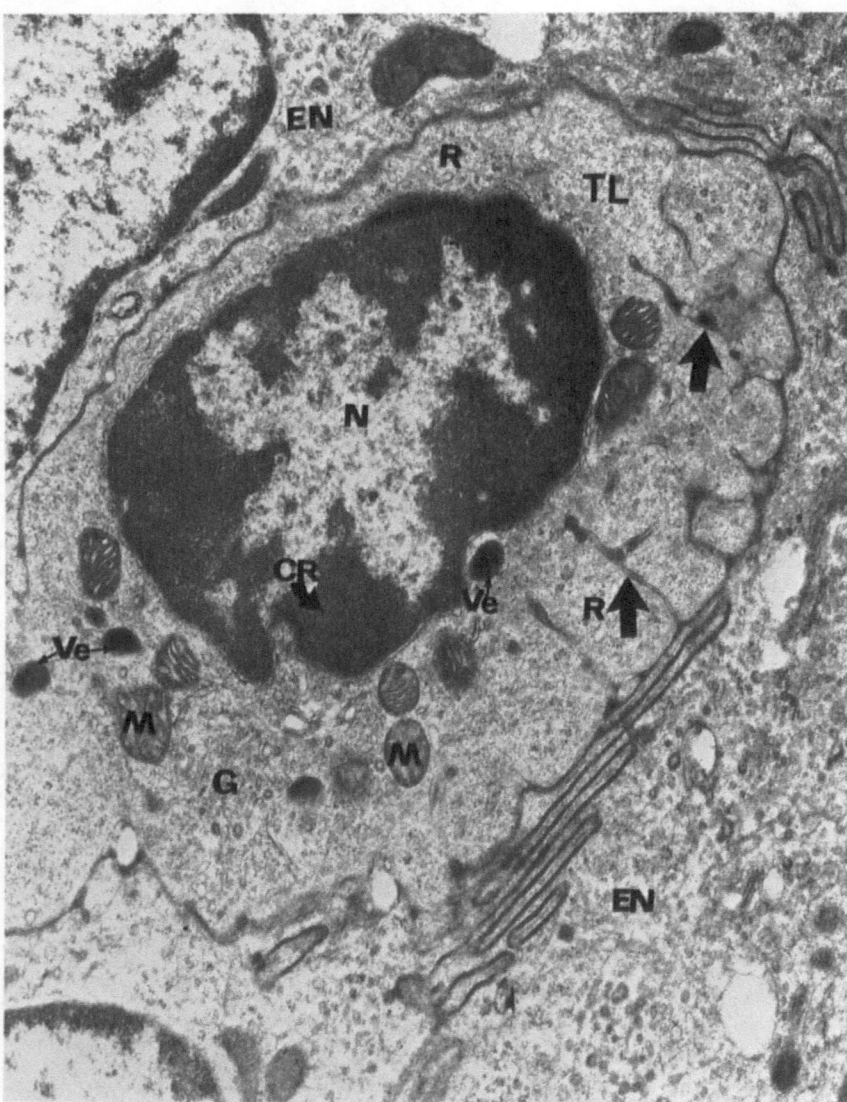

1.36b. Interepithelial cell (*TL*) surrounded by enterocytes (*EN*). The nucleus (*N*) contains heavy chromatin material (*CR*). The cytoplasm, apart from showing mitochondria (*M*), Golgi vesicles (*G*), ribosomes and polysomes, contains pinocytotic membranous invaginations of the cell membrane filled with homogeneous electron-dense material (*arrows*) (?antigen) which is also seen in membrane-bound intracytoplasmic vesicles (*Ve*). Compare with Figs. 1.35 and 1.36a. (×17 010)

The lamina propria (see Fig. 1, p. 1)

The lamina propria is a histological term denoting the space occupied by connective tissue and its cellular content between the basal laminae of the villous epithelium and the muscularis mucosae. The various cell types of interest are:

1) the infiltrating (inflammatory or non-attached) cells
2) the Schwann cells and nerve fibres
3) the endothelial cells of small blood vessels and lymphatics
4) the fibrocytes and their processes (including collagen).

Cells infiltrating the lamina propria

Since the lymphocytes, plasma cells, macrophages, histiocytes, mast cells and possibly eosinophils are normal constituents of the mucosal lamina propria, the descriptive term of 'infiltrating, inflammatory or non-attached' for these cell types is misleading. Only the polymorphonuclear leucocyte might be thought of as outside the normal cellular constituents of the lamina propria.

The *lymphocyte* of the lamina propria may be small or large (Figs. 1.37, 1.38) with convoluted or round nuclei and relatively little cytoplasm. The nucleus may contain a nucleolus. The nuclear chromatin is arranged as dense aggregates, similar to the cart-wheel pattern of the plasma cell nucleus. The

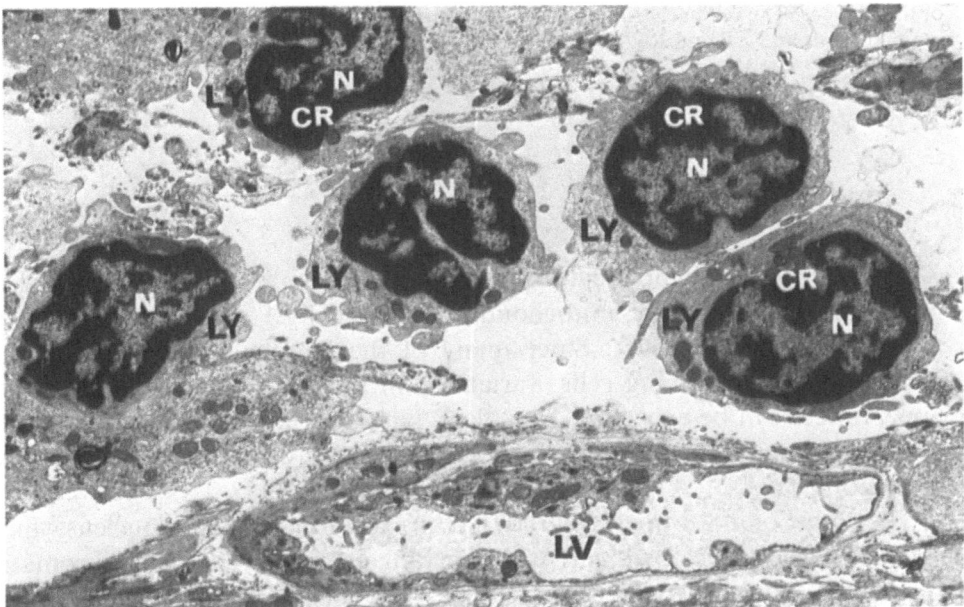

Fig. 1.37. Lymphocytes (*LY*) in the lamina propria, containing convoluted nuclei (*N*) with heavy and dense chromatin material (*CR*) and a small amount of cytoplasm rich in free ribosomes and relatively poor in other organelles except mitochondria. *LV*, lymph vessel. (× 5950)

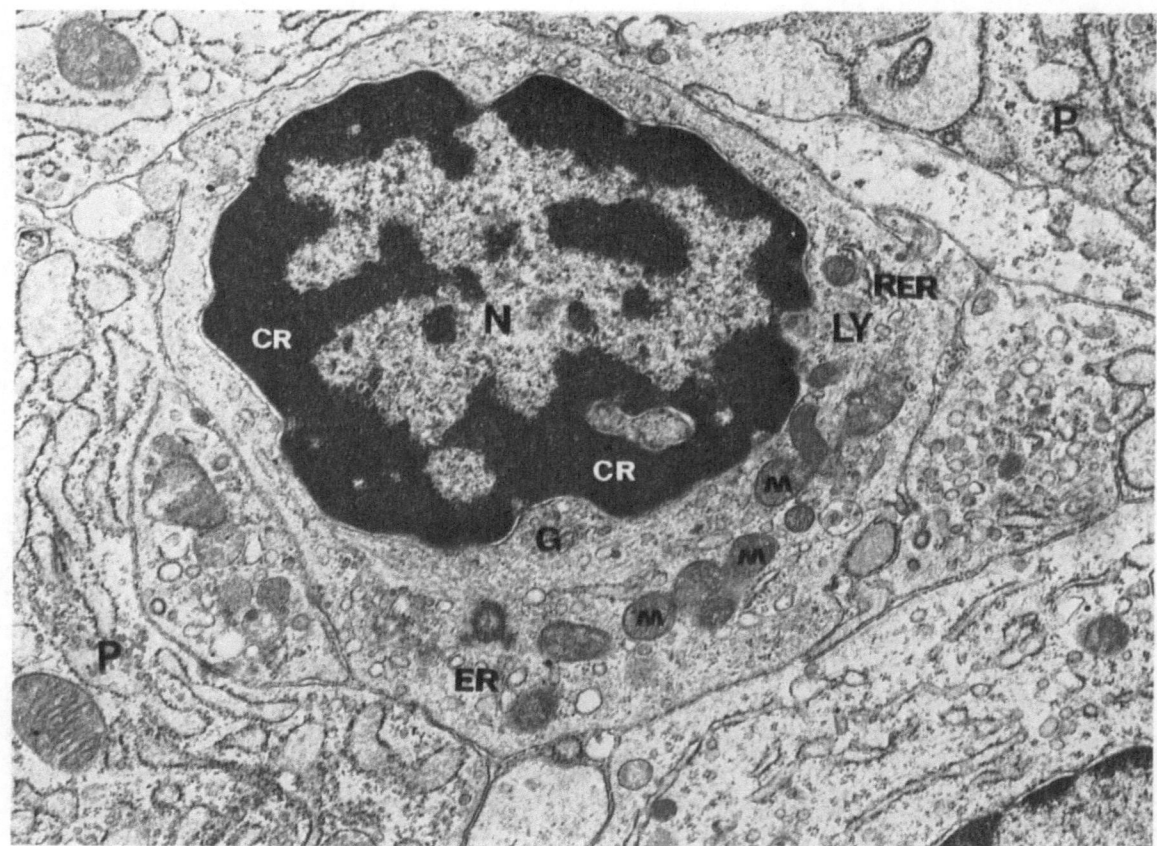

Fig. 1.38. Lymphocyte (*LY*) surrounded by plasma (*P*) in the lamina propria. The nucleus (*N*) is larger and round and contains a dense band of peripherally arranged chromatin (*CR*) which also extends into the interior of the nucleus. The relatively small amount of cytoplasm contains fewer free ribosomes, but mitochondria (*M*) are numerous and *ER* and *RER* is increased. *G*, Golgi (× 10670)

cytoplasm of the lymphocyte contains a variable variety of organelles, including Golgi complex, mitochondria, ER and RER and often numerous ribosomes and polysomes. Since many of the lymphocytes of the lamina propria are transforming cells, variations in their nuclear and cytoplasmic appearances can be expected. The 'blast' lymphocyte (Fig. 1.39) shows little nuclear chromatin and its cytoplasm contains mainly free ribosomes and few mitochondria.

The young or maturing *plasma cell* has an excentrically placed nucleus which shows a well developed cart-wheel arrangement of clumped chromatin (Fig. 1.40). Adjacent to the nucleus, the cytoplasm is rich in Golgi vesicles and other organelles such as mitochondria, ribosomes and ER, forming the light microscopist's so-called Hof. Near the periphery of the cell is an abundance of cisternae lined with RER. These cisternae are arranged in parallel fashion to each other and to the cell membrane and dilate with

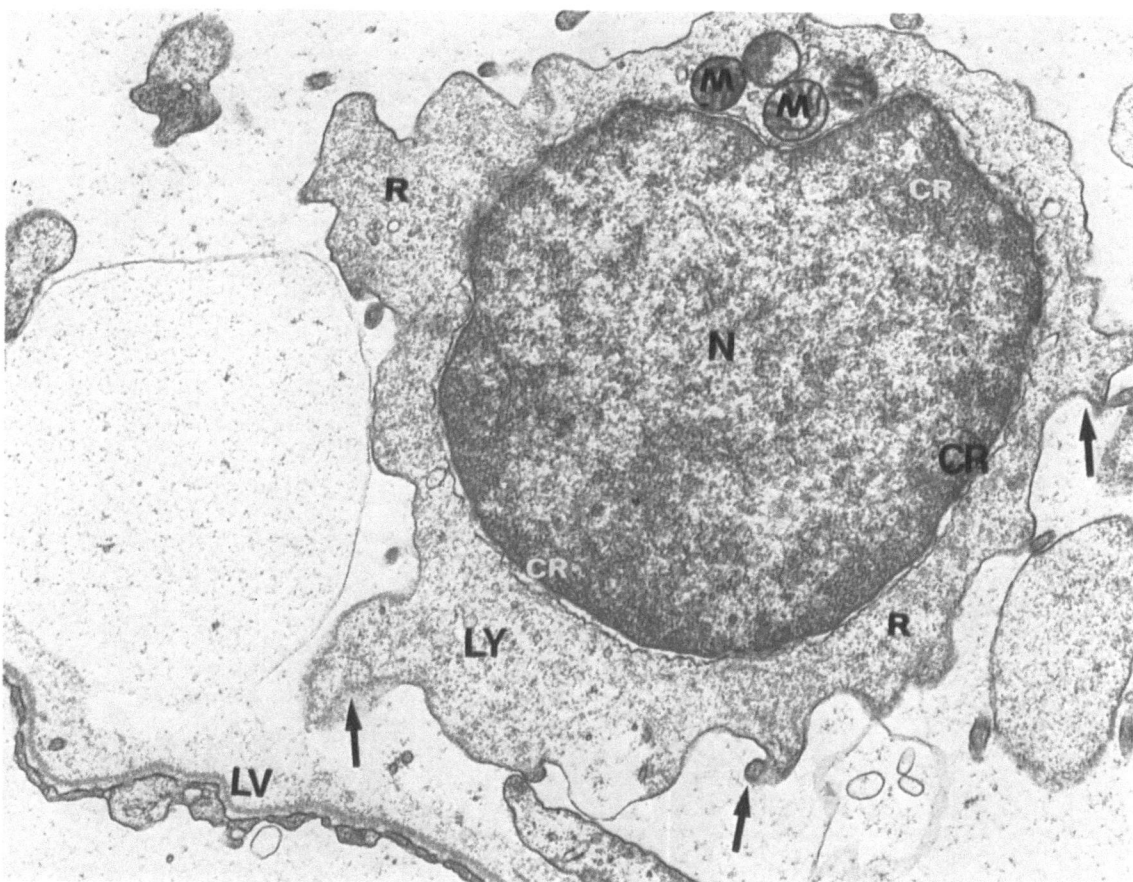

Fig. 1.39. 'Blast' lymphocyte (*LY*) (compare with Fig. 1.39) in the lamina propria near a lymph vessel (*LV*) showing a large nucleus (*N*) with sparse chromatin (*CR*), large numbers of cytoplasmic (free) ribosomes (*R*) and few mitochondria (*M*). The cell membrane is thrown into folds with cytoplasmic extensions (*arrow*). (× 15 500)

increasing ribosomal activity, which results in the formation of intracisternal immunoglobulin. As the plasma cell matures, more and more of its cytoplasmic space is taken up by RER-bound cisternae (Fig. 1.41) so that the Golgi complex and mitochondria become inconspicuous. Eventually the plasma cell is seen as possessing an excentric nucleus and a cytoplasmic space which is almost entirely taken up by more or less dilated cisternae lined by RER (Fig. 1.42). The plasma cell is the most numerous cell type seen in the normal lamina propria, and the cells will be seen in different stages of activity depending on their maturity and stimulation for immunoglobulin production. The mode of discharge of the immunoglobulin material from the normal plasma cell is not understood. The nuclear chromatin becomes somewhat paler towards the end of the life span of the plasma cell, and phagocytic vacuoles may appear in the cytoplasm. Cell death is seen when the nucleus undergoes necrobiosis, but this is not a common observation.

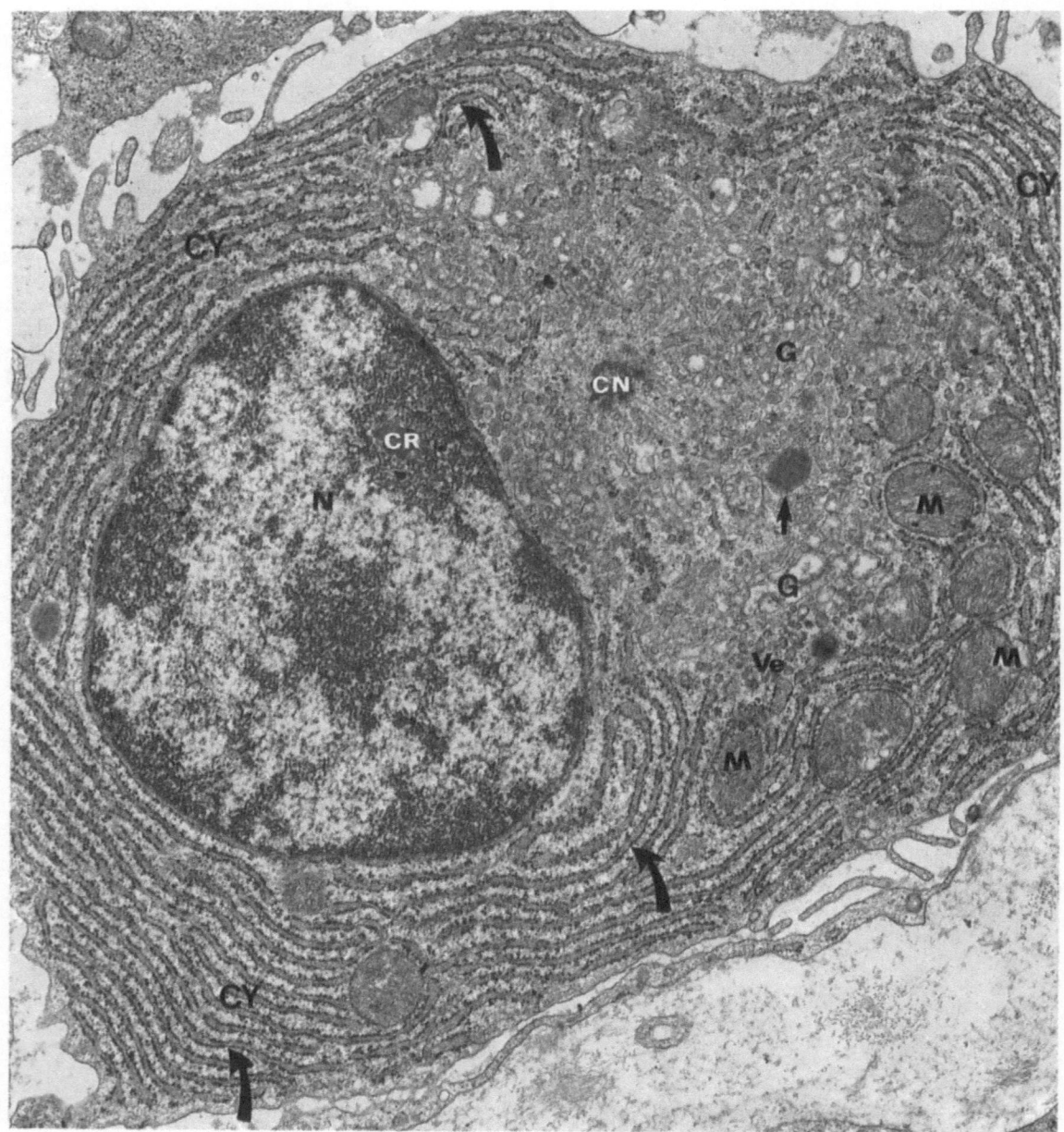

Fig. 1.40. Maturing plasma cell with excentrically placed nucleus (*N*) in which the chromatin material (*CR*) is arranged in the well-known cart-wheel pattern. To one side of the nucleus the cytoplasm is rich in organelles— ER, Golgi (*G*) and other small vesicles (*Ve*), a centriole (*CN*) and a dense body (*arrow*). The cytoplasmic cisternae (*CY*) occupy a large part of the cell and are arranged peripherally towards the cell membrane. The cisternae are arranged in parallel fashion to each other, are lined by RER (*curved arrow*) and contain moderately dense finely granular material, the immunoglobulin. Interspersed amongst the cisternae are a few mitochondria (*M*). The cell membrane has an oval shape and shows cytoplasmic extensions on its outer surface. (× 35 370)

Fig. 1.41. Part of the cytoplasm of a mature plasma cell showing dilated cisternae (*CY*) surrounded by *RER*   ▷ and filled with finely granular material (*arrow*) which is more electron dense than the surrounding cytoplasm. Free ribosomes (*R*) can be observed. (× 100 835)

Fig. 1.42. The mature plasma cell with a central nucleus (*N*) in which the chromatin (*CR*) is relatively sparse.   ▷ The cytoplasm contains only a few mitochondria (*M*). Most of the cytoplasmic space is taken up by moderately dilated cisternae (*CY*) filled with floccular immunoglobulin. (× 20 960)

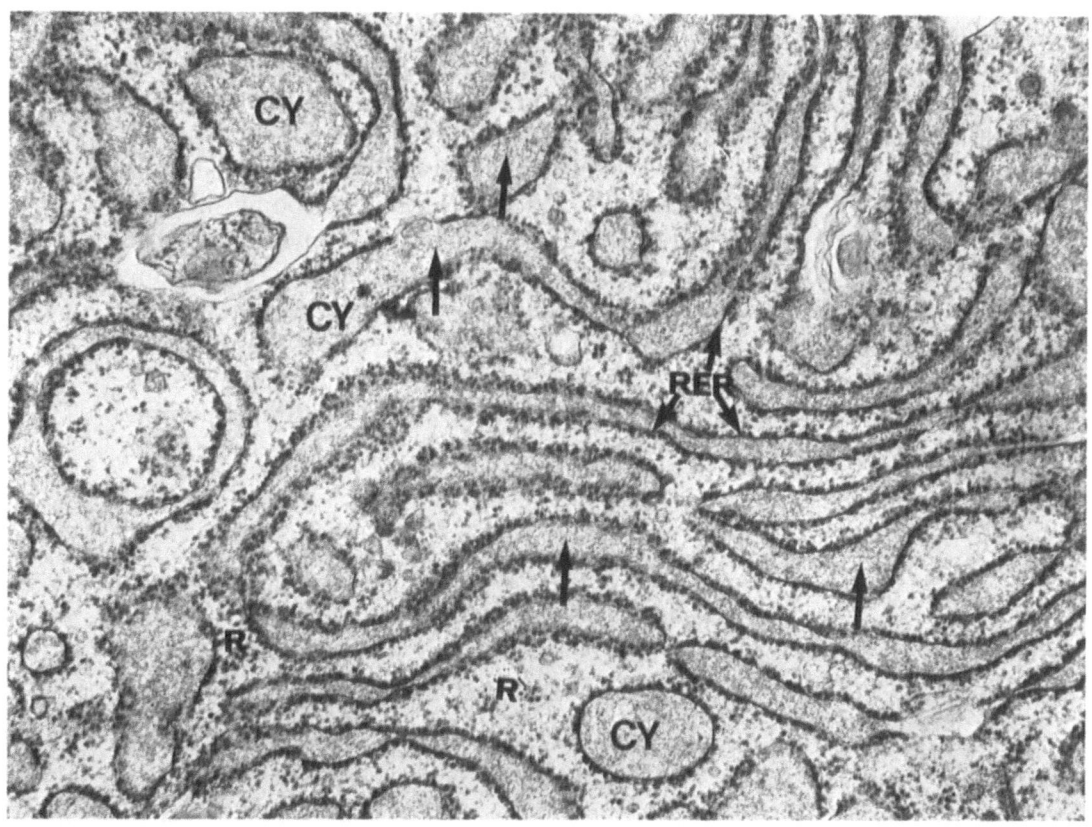

Fig. 1.41. △   Fig. 1.42. ▽

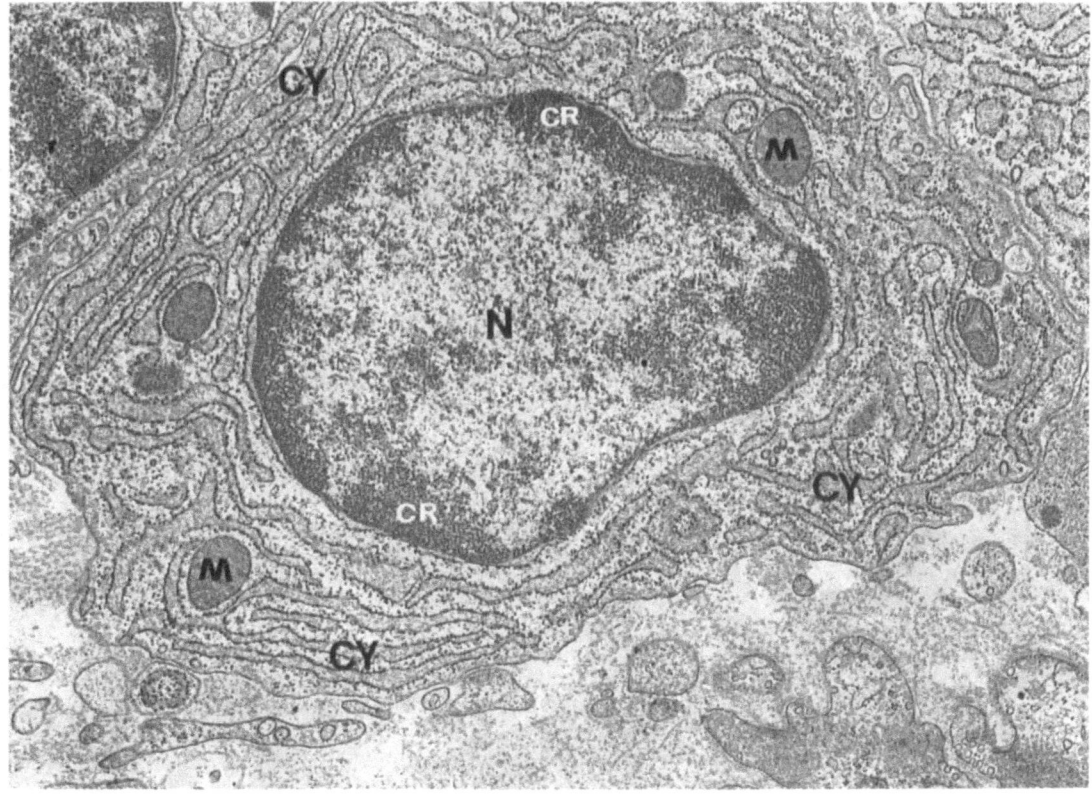

The *macrophages* are large cells with a relatively small excentric nucleus and a large amount of cytoplasm. The nucleus may appear round, oval, indented or kidney shaped and contains lightly coloured granular material and a fine rim of chromatin arranged parallel to the nuclear membrane (Figs. 1.43, 1.44). The cytoplasm is rich in organelles of which the phagolysosomes are the most characteristic (Fig. 1.44). These are dense, often heterogeneous bodies varying greatly in size and activity and are bound by a single smooth membrane. The cytoplasm also contains smooth-membraned vesicles and vacuoles containing a clear material, RER-bound cisternae which may be arranged in parallel stacks (but are not dilated like plasma cell cisternae), one or more Golgi complexes, numerous mitochondria and free-lying ribosomes or polysomes. Macrophages fulfil the important function of phagocytosis within the lamina propria and are particularly rich in acid hydrolases. They also play a role in the

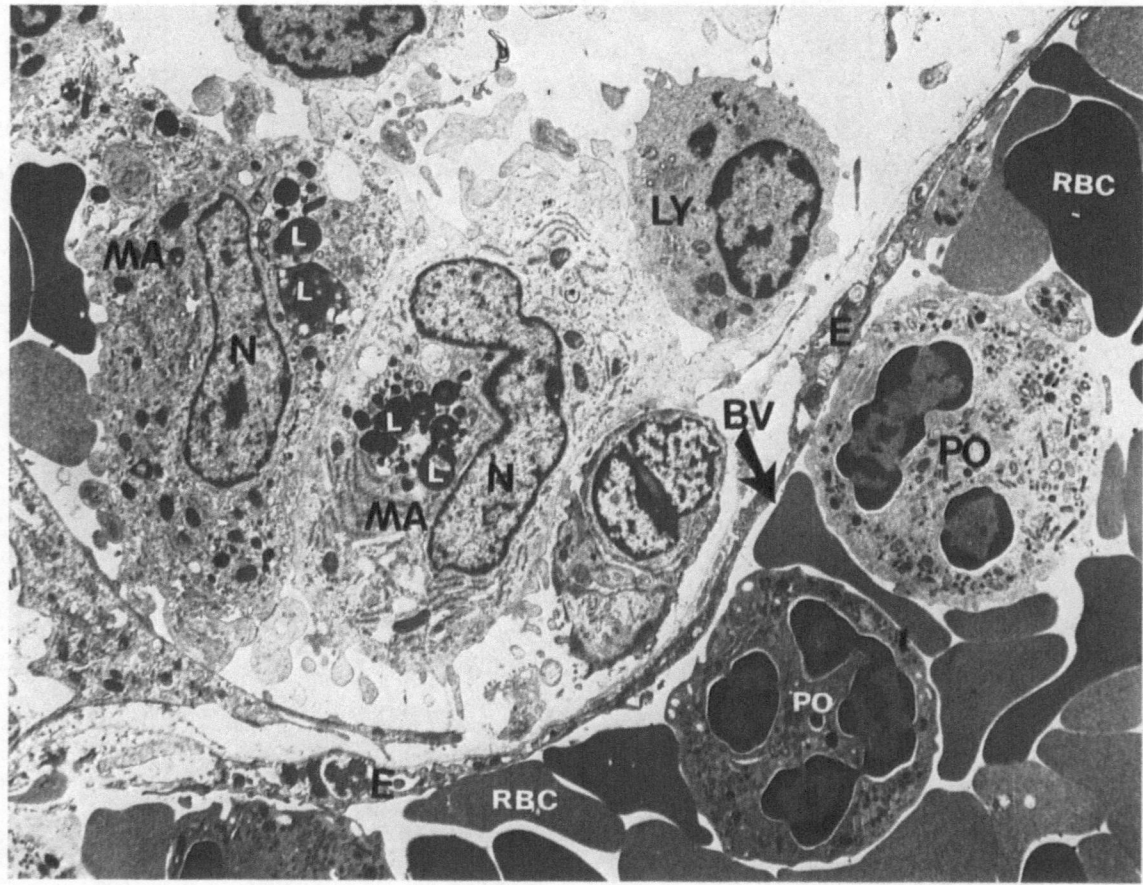

Fig. 1.43. Two macrophages (*MA*) within the lamina propria characterised by their relatively large size, lightly coloured nucleus (*N*) which has only a fine peripheral rim of chromatin, and numerous cytoplasmic phagolysosomes (*L*). The macrophages show numerous cytoplasmic extensions from their surfaces which appear to make contact with other cells, e.g. lymphocytes (*LY*). Note the close proximity of a large blood vessel (*BV*) lined by endothelial cells (*E*) and containing numerous red blood cells (*RBC*) as well as two polymorphs (*PO*). (×1935)

stimulation of local plasma cells. The macrophage can be thought of as a filter, ingesting and denaturing exogenous material, viruses, bacteria, and cellular material from surrounding disintegrating cells. Large fat globules are often seen within macrophage cytoplasm after fat ingestion. The *histiocytes* are rarer cell types of the normal lamina propria and resemble macrophages; indeed they may be the precursors of the macrophage. The nucleus is similar to the macrophage nucleus but is large in relation to the cytoplasmic area and shows one or more indentations (kidney shape) (Fig. 1.45). The cytoplasm often contains fewer organelles than the macrophage and the phagolysosomes in particular are poorly developed and contain few dense bodies. Though the histiocytes are thought of as precursor cells it is not clear whether the definitive cell is the macrophage or the lymphocyte.

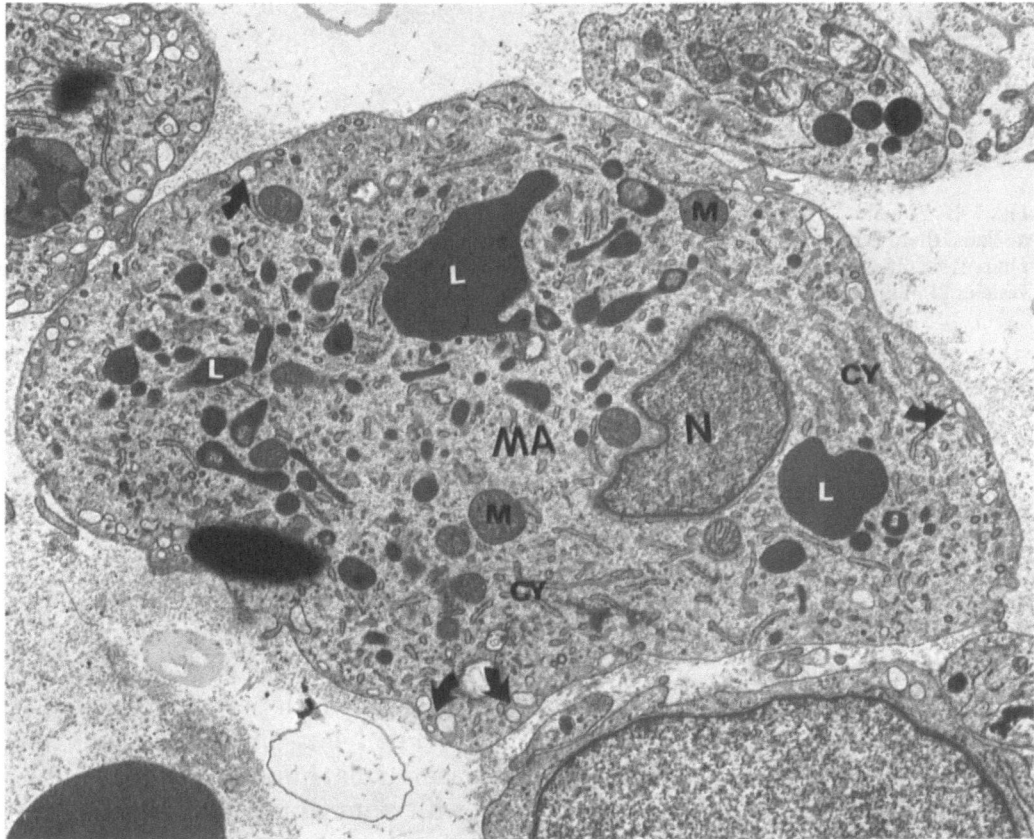

Fig. 1.44. Higher magnification of a macrophage (*MA*) in which the nucleus (*N*) is seen in an excentric position, surrounded by numerous organelles within the cell cytoplasm. Most conspicuous are the intensely electron-dense phagolysosomes (*L*), small and large, which contain heterogeneous material. The cytoplasm is also rich in small cisternae (*CY*) lined by RER. Vacuoles, which may be pinocytotic since they are located immediately beneath the cell membrane (*arrow*), are seen as well as mitochondria (*M*). (× 11 490)

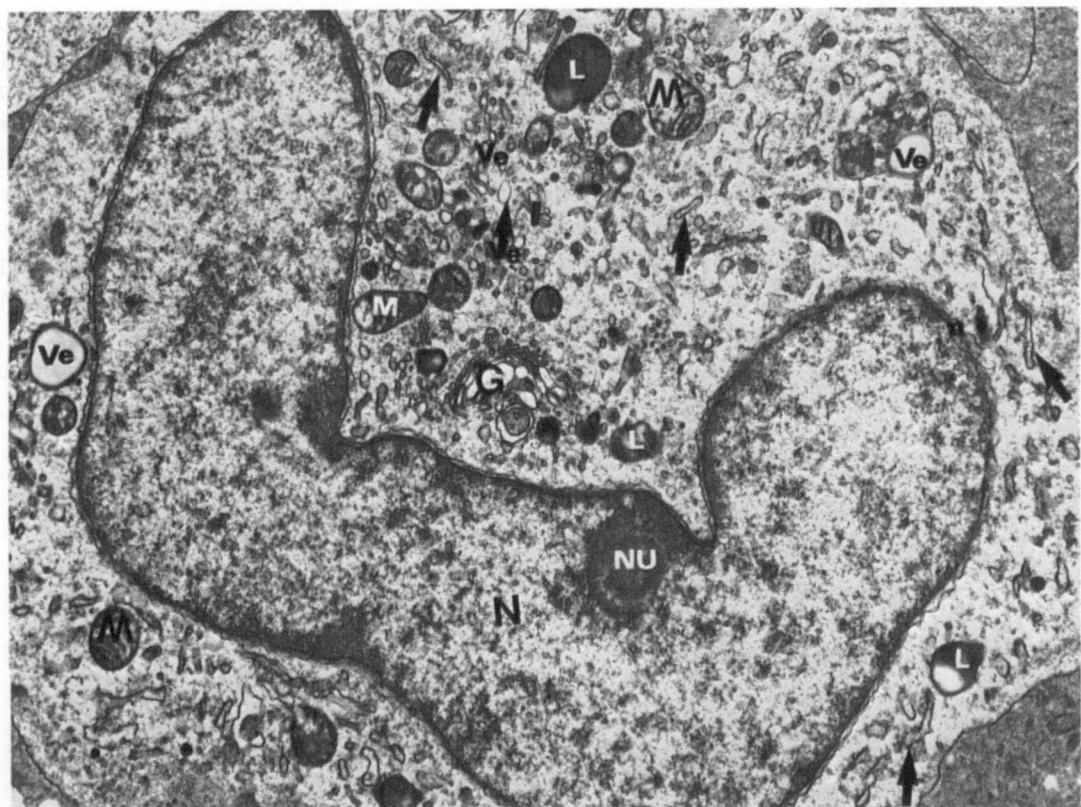

Fig. 1.45. A histiocyte showing a large indented nucleus (*N*) with a nucleolus (*NU*). Like the macrophage nucleus, there is only a sparse amount of nuclear chromatin. The cytoplasm contains fewer phagolysosomes (*L*), a small Golgi complex (*G*), few mitochondria (*M*), but numerous small and large vesicles (*Ve*) lined by smooth ER, as well as RER (*arrows*). (×11 780)

The *mast cells* are also normal constituents of the mucosal lamina propria but are few in number compared to the submucosa. They are round or oval cells (Fig. 1.46a) often showing numerous cytoplasmic projections from their cell surfaces. They possess a single round nucleus which takes up a central position within the cell and contains peripherally clumped chromatin material. The distinguishing features of the mast cell are the cytoplasmic vacuoles, composed of smooth membrane, containing material which may be seen as granular Fig. 1.46b), whorl-like or scroll-shaped (Fig. 1.46c). The vacuoles are round bodies which take up most of the cytoplasm so that other organelles are sparsely represented . They may appear filled with material rich in vasoactive and tissue damage mediators, or after stimulation empty as 'ghosts'. Usually both material containing and empty vacuoles can be recognised in any mast cell. Mast cells take part in reaginic reactions, are said to carry receptors for IgE on their surface membranes, discharge their granules on antigenic stimulation and attract eosinophils and also polymorphs into the lamina propria by the action of chemotactic mediators [12].

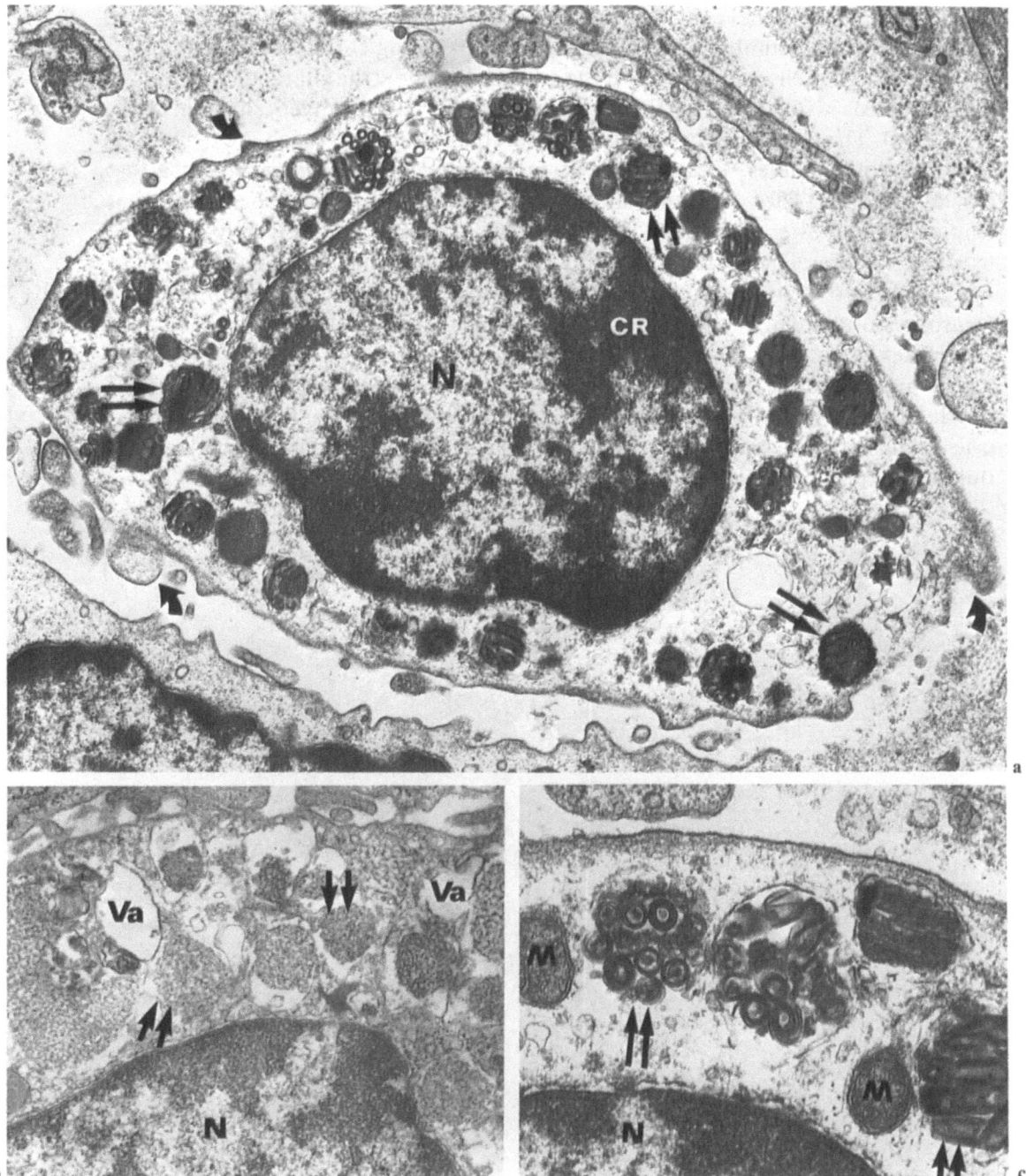

Fig. 1.46a. A typical mast cell showing irregular membrane-bound surfaces due to cytoplasmic projections (*arrows*) and a centrally placed nucleus (*N*) displaying thick chromatin material (*CR*). The main cytoplasmic features are the large inclusion bodies bound by smooth membrane (*double arrows*). These bodies are of various sizes and shapes and their inclusions may contain granular (**b**), whorl-like or scroll-like material (**c**) (*double arrows*). Several of the vacuoles (*Va*) are clear of material whilst others are only half-filled (**a, b**), indicating that there is a constant discharge of their contents. *M*, mitochondria. (**a** ×12 722; **b** ×24 980; **c** ×31 460)

The *eosinophils* are never absent from the normal lamina propria and may be found in increased number without any obvious pathological alteration within the mucosa. The cells are relatively large and usually show the characteristic bi-lobed nucleus with its dense thick rim of peripherally arranged chromatin (Fig. 1.47). The cytoplasm contains the eosinophil 'granules' which are dense, round or oval bodies, surrounded by membrane, and showing a central crystalloid core. These granules are not homogeneous and may be seen as empty vacuoles after discharge. The remainder of the cytoplasm is rich in the usual organelles. The eosinophil granules contain acid and other hydrolases and are therefore considered part of the lysosomal system, forming secondary lysosomes after phagocytosis of foreign material, such as antigen–antibody complexes.

The *membranes* of the cells of the lamina propria have important functions in relation to the metabolic activity of the cell and deserve special mention. All cells of the lamina propria possess a variety of cell processes which may extend outwards (pseudopodia), thus aiding locomotion of the cell as well as

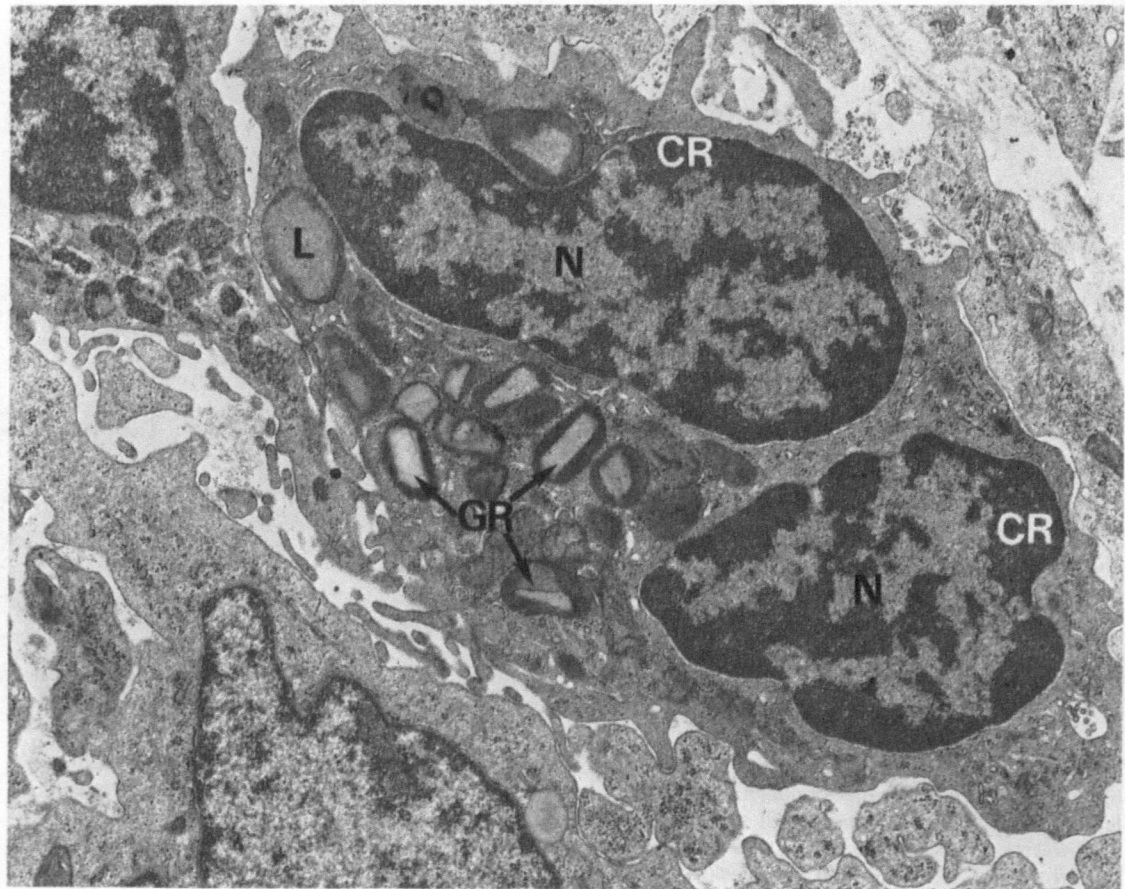

Fig. 1.47. An eosinophil showing a bilobar nucleus (*N*) which contains heavy chromatin material (*CR*) at the periphery. The nuclear contours are usually smooth, round or oval. The characteristic cytoplasmic features are the densely staining granules (*GR*) with a central lighter staining core of homogeneous crystalloid bodies appearing as rectangles or squares. The granules are surrounded by smooth membrane. *L*, lysosomes. (× 13 400)

phagocytosis, or inwards, whereby the cell membrane invaginates to form the endocytic or pinocytotic vacuoles or vesicles. External cell processes are particularly evident in macrophages, eosinophils, mast cells and, if present, neutrophils. Apart from locomotion these processes serve to establish contact with other infiltrating cells (Fig. 1.48) and it is assumed that in this way important information is passed from one cell to another. Thus two or more cells can be observed to be in intimate contact, separated by their respective cell membranes. Transport by exocytosis, whereby cellular material is passed outwards through vesicles or vacuoles derived from the endoplasmic reticulum, is accomplished by fusion of ER with the cell membranes. Endocytotic vacuoles are particularly evident in endothelial cells (micro-pinocytosis) and consist of small sacs with membranes derived from the cell membrane (see Figs. 1.53, 1.54). In other infiltrating cells like the macrophage, numerous small and large smooth-membraned vacuoles can be seen immediately internal to the cell membrane but not attached to it. These vacuoles may contain phagocytosed material which necessitates fusion with primary

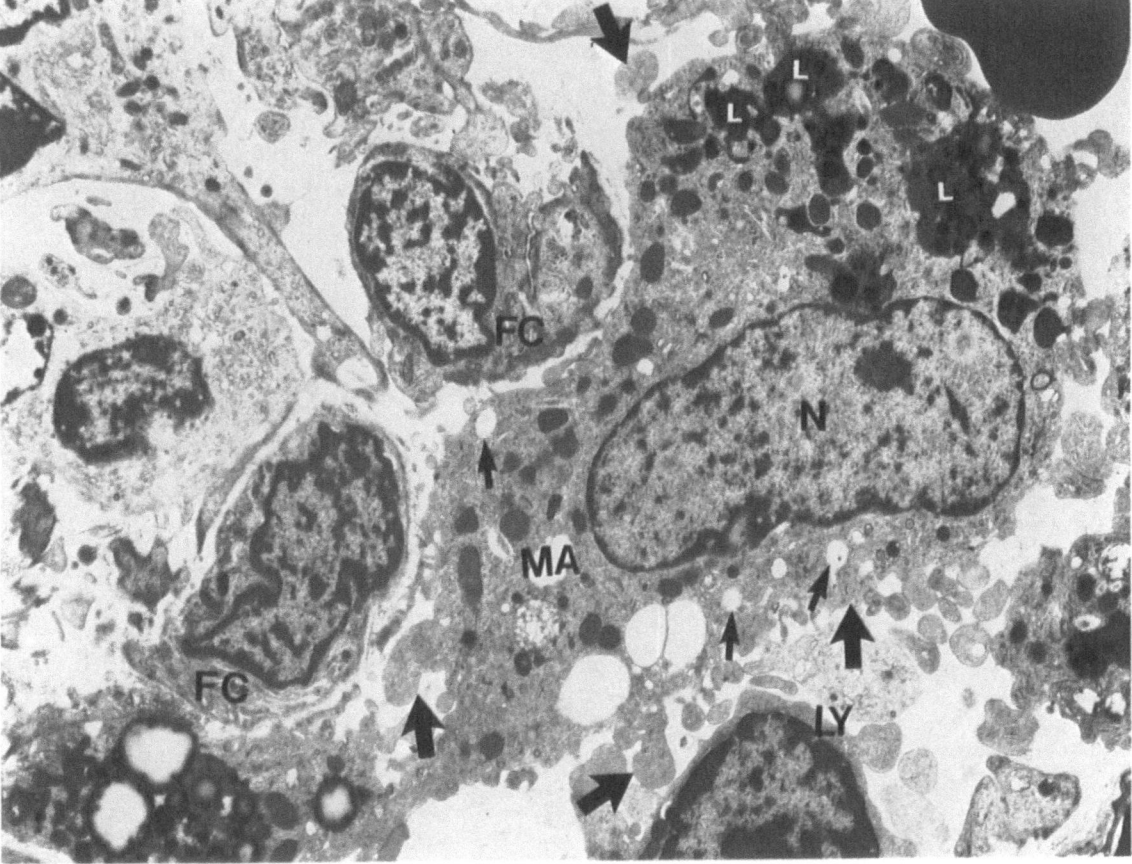

Fig. 1.48. A macrophage (*MA*) with its nucleus (*N*) showing numerous cytoplasmic processes (*thick arrows*) on its outer surface. These processes are surrounded by the cell membrane and appear to make contact with adjacent cells, such as a lymphocyte (*LY*) on the right and two fibrocytes (*FC*) on the left. The cytoplasmic processes also serve for locomotion. Immediately internal to the limiting membrane of the macrophage are cytoplasmic vacuoles (*thin arrows*) which may eventually form part of the lysosomal system (*L*). (× 3930)

cytoplasmic lysosomes to form phagolysosomes. Thus contact between the external environment and the phagocytic system within the cell cytoplasm is established. All surface cell membranes also carry immune receptors.

Schwann cells and unmyelinated nerve fibres

The lamina propria is rich in small nerve fibrils which can be found in the connective tissue of the villi, in the glandular region and particularly in the smooth muscle fibres of the muscularis mucosae. It is more common to see bundles of axons carried within the Schwann cell sheath but occasionally this cell is cut at the nuclear level (Fig. 1.49) when individual axons will be clearly seen in cross-section in their own grooves formed by invaginations of the Schwann cell membrane. Outside of this the cell is surrounded by a basal lamina. In the axoplasm of the individual axons there are mitochondria, numerous vesicles, small dense bodies, neurotubules and neurofibrils (Figs. 1.50, 1.51).

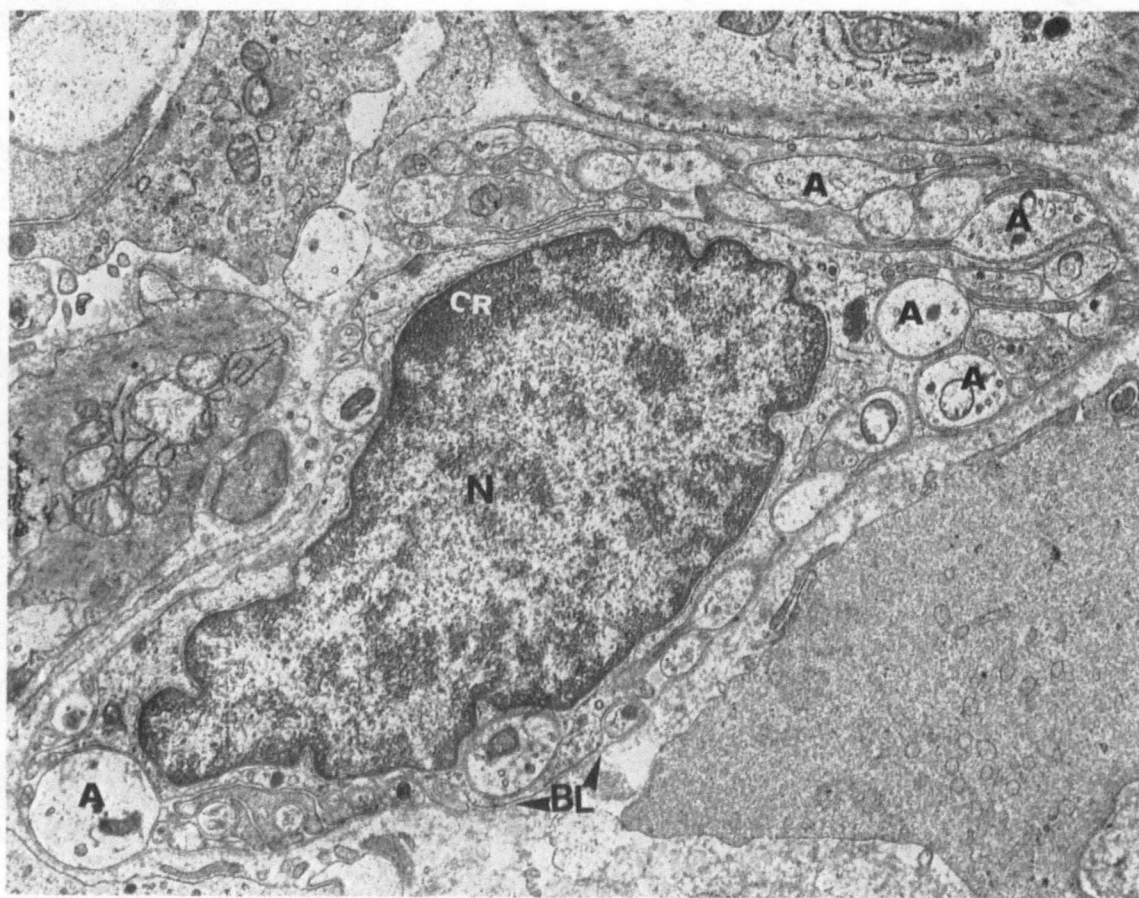

Fig. 1.49. A Schwann cell and its processes (axons) at the nuclear level. The nucleus (*N*) has an irregular outline and relatively sparse chromatin (*CR*). The cytoplasm is sparse and surrounded by numerous cytoplasmic processes which form the nerve axons (*A*). *BL*, basal lamina (× 11 070)

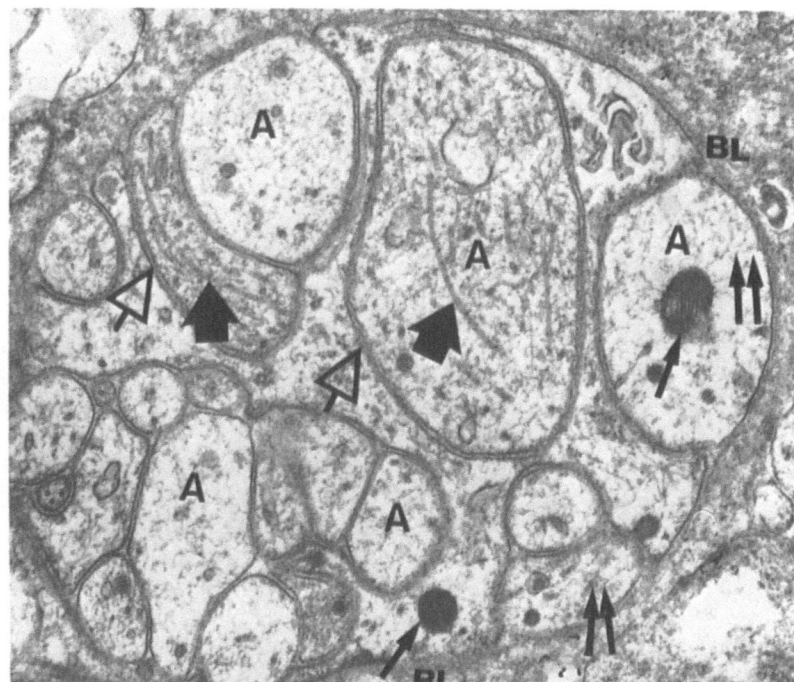

Fig. 1.50. Cross-section of several axons (*A*) surrounded by a sheath derived from the Schwann cell (*open arrows*). The axons are carried in bundles within their own limiting membrane and that derived from the sheath membrane. The latter has a basal lamina on its outer surface (*BL*). The axoplasm contains small dense bodies (*thin arrows*), neurotubules (*thick arrows*) and neurofibrils (*double arrows*). (× 20 400)

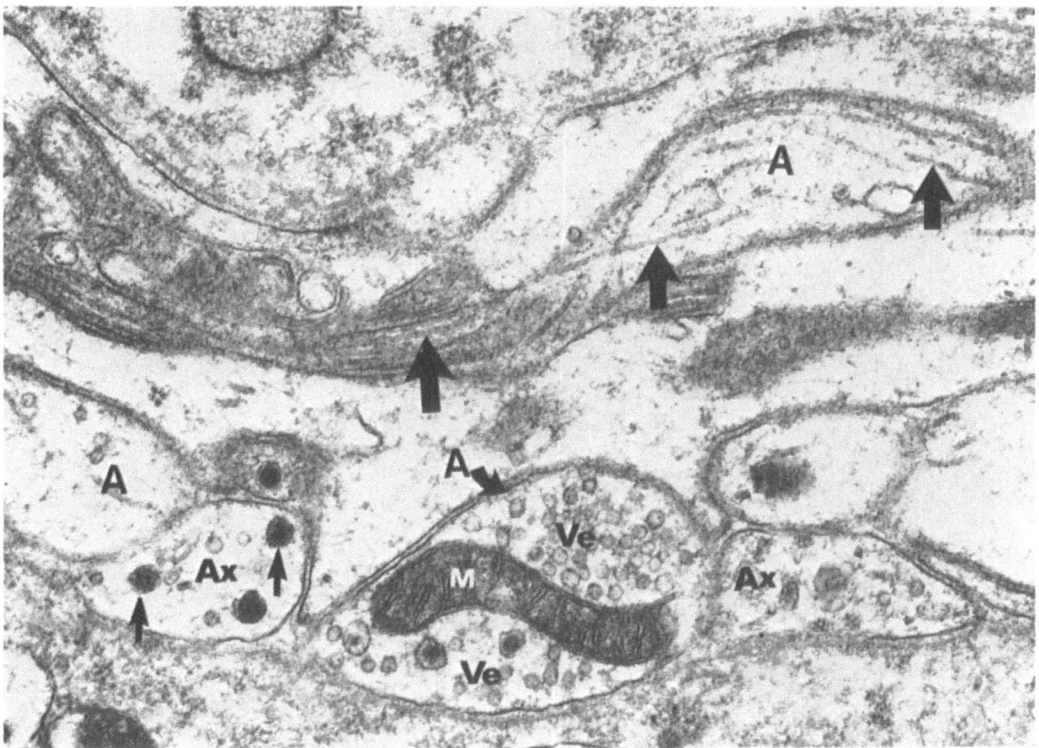

Fig. 1.51. Oblique sections of axons (*A*) showing certain other organelles of the axoplasm (*Ax*) such as mitochondria (*M*), numerous vesicles (*Ve*) as well as dense bodies (*arrows*) and neurofibrils (*thick arrows*). (× 26 000)

Endothelial cells

The walls of the small capillaries of the lamina propria are composed of endothelial cells (Figs. 1.52, 1.53). These surround a lumen within which light, flocculent material, one or more dense, homogeneous red blood corpuscle,

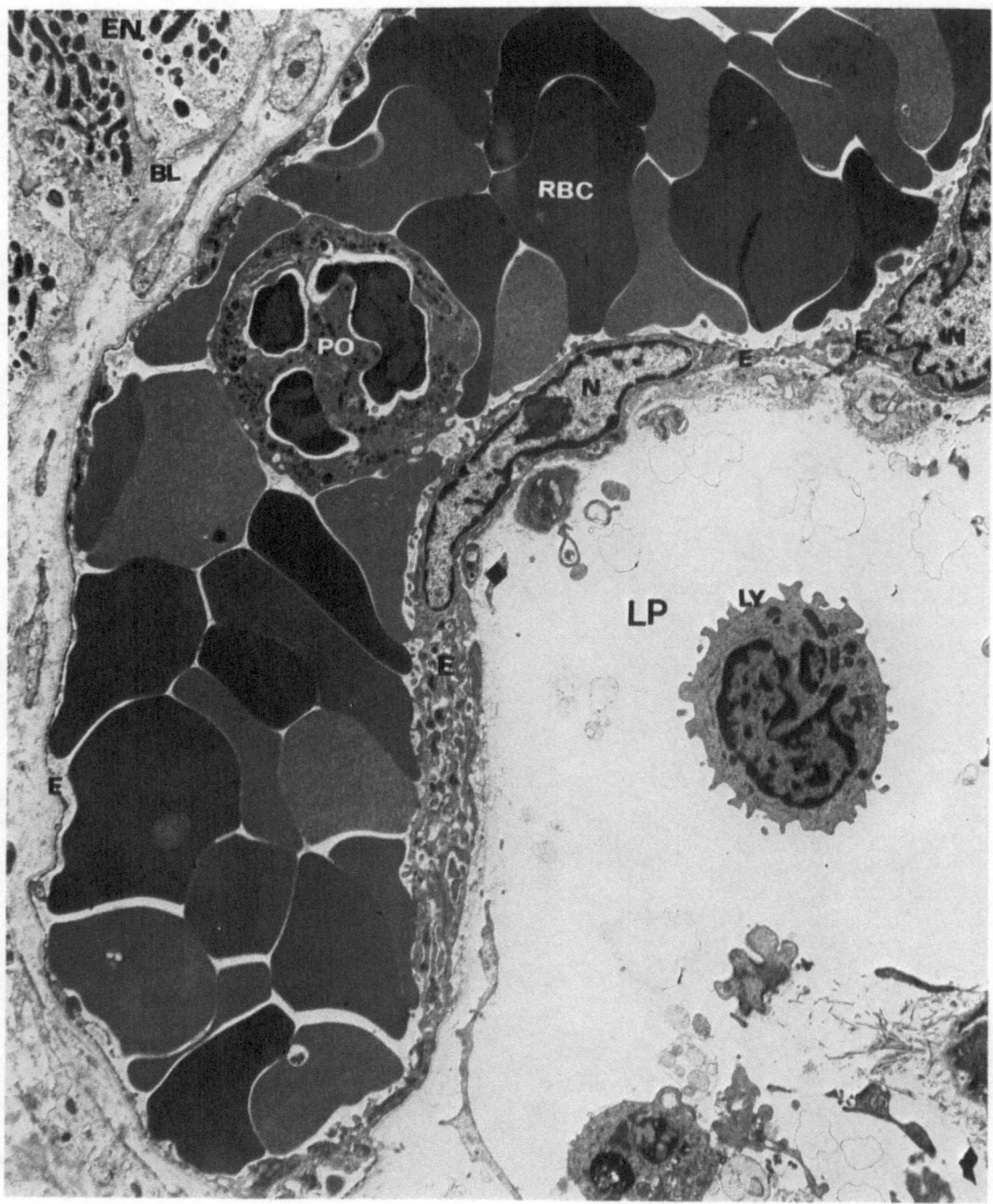

Fig. 1.52. Small blood vessel situated immediately beneath the basal lamina (*BL*) of enterocytes (*EN*) and containing numerous red blood cells (*RBC*) as well as a polymorphonuclear cell (*PO*). The vessel is lined by the endothelial cell (*E*) with its nucleus (*N*). *LY*, lymphocyte in the lamina propria (*LP*). (× 2580)

and occasionally lymphocytes, eosinophils, neutrophils and platelets are found. The endothelial cells are usually seen as thin cytoplasmic processes which become voluminous only at the nuclear level where the cytoplasmic organelles are concentrated (Fig. 1.53). The cytoplasmic process of one cell displays special junctional complexes with those of its neighbouring cell. In addition there are numerous pores or fenestrations where the membranes of endothelial cell processes thin out to give a 'sausage like' appearance (Fig. 1.53). They may therefore be seen as a discontinuous structure through which exchange of material takes place between the lumen and the exterior. A similar function has been attributed to the numerous micropinocytotic vesicles and marginal folds (Figs. 1.53, 1.54) formed by invaginations and outgrowths of the cell membranes. External to the cell membranes of the endothelial cells a continuous fine basal lamina can be seen surrounding the capillary (Fig. 1.53).

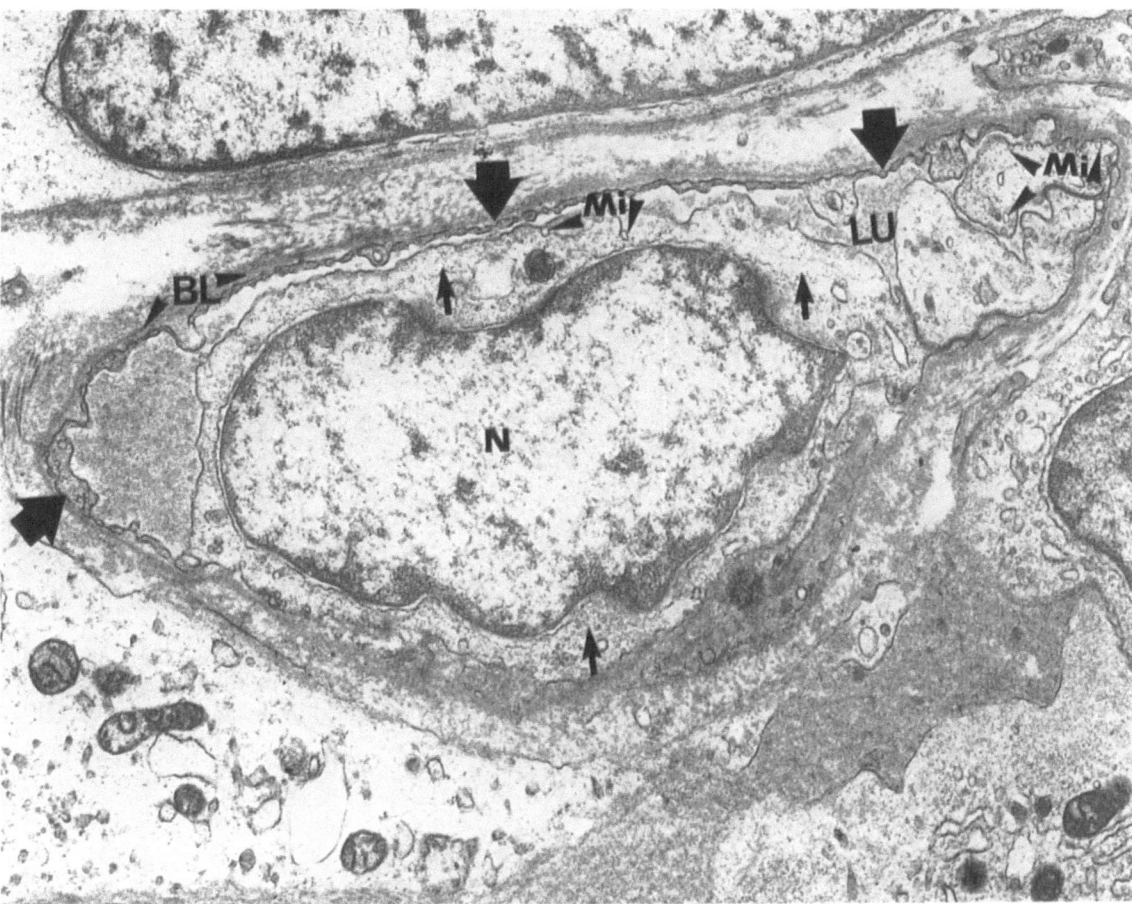

Fig. 1.53. Small blood vessel lined by an endothelial cell. The nucleus (*N*) of this cell contains a thin rim of chromatin and is surrounded by sparse cytoplasm (*arrows*). At the nuclear level the endothelial cell appears to bulge into the vessel lumen (*LU*). Cytoplasmic processes in the form of linear 'sausage shaped' extensions surround the lumen (*thick arrows*). *Mi*, micropinocytotic vesicles; *BL*, basal lamina. (× 12 770)

At times platelets (Fig. 1.55) can be seen aggregated in the lumen of the blood vessel. The endothelium lining the lymph vessels (Fig. 1.56) in the lamina propria is indistinguishable from the capillary endothelium except that fenestrations are absent.

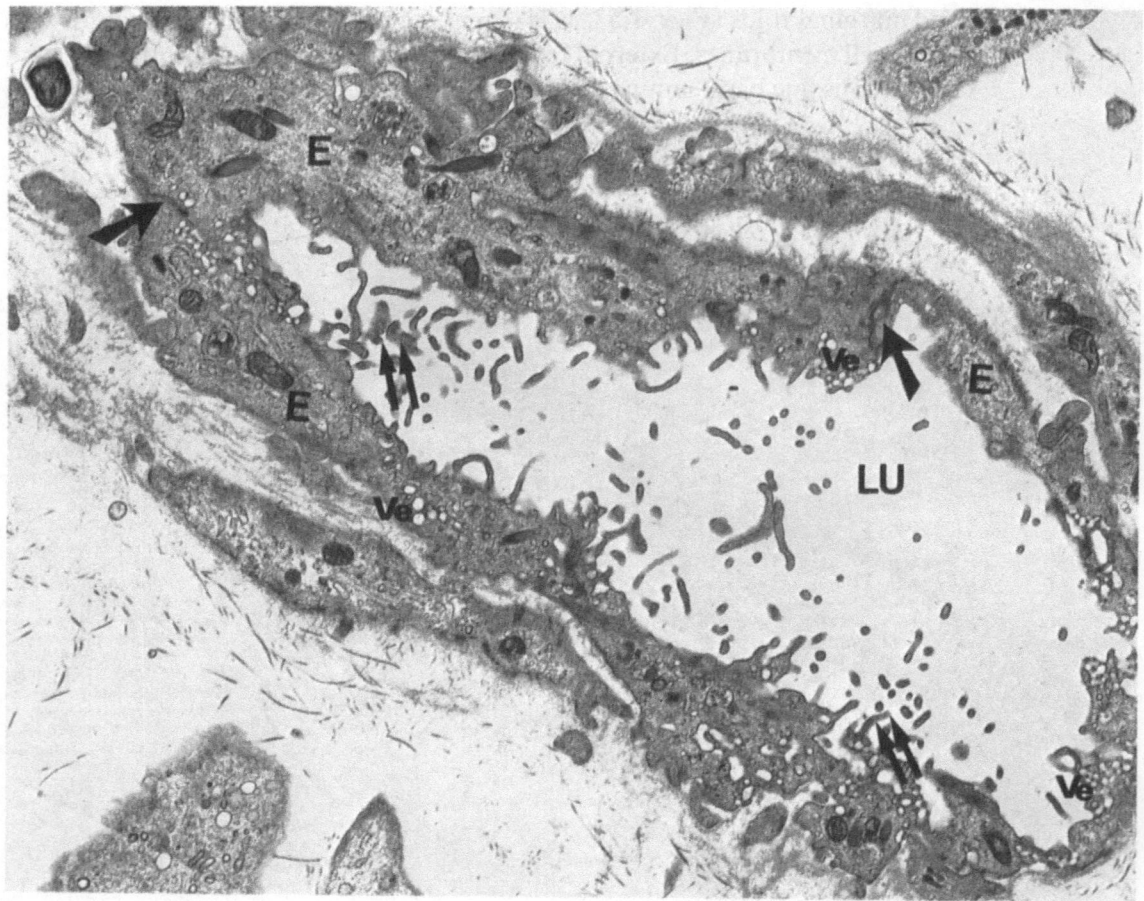

Fig. 1.54. Small blood vessel showing cytoplasmic processes or marginal folds (*double arrows*) of endothelial cells (*E*) extending into the lumen (*LU*). The individual endothelial cells are joined by specialised cell junctions (*thick arrows*). Numerous clear small cytoplasmic vesicles (*Ve*) are seen, formed by invaginations of the cell membrane. (× 10 950)

Fig. 1.55. Small blood vessel lined by cytoplasmic extensions of endothelial cells (*E*) which show occasional   ▷
discontinuations or fenestrations (*arrow*). The lumen (*LU*) contains several platelets (*PL*). These are small cells, surrounded by membrane, containing cytoplasm but no nucleus. The cytoplasm of the platelets shows many granular bodies (*GR*) surrounded by ER as well as numerous vacuoles (*Va*). *M*, mitochondria. (× 18 950)

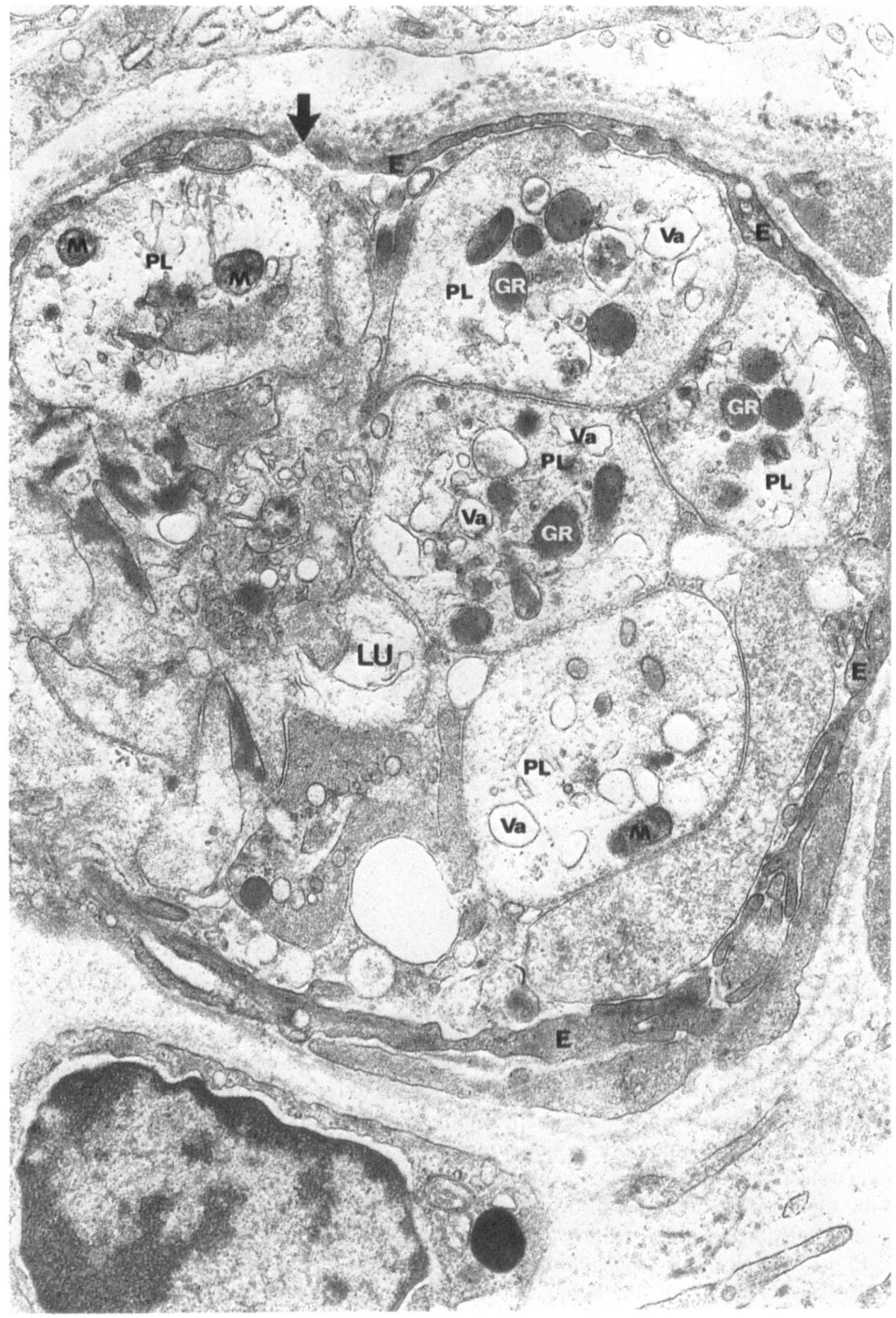

Fig. 1.55.

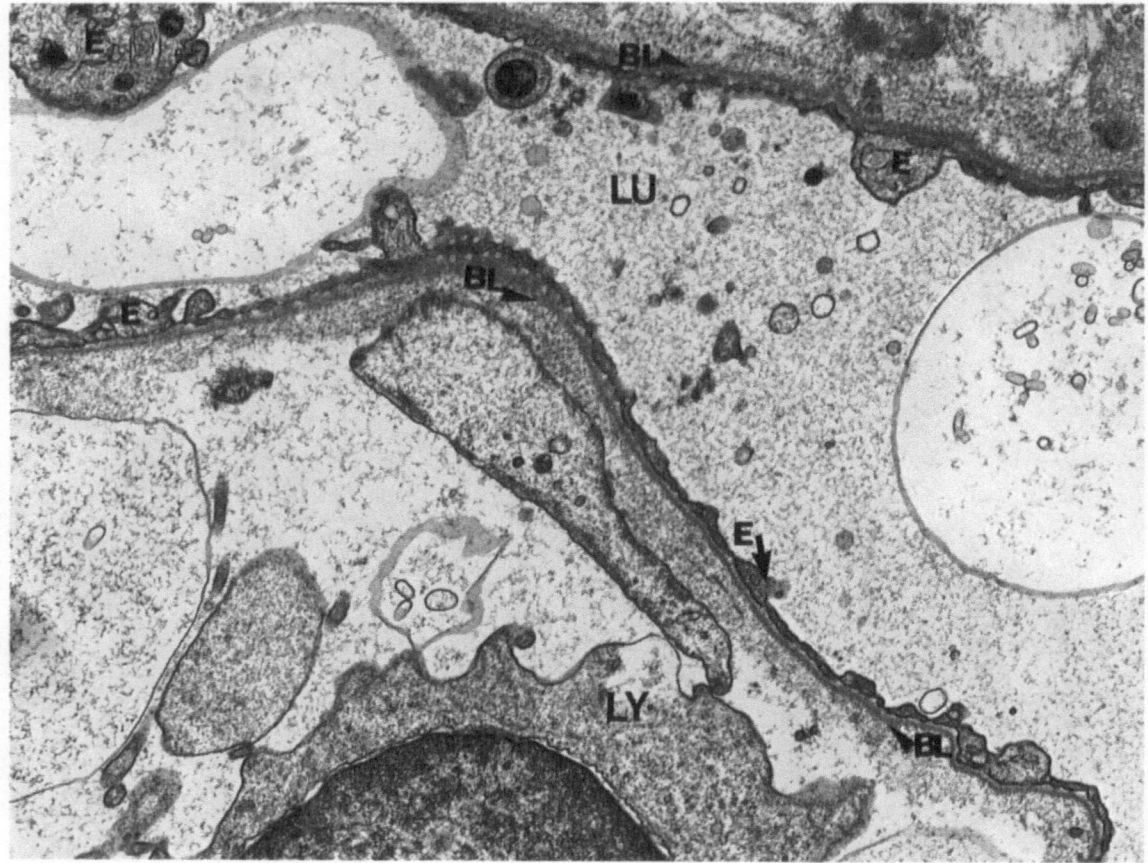

Fig. 1.56. Endothelial lining (*E*) of a lymph vessel with a well-defined basal lamina (*BL*). *LU*, lumen. Part of a lymphocyte (*LY*) is seen near and outside the vessel. (× 14 150)

Fibrocytes and their fibrillar processes

The fibroblast [11] or fibrocyte (Fig. 1.57) forms both the fine connective tissue fibrils and the collagen fibres. The cell has an elongated structure and the cytoplasm may extend on either side of the nucleus to form long processes. The nucleus is elongated and sparse in chromatin material, which is arranged close to the inner nuclear membrane. The cytoplasm is rich in RER and ER as well as vacuoles. The mitochondria and Golgi complexes are usually arranged around the nucleus. The collagen fibres are distinctive structures displaying a transverse periodicity of dense lines, each repeating period measuring about 640 A (Fig. 1.58). Normally the lamina propria contains a fine connective tissue fibrillar network and few collagen fibres. In many pathological conditions affecting this area there is an increase in both types of fibres, though this does not seem to be related to any particular clinical disease.

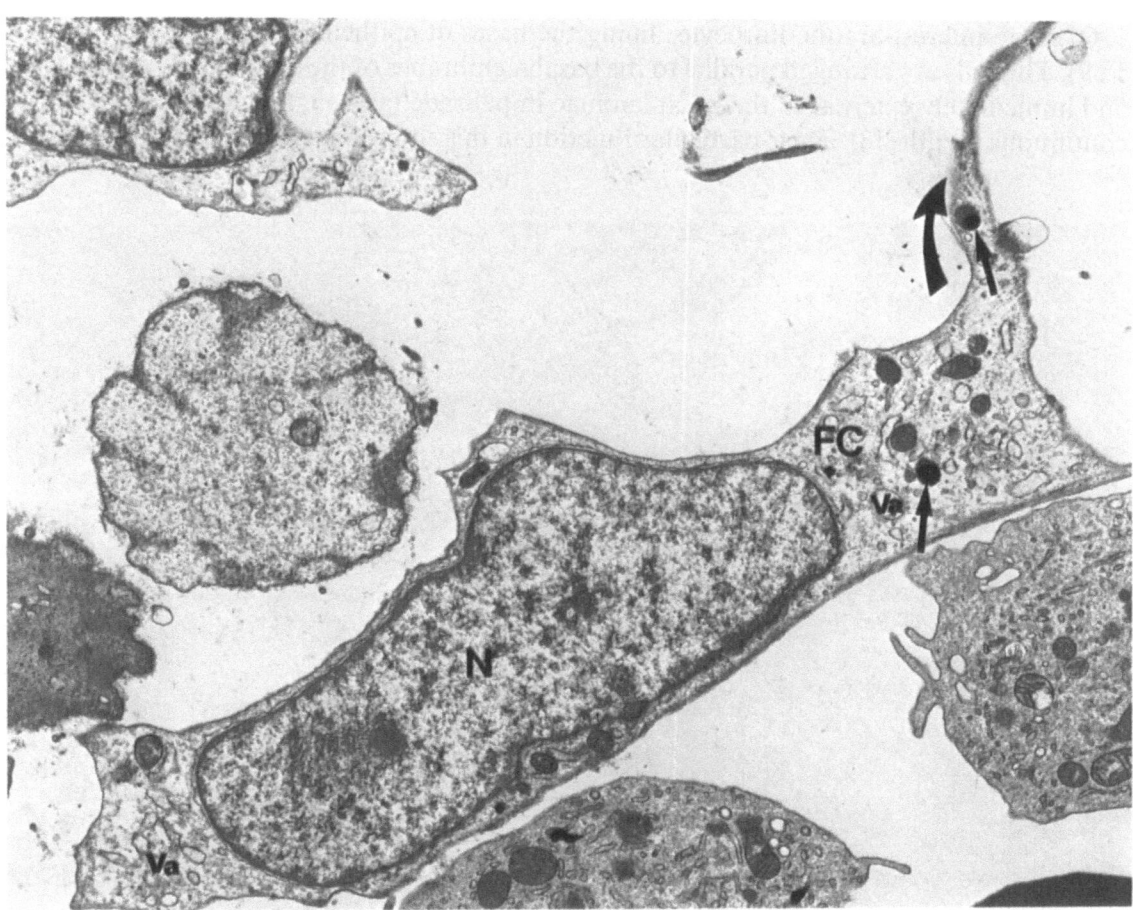

Fig. 1.57. A Fibrocyte (*FC*) showing an elongated nucleus (*N*) with sparse chromatin close to the nuclear membrane. The cytoplasm contains many vacuoles (*Va*) and small dense bodies (*arrows*). Characteristic cytoplasmic processes extend outwards (*thick arrow*) to form the fibrillar network of the lamina propria. (× 12 760)

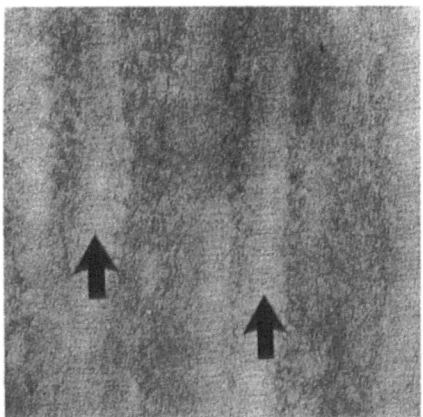

Fig. 1.58. Several collagen fibres in the lamina propria. These fibres are wider than the connective tissue fibres and show transverse striation of regular periodicity (*arrows*). (× 98 000)

Of some interest are the fibrocytes lining the bases of epithelial cells (Fig. 1.59). The cells are arranged parallel to the basal membranes of the epithelium and immediately external to the basal laminae in palisade fashion, forming a continuous sheath [13]. Their particular function in this situation is unknown.

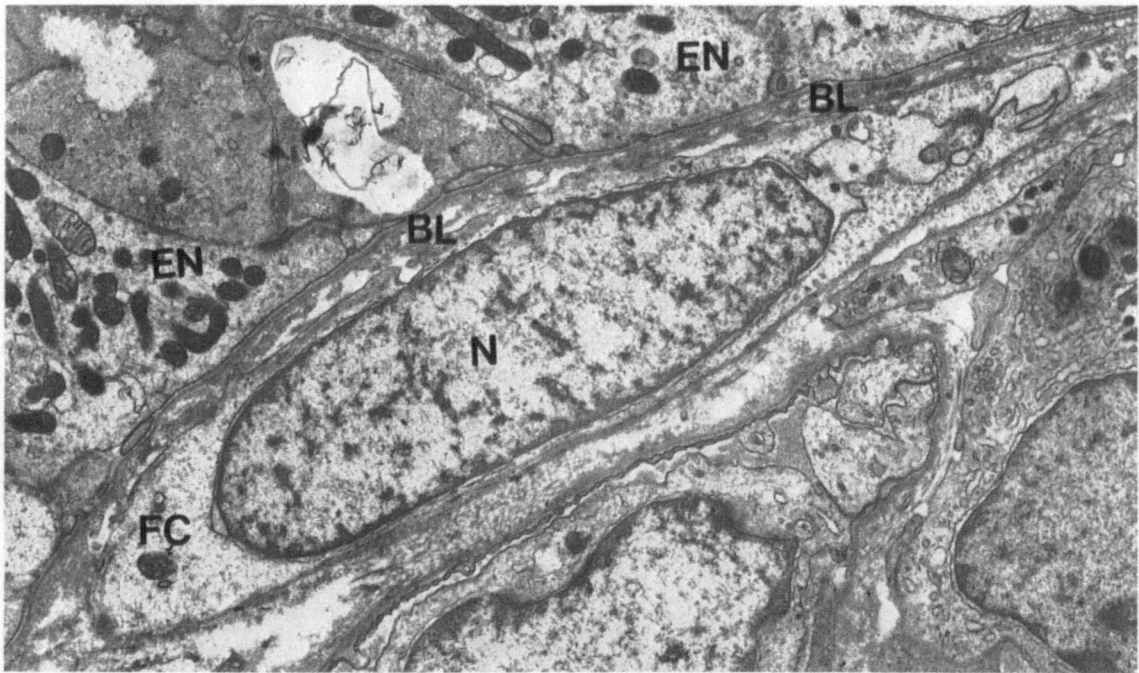

Fig. 1.59. Fibrocyte (*FC*) 'palisading' the bases of enterocytes (*EN*). They are arranged with their long axis immediately below and parallel to the basal laminae (*BL*) of the enterocytes. *N*, nucleus of fibrocyte. (× 8770)

References

1. Bohane TD, Cutz E, Hamilton JR, Gall DG (1977) Acrodermatitis enteropathica, zinc and the Paneth cell. A case report with family studies. Gastroenterology 73:587–592
2. Collan Y (1972) Characteristics of non-epithelial cells in the epithelium of normal rat ileum. Scand J Gastroenterol 7 [Suppl 18]:5–66
3. Crane RK (1968) Digestive-absorptive surface of the small bowel mucosa. Ann Rev Med 19:57–68
4. Erlandsen SL, Parsons JA, Taylor TD (1974) Ultrastructural immunocytochemical localisation of lysozyme in the Paneth cells of man. J Histochem Cytochem 22:401–413
5. Fichtelius KE (1968) The gut epithelium—a first level lymphoid organ? Exp Cell Res 49:87–104
6. Gray GM, Cooper HL (1971) Protein digestion and absorption. Gastroenterology 61:535–544
7. Ito S (1974) Form and function of the glycocalyx on free cell surfaces. Philos Trans R Soc Lond (Biol) 268:55–66

8. Marsh MN (1975) Studies of intestinal lymphoid tissue. 1. Electron microscopic evidence of 'blast transformation' in epithelial lymphocytes of mouse small intestinal mucosa. Gut 16:665–674

9. Marsh MN, Swift JA (1969) A study of small intestinal mucosa using the scanning electron microscope. Gut 10:940–949

10. Mooseker MK, Tilney LG (1975) Organisation of an actin filament-membrane complex. Filament polarity and membrane attachment in the microvilli of intestinal epithelial cells. J Cell Biol 67:725–743

11. Movat HZ, Fernando NVP (1962) The fine structure of connective tissue. 1. The fibroblast. Exp Mol Pathol 1:509–534

12. Padawer J (1979) Mast cell structure. In: Pepys J, Edwards AM (eds) The mast cell—its role in health and disease. Pitman Medical, London, pp 1–8

13. Parker FG, Barnes EN, Kaye GI (1974) The pericryptal fibroblast sheath. IV. Replication, migration and differentiation of the subepithelial fibroblasts of the crypt and villus of the rabbit jejunum. Gastroenterology 67:601–621

14. Pearse AGE, Polak JM, Bloom SR (1977) The newer gut hormones. Cellular sources, physiology, pathology and clinical aspects. Gastroenterology 72:746–761

15. Pink IJ, Croft DN, Creamer B (1970) Cell loss from small intestinal mucosa; a morphological study. Gut 11:217–222

16. Selby WS, Janossy G, Jewell DP (1981) Immunohistological characterization of intra-epithelial lymphocytes of the human gastrointestinal tract. Gut 22:169–176

17. Shiner M, Birbeck MSC (1961) The microvilli of the small intestinal surface epithelium in coeliac disease and in idiopathic steatorrhoea. Gut 2:277–284

18. Toner PG, Ferguson A (1971) Intraepithelial cells in the human intestinal mucosa. J Ultrastruct Res 34:329–334

Select bibliography

Books

Bessis M (1973) Living blood cells and their ultrastructure. Springer-Verlag, Berlin, Heidelberg, New York

Fawcett DW (1966) An atlas of fine structure. The cell. Saunders, Philadelphia, London

Grossman MI, Brazier MAB, Lechapo J (eds) (1981) Cellular bases of chemical messengers in the digestive system (UCLA forum in medical sciences, no 23) Academic, New York

Johannessen JV (1980) Electron microscopy in human medicine. Digestive system, vol. 7. McGraw-Hill, London

Pfeiffer CJ, Rowden G, Weibel J (1975) Gastrointestinal ultrastructure. Thieme, Stuttgart, pp 208–253

Polak JM, Bloom SR (1980) Regulatory peptides of the gut: the essential mechanism of gut control. In: Wright R (ed) Recent advances in gastrointestinal pathology. Saunders, London, Philadelphia, Toronto, pp 23–46

Toner PG, Carr KE, Wyburn CM (1971) The digestive system. An ultra-structural atlas and review. Butterworths, London

Articles

Creamer B (1967) The turnover of the epithelium of the small intestine. Br Med Bull 23:226–230

Creamer B (1974) Intestinal structure in relation to absorption. Biomembranes 4A:1–42

Gardner JD, Brown MS, Laster L (1970) The columnar epithelial cell of the small intestine: digestion and transport. N Engl J Med 283:1196–1202

Merker MJ (1969) Electron microscopic morphology of intestinal absorption. Verh Dtsch Ges Pathol 53:57–79

Orlic D, Lev R (1977) An electron microscopic study of intraepithelial lymphocytes in human fetal small intestine. Lab Invest 37:554–561

Osaka M, Sasagawa T, Fujita T (1973) Endocrine cells in human jejunum and ileum: an electron microscope study of biopsy materials. Arch Histol Jpn 35:235–248

Otto HF (1973) The intestinal Paneth cell. Cytomorphology, ultrastructural pathology and function. A contribution to the lysozyme theory. Veroeff Morphol Pathol 94:1–75

Repassy G, Lapis K (1979) Ultrastructural characteristics, secretory and phagocytotic activity of Paneth cells. Acta Morphol Acad Sci Hung 27:21–24

Riecken EO, Martini GA (1973) The classification of abnormal small intestinal mucosal appearances. Morphology function and diagnostic significance. Ger Med 3:120–127

Toner PG, Carr KE, Ferguson A, Mackay C (1970) Scanning and transmission electron microscopic studies of human intestinal mucosa. Gut 11:471–481

Trier JS, Rubin CE (1965) Electron microscopy of the small intestine: a review. Gastroenterology 49:574–603

Chapter 2

Coeliac Disease

A clinical intolerance, with histological changes, to the ingestion of gluten products characterised by a 'flat' mucosal lesion in the proximal small intestine which reverses on treatment with a gluten-free diet and relapses on gluten challenge [3, 17].

Untreated (48 patients)

Cytopathological changes are seen in many cells of the jejunal mucosa. Whereas on light microscopy these changes are most obvious within the villi and their epithelial components (see Fig. 2a, p. 2), the EM enables us to study not only the detailed fine structural abnormalities of these cells but also those involving various other cell types of the lamina propria.

The *enterocytes* are shorter and more cuboidal than normal when examined by light microscopy (Figs. 2.1a, b). Their microvillous (brush) border is histologically ill defined and the nuclei are irregularly arranged within the cells.

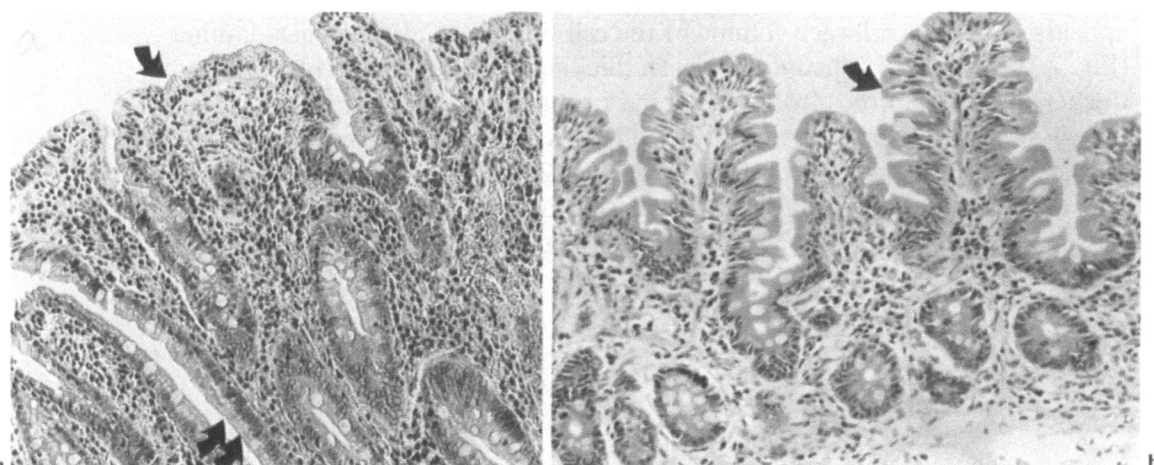

Fig. 2.1. a Light microscopic appearance of part of the mucosa in untreated coeliac disease showing short cuboidal or stratified-type enterocytes covering the surface (*arrow*) and columnar-type epithelium lining the deep crypts (*double arrows*). (H & E × 100). **b** Normal, columnar enterocytes (*arrow*) in the same patient after treatment. (H & E × 150)

The shortest cells are seen on the luminal surface and they become more columnar towards the crypt–villous junction. Mitosis is increased in the crypt epithelium. Ultrastructurally (Fig. 2.2) the enterocytes facing the lumen of the bowel also show the most severe changes, though they vary from cell to cell. The microvilli in untreated coeliac disease (Fig. 2.3) are uneven in height and often joined at their bases, appearing to arise in common as a heaped-up projection of the cell before branching out into the lumen (compare with normal microvilli (Fig. 2.4)). Between two and five microvilli may be seen to arise from a common base. The microvilli of the cells lining the surface and facing the lumen of the bowel are the most severely affected (Fig. 2.5) whereas those near the mouth of the crypts resemble the normal relatively un-differentiated crypt cell type (Fig. 2.6). Little is known about the changes in the internal filaments of the microvilli or those of the terminal web. The glycocalyx may appear denser than normal, or, if the microvilli are particularly sparse, very little of that coating material may be seen. Technical causes for these inconsistencies cannot be ruled out. The intracellular organelles show changes which could be attributed to a combination of cellular immaturity and shortened life span leading to early destruction [26]. Thus the cytoplasm of the surface cells may show relatively less RER and more free ribosomes and polysomes (Fig. 2.7). Smooth-membraned vacuoles are abundant (Fig. 2.5) and often dilated with unidentified retained material. The orderly arrangement of RER to mitochondria is no longer apparent. The mitochondria are often swollen, with disruption of the cristae mitochondrales (Figs. 2.7, 2.8). Lysosomes are usually increased (Figs. 2.2, 2.7, 2.8) and may contain recognisable parts of organelles such as mitochondria (Fig. 2.7). They are thus autolysosomes but may also have heterolysosomal activity. The Golgi complex appears active, showing dilation of its sacs and cisternae (Fig. 2.8). The nucleus may be displaced more centrally within the enterocyte and is usually larger and rounder than normal (Fig. 2.2), often with irregular contours (Fig. 2.9). It thus appears to occupy a larger volume of the cell than normal. The basal lamina (Fig. 2.10) is usually indistinct, varies in thickness and appears to blend with a thickened band of fibres from the lamina propria.

It is important to state that although there is general agreement on the ultrastructural changes in coeliac disease [21,25,27], none of the enterocyte appearances described are invariably present or are a constant feature of all cells. Nor should these changes be regarded as specific for untreated coeliac disease [25].

Fig. 2.2. Untreated coeliac disease: ultrastructure of enterocytes (*EN*) facing the lumen (*LU*) of the bowel. The ▷ cells are short and the large round nucleus (*N*) occupies more than one-third of the cell volume. The microvilli (*MI*) are short and branched. There is an increase in free ribosomes (*R*) and in lysosomes (*L*) and some disruption of the cristae mitochondrales (*arrows*) (see also Fig. 2.5). Numerous Golgi complexes (*G*) are seen. (× 20 490)

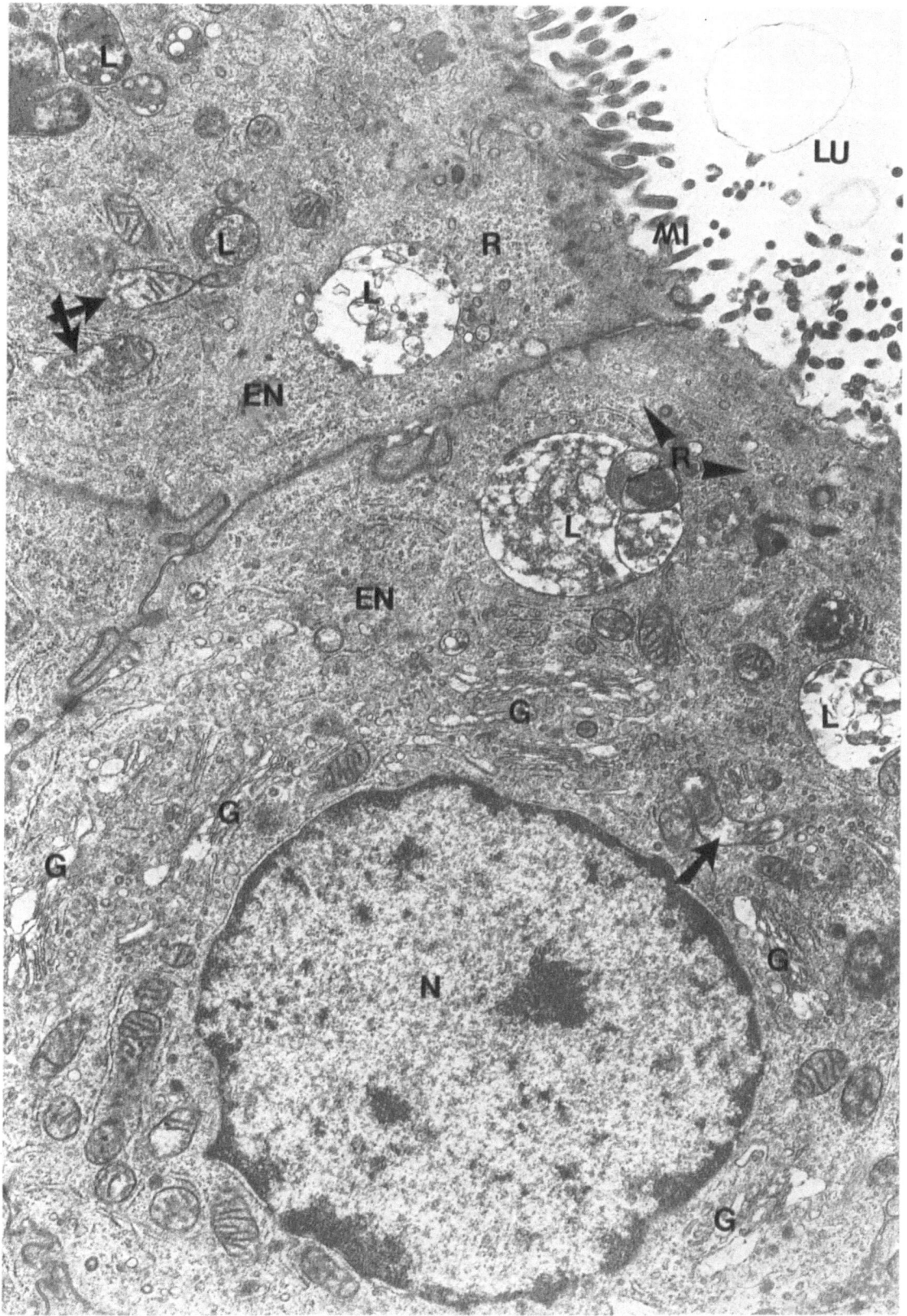

Fig. 2.2.

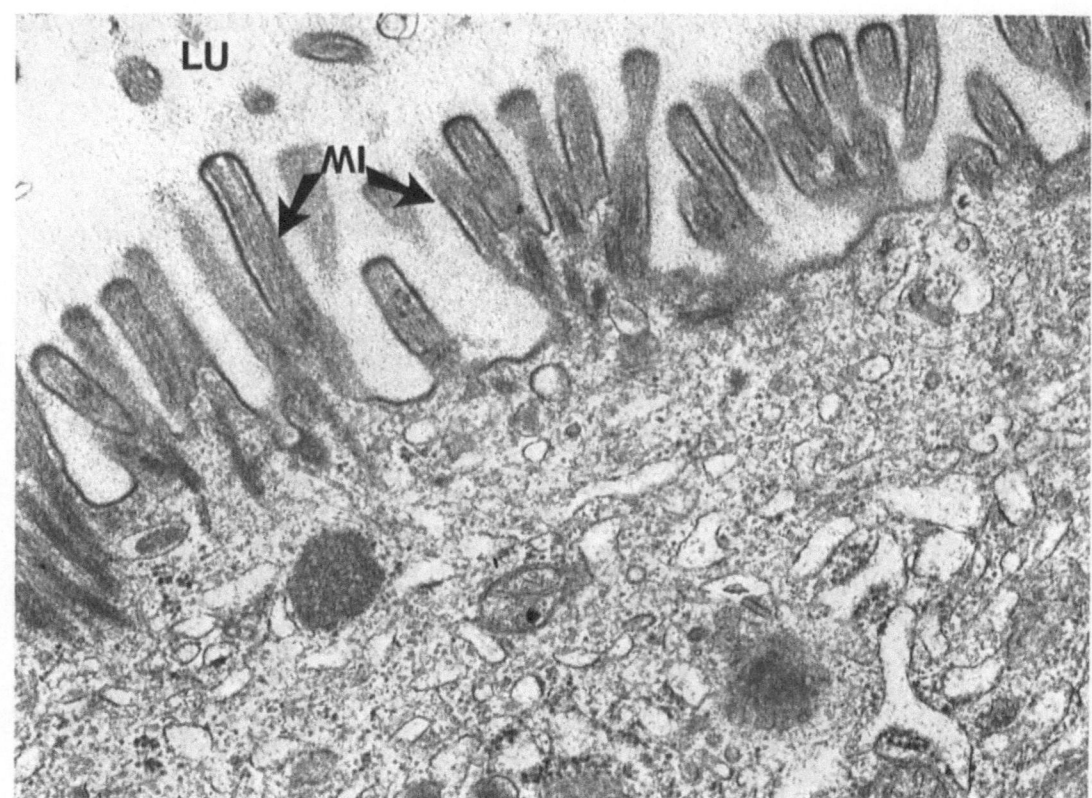

Fig. 2.3. △   **Fig. 2.4.** ▽

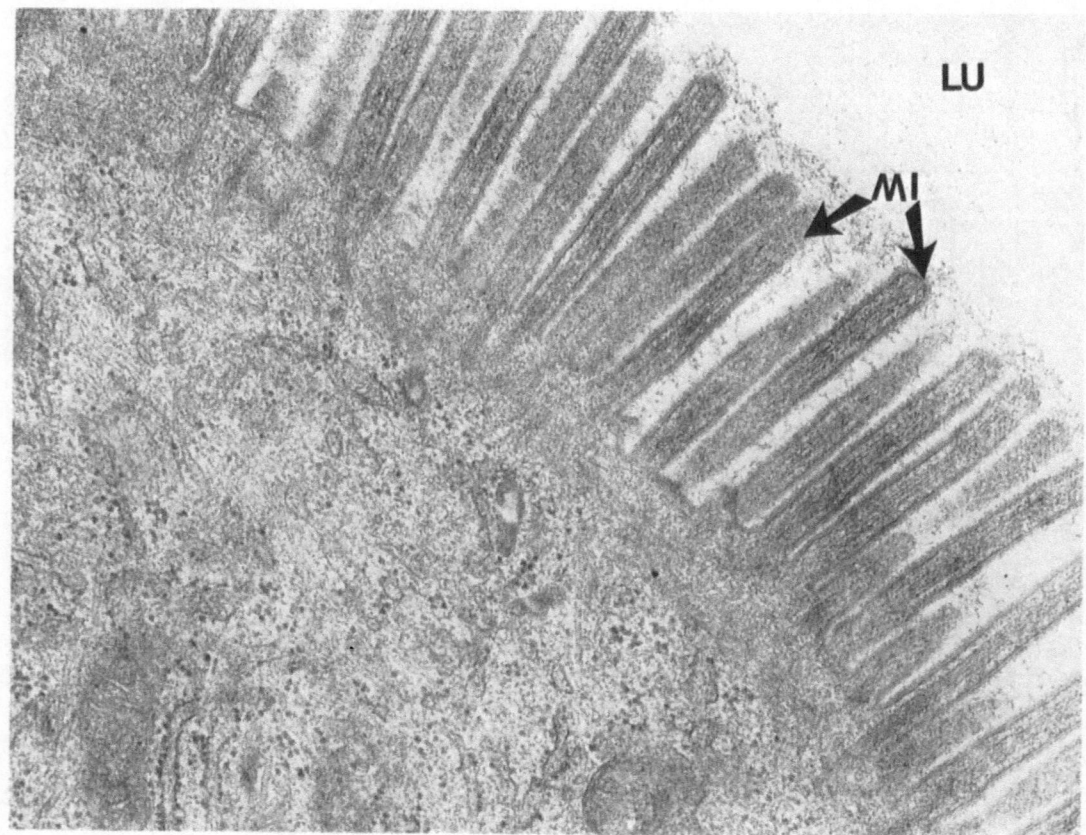

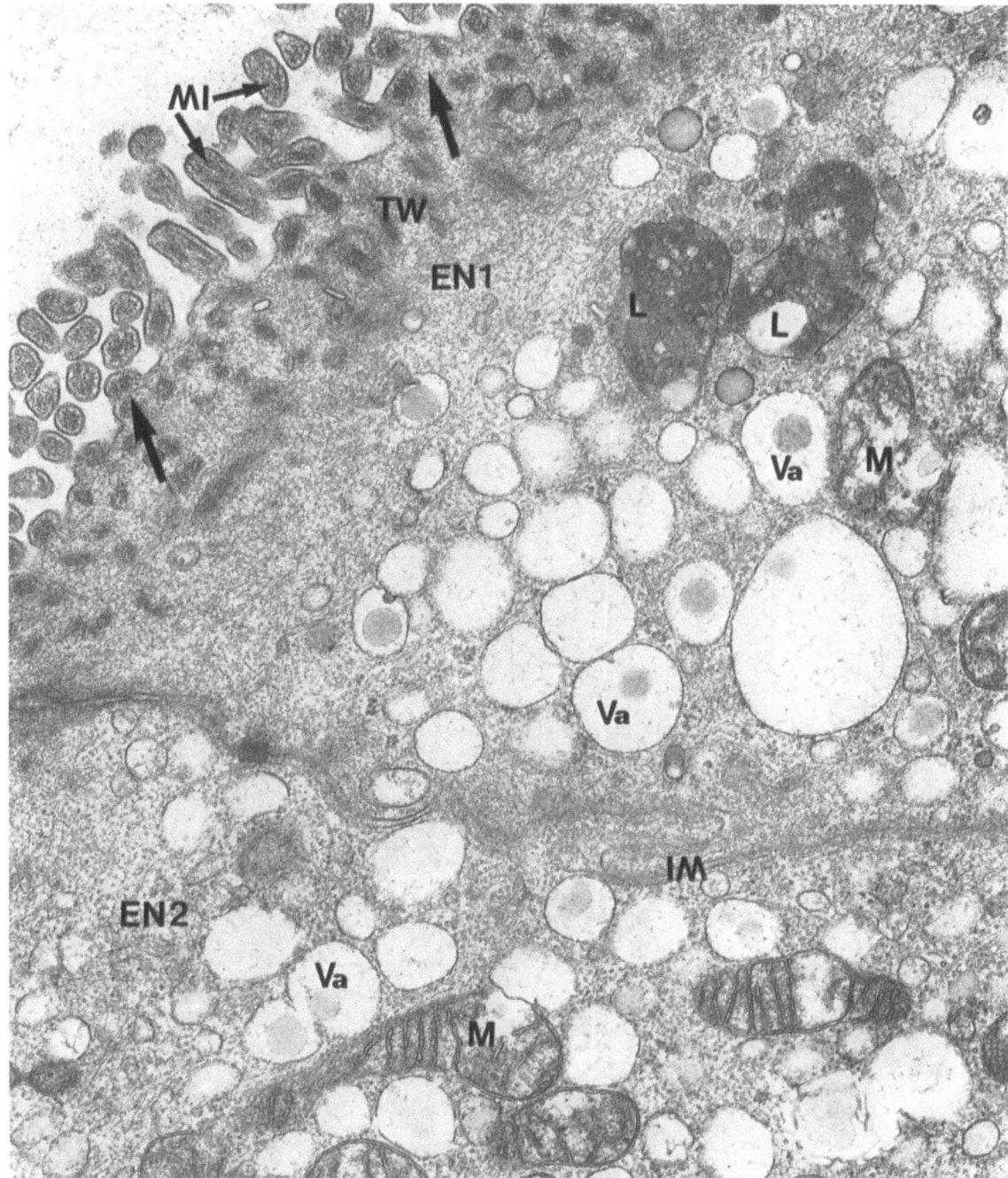

Fig. 2.5. Untreated coeliac disease: upper parts of two enterocytes (*EN 1* and *EN 2*) facing the lumen of the bowel. The microvilli (*MI*) are irregular, short and broad. The limiting membrane at the surface of the cell appears heaped up (*arrows*). The fibres of the terminal web (*TW*) are irregularly arranged (compare with Fig. 1.6). The cytoplasm of the cell contains numerous large, smooth-membraned vacuoles (*Va*) enclosing unidentified (probably ingested) granular material and two large lysosomes (*L*). *IM*, intercellular membranes; *M*, mitochondria. (× 35 440)

◁ **Fig. 2.3.** Untreated coeliac disease: microvilli (*MI*) of surface enterocytes, appearing shorter, branched and less densely spaced. *LU*, lumen of bowel. (× 36 360)

◁ **Fig. 2.4.** Normal microvilli from a control biopsy. (Compare with Fig. 2.3.) *LU*, lumen of bowel. (× 41 800)

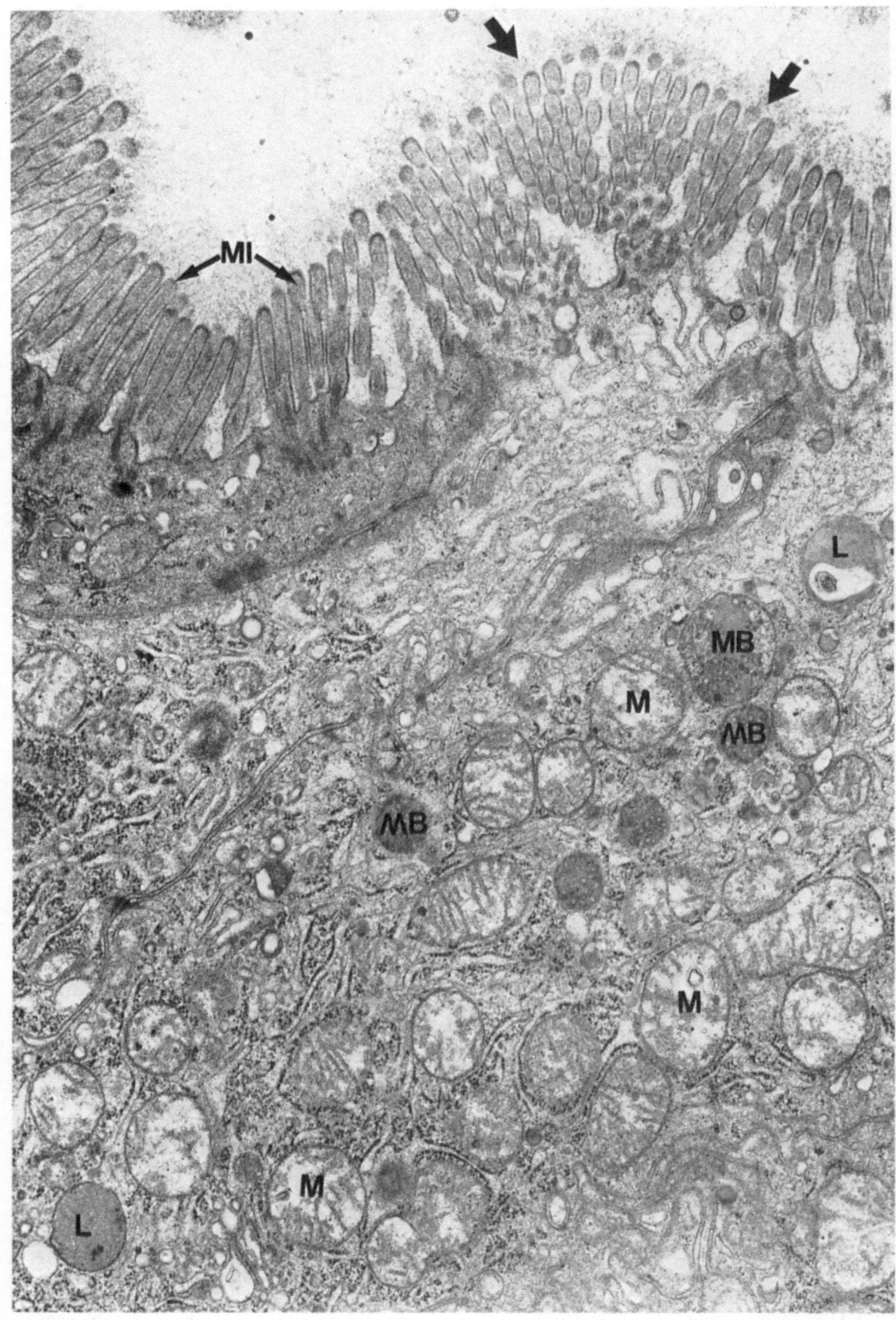

Fig. 2.6.

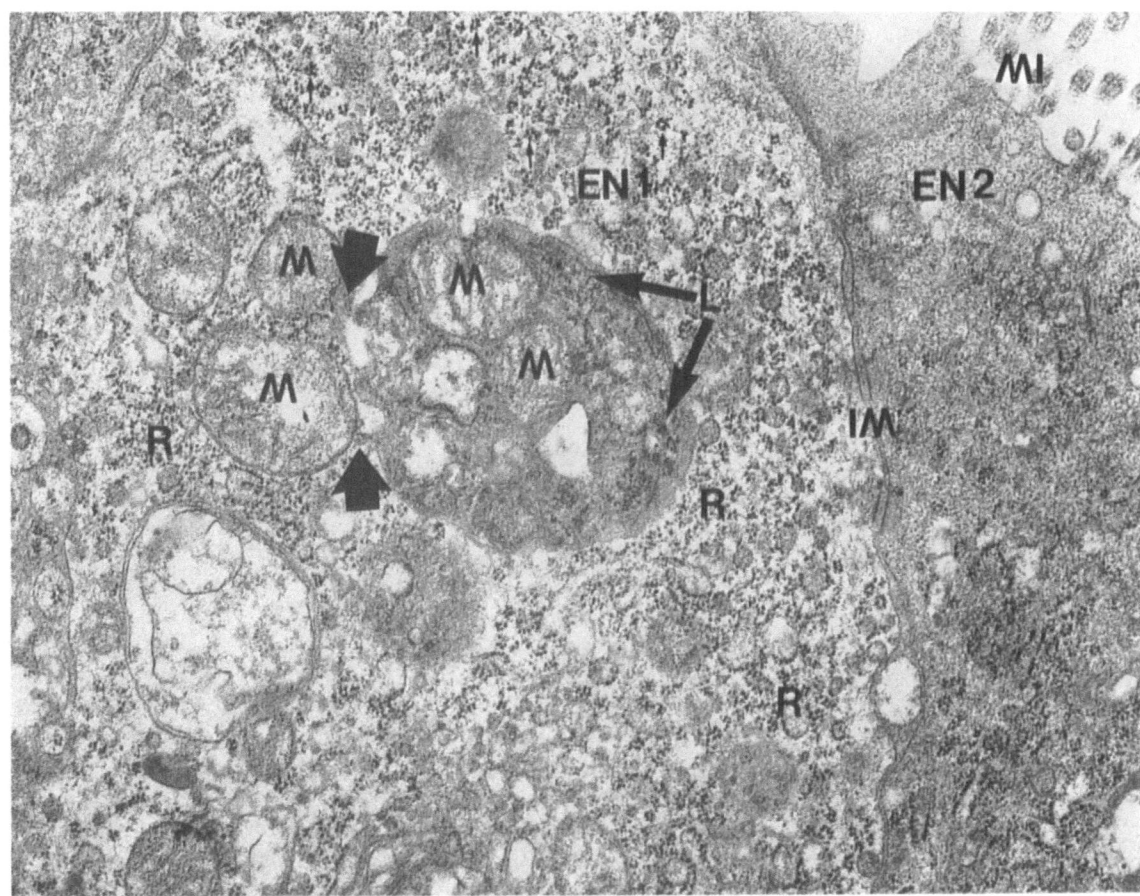

Fig. 2.7. Untreated coeliac disease: upper parts of two enterocytes (*EN1* and *EN2*) facing the lumen of the bowel. Irregular microvilli (*MI*) can be seen in the upper right hand of the cell EN2. Enterocyte EN1 (left of the intercellular membrane (*IM*)) contains numerous ribosomes (*R*) and polysomes (*arrows*) in the cytoplasm, with little ER and RER. In the centre is a large autophagic lysosome (*L*) containing two mitochondria (*M*). This lysosome appears to make contact with at least two other mitochondria (*thick arrows*) which show disruption of their cristae. (× 18 900)

◁ **Fig. 2.6.** Untreated coeliac disease: epithelial cells from the junction of crypts and short villi. The microvilli (*MI*) on the left appear normal but those on the right, though long and narrow, show branching and are therefore obliquely positioned (*arrows*). The cytoplasmic appearances of the cells are typical of differentiating crypt cell epithelium (compare with Figs. 1.28 and 1.29) except for increase in lysosomes (*L*) and multivesicular bodies (*MB*) and some disruption of the cristae of the mitochondria (*M*). (× 17 000)

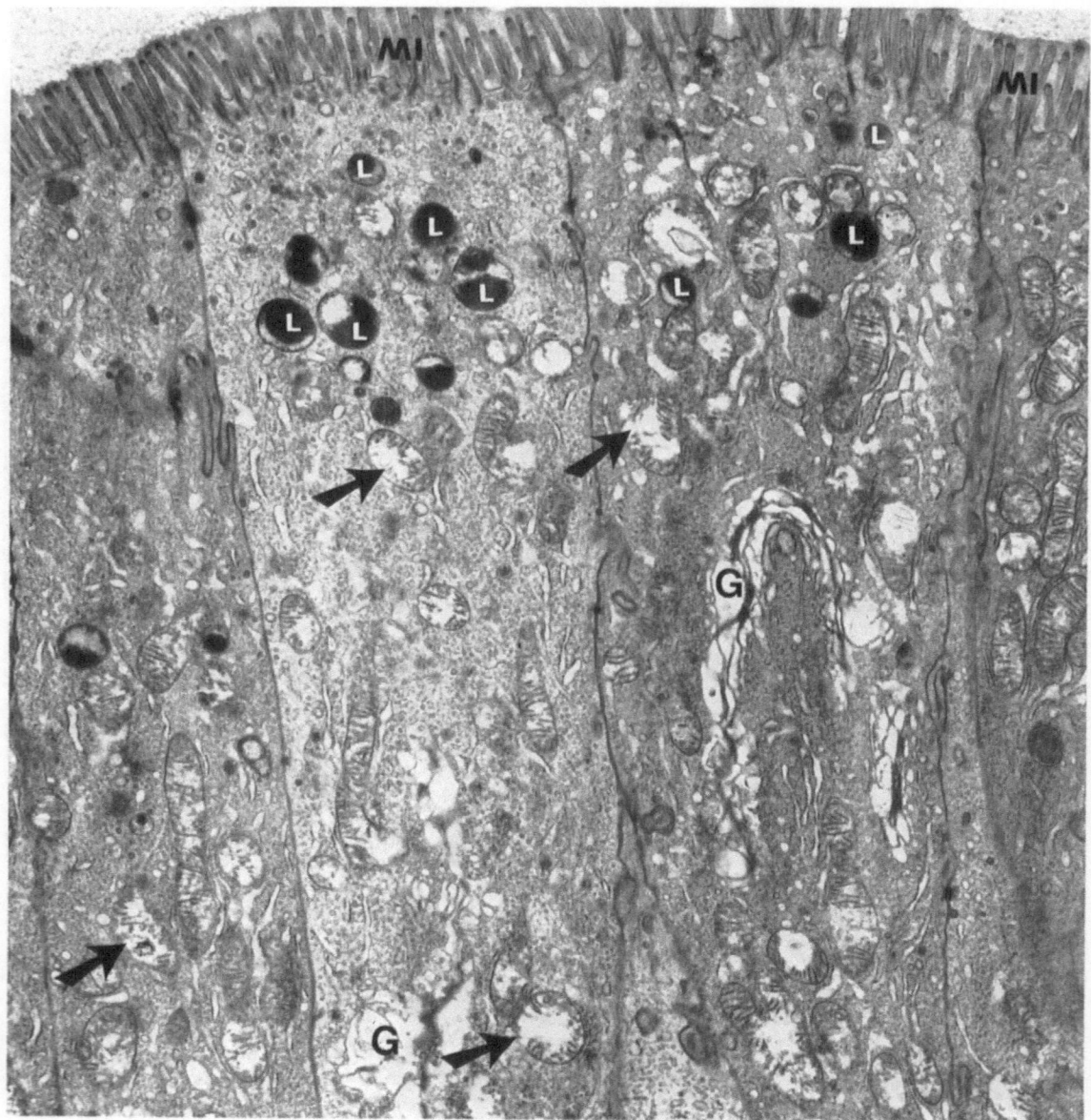

Fig. 2.8. Untreated coeliac disease: longitudinal section of upper parts of several enterocytes nearer the crypt–villous junction. The microvilli (*MI*) are short and display typical branching. Within the cytoplasm numerous small and large lysosomes (*L*) are seen. Many of the mitochondria show swelling and disruption of the cristae (*arrows*). The Golgi complex (*G*) is dilated, indicating increased activity. (× 10 720)

Fig. 2.9. Untreated coeliac disease: the enterocyte nucleus (*N*) is large, oval and has irregular contours. A ▷ prominent nucleolus (*NU*) is situated centrally within the nucleus. See also Fig. 2.2. (× 21 500)

Fig. 2.10. Untreated coeliac disease: the basal membranes (*BM*) and basal laminae (*BL*) of several enterocytes ▷ (*EN*). The fine fibres of the basal laminae are indistinct and appear to blend with fibres of the supporting connective tissues of the lamina propria, which are increased in density. *FC*, fibrocyte; *BV*, blood vessel. (× 8480)

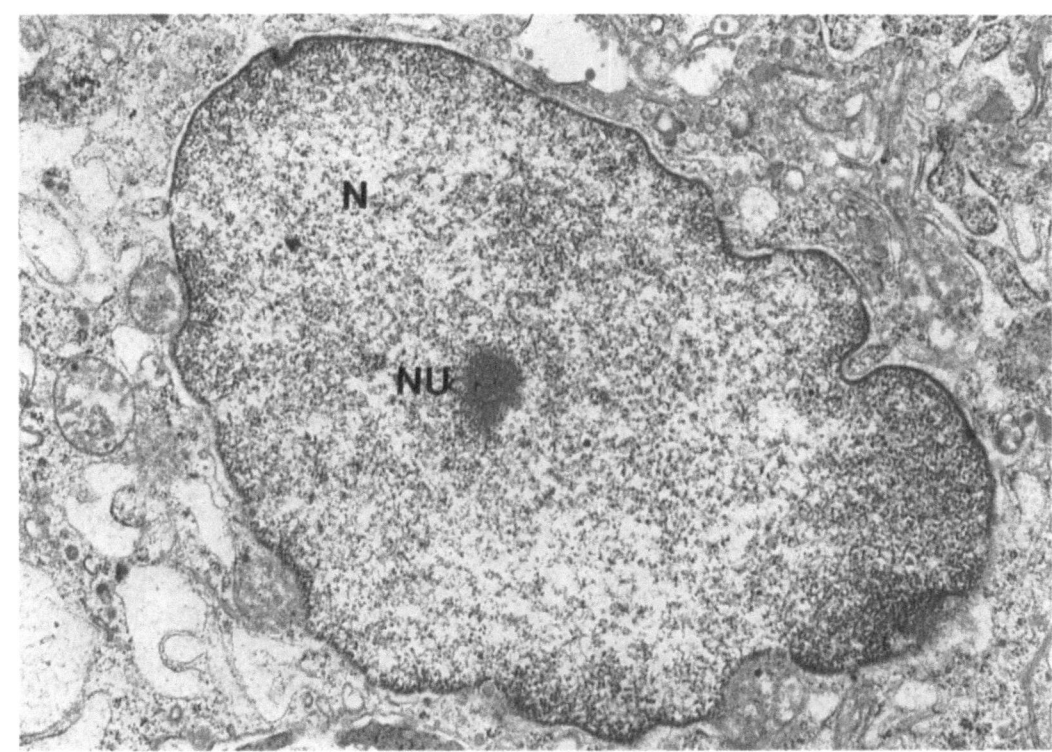

Fig. 2.9. △   **Fig. 2.10.** ▽

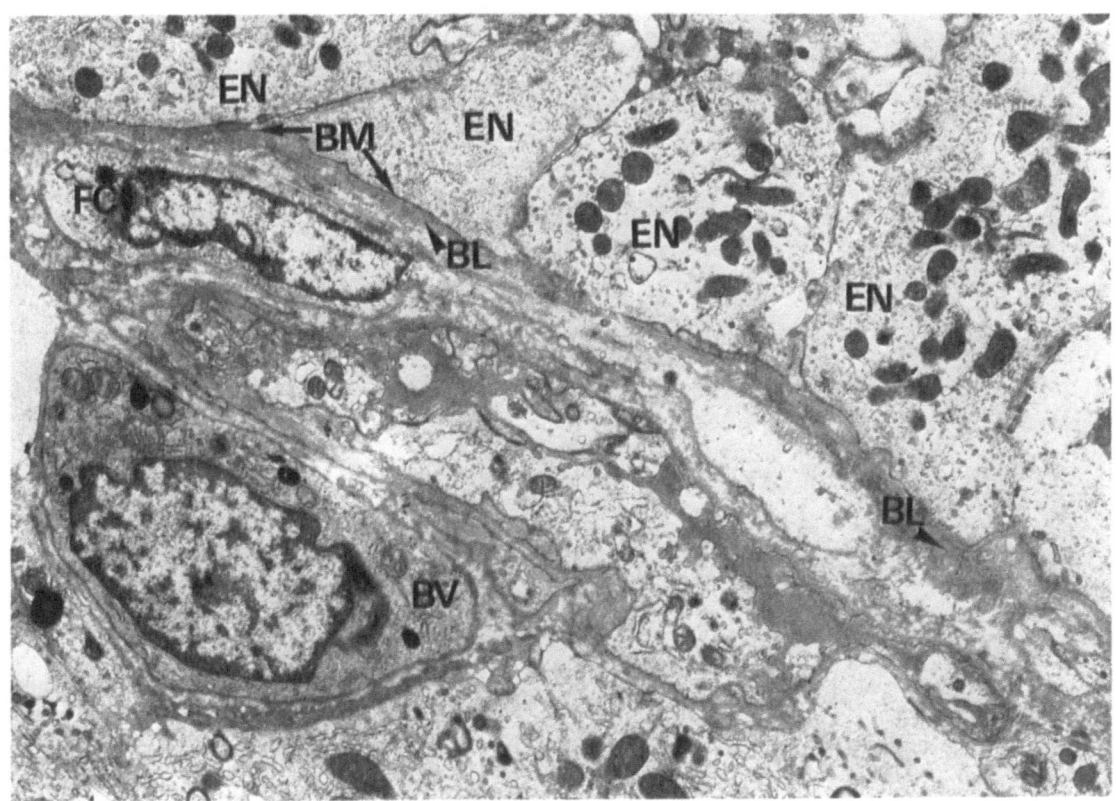

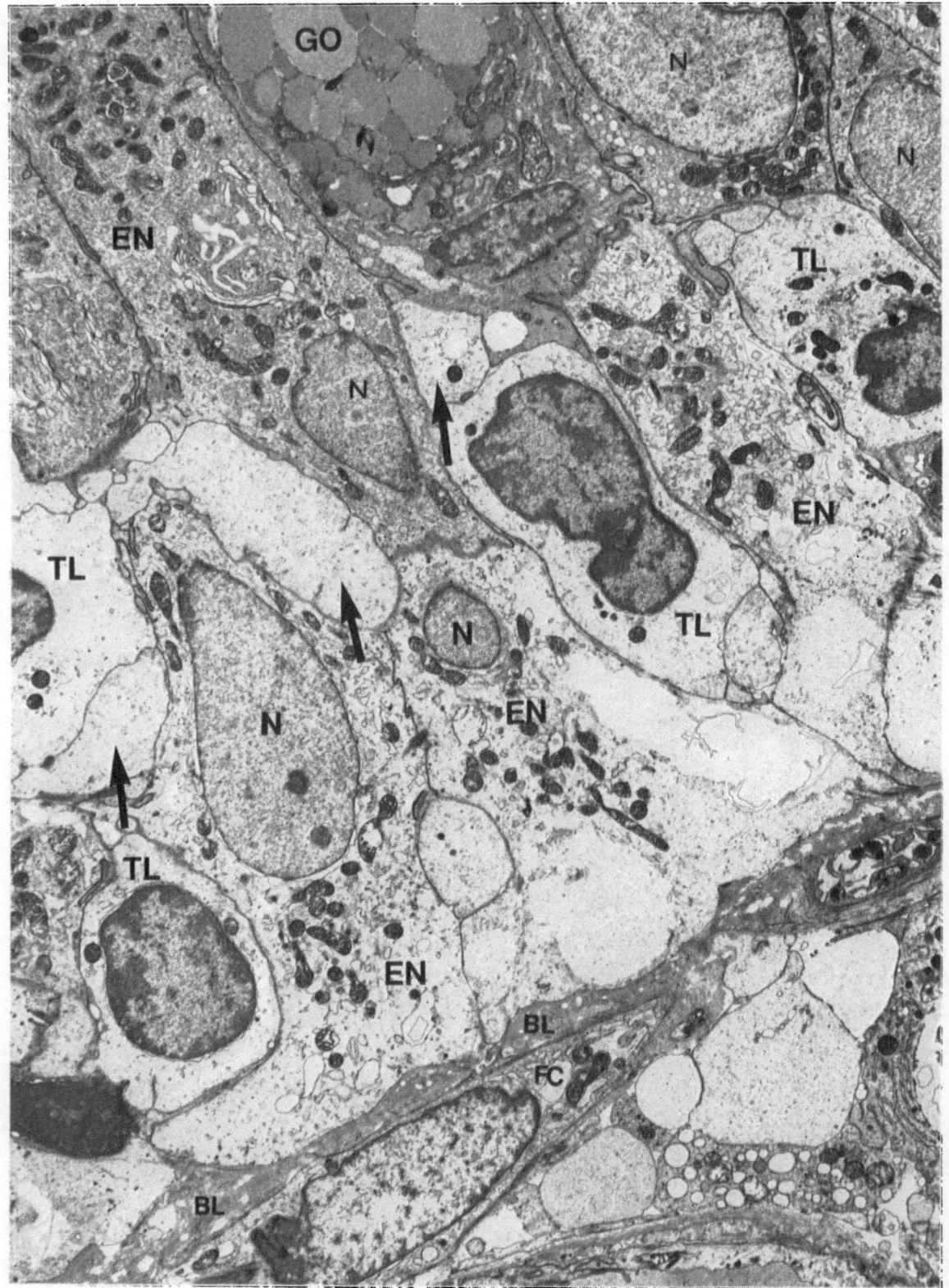

Fig. 2.11.

The *theliolymphocytes* are invariably increased in untreated coeliac disease [16] (Fig. 2.11). This increase is probably greater than in most other diseases affecting the small intestinal mucosa. Expressed as a ratio, the number of theliolymphocytes to epithelial cells is 0.5–1:1 (normal = <1:3) [27]. This is clearly seen with the EM, though it may vary from field to field. These cells are found occupying the spaces between the enterocytes, usually in their lower halves, but very rarely a theliolymphocyte may be seen at the level of the terminal bar of the enterocyte and even more rarely in the lumen of the bowel. This escape of the theliolymphocyte may only be possible with increased cell death of enterocytes. Ultrastructurally (Fig. 2.12) the nuclei of the theliolymphocytes do not appear different from those seen in the normal mucosa (Figs. 1.34–1.36) and their cytoplasm contains large numbers of ribosomes and a few other organelles. Some of the theliolymphocytes are larger cells with irregularly shaped nuclei containing little chromatin material. They show increased cytoplasmic ER, RER and mitochondria as well as other organelles consisting of vesicles which contain light-coloured homogeneous material (Fig. 2.13 and inset). Their function is not clear, but they do not resemble blast cells [15] and could be macrophages.

◁ **Fig. 2.11.** Untreated coeliac disease: several theliolymphocytes (*TL*) amongst enterocytes (*EN*) facing the bowel lumen. Note that the theliolymphocytes are confined to the intercellular spaces of the lower half of the enterocytes. They resemble small and large lymphocytes. Some of the membrane-bound spaces (*arrows*) contain ribosomes but no nucleus and may well be other theliolymphocytes that are not cut at their nuclear level or may represent cytoplasmic processes of theliolymphocytes. *MI*, microvilli; *GO*, goblet cell; *N*, nuclei of enterocytes; *BL*, basal lamina; *FC*, fibrocyte. (× 5474)

Overleaf (pages 72–73):

Fig. 2.12. Untreated coeliac disease: several theliolymphocytes (*TL*) occupying spaces between enterocytes ▷ (*EN*) which are seen in oblique section at their nuclear level (*N*). The theliolymphocytes are of small and large type and their cytoplasm contains numerous ribosomes (*R*), few mitochondria (*M*) and a small Golgi complex (*G*). (× 8400)

Fig. 2.13. Untreated coeliac disease: two theliolymphocytes (*TL1* and *TL2*) amongst enterocytes (*EN*). TL1 is ▷ a large cell with an oval nucleus (*N*) which contains little chromatin (compare with TL2). Its cytoplasm is rich in ribosomes (*R*) as well as other organelles, such as small and large vesicles (*Ve*) which contain light-coloured, homogeneous material (*see inset*). This cell resembles a macrophage morphologically. *G*, Golgi; *M*, mitochondria. (× 15 470)

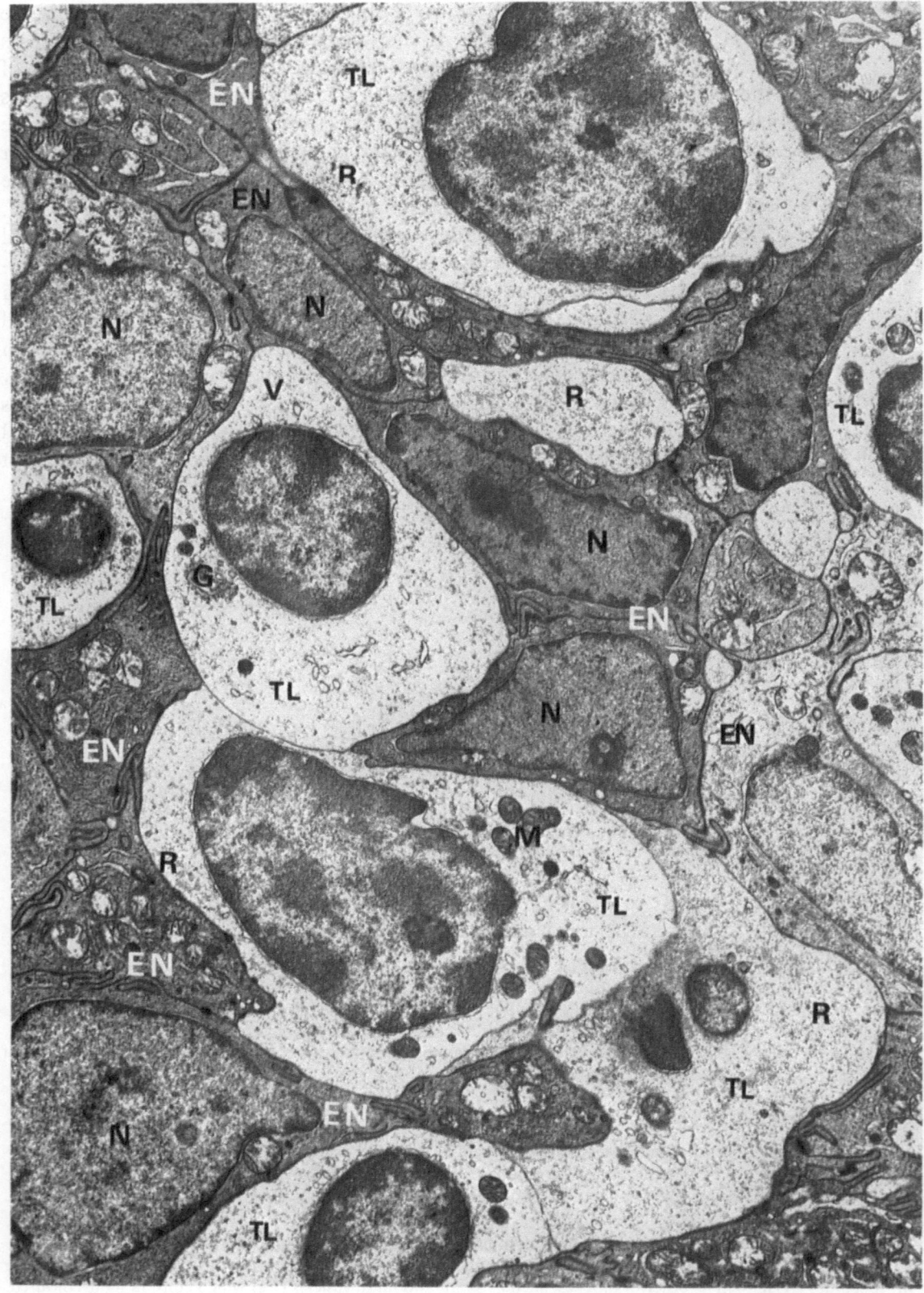

Fig. 2.12.

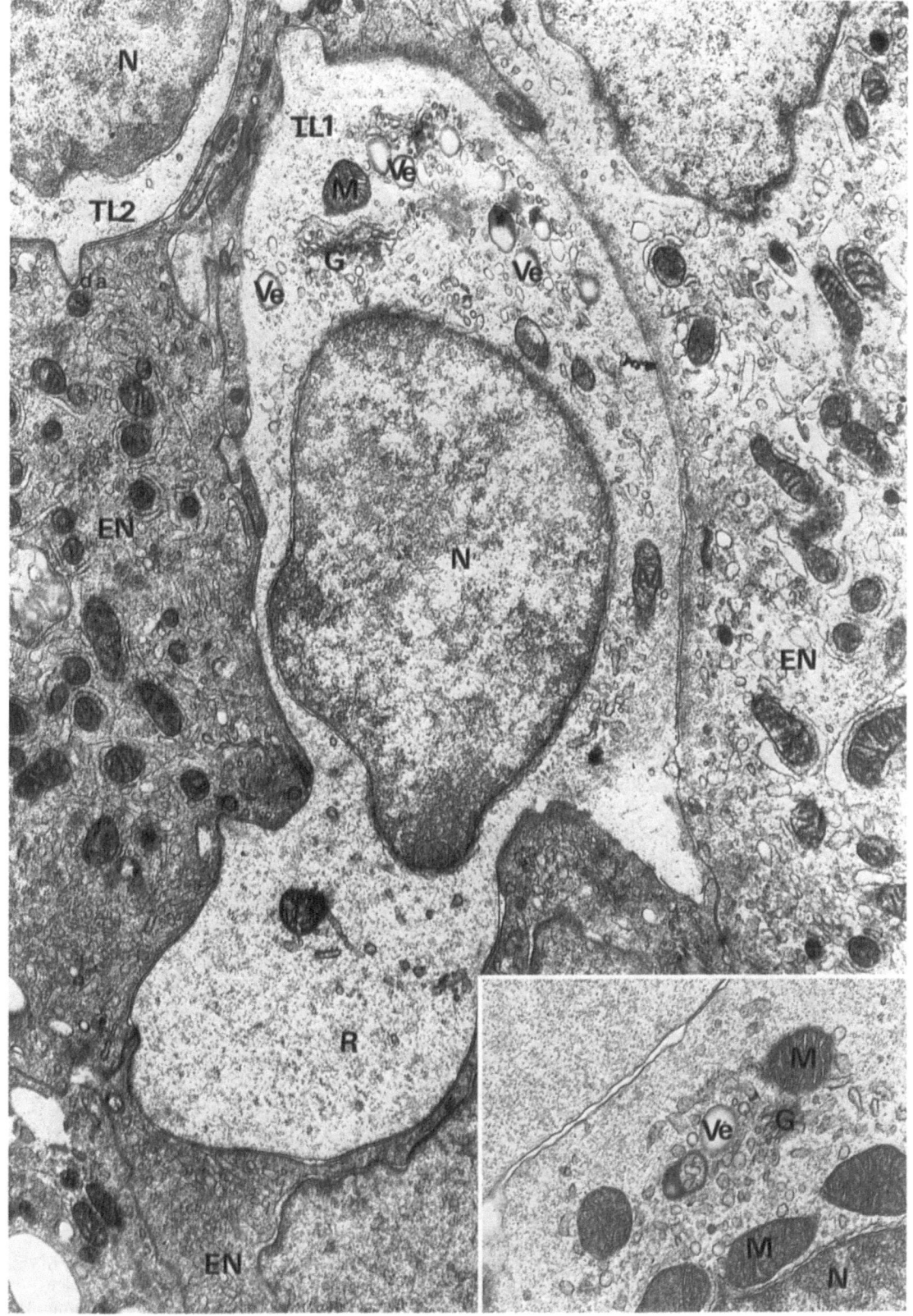

Fig. 2.13.

The cells and fibres of the *lamina propria* show significant abnormalities. The connective tissue fibrils may be either widely spaced due to oedema (Fig. 2.14) or more commonly may show increased density and are interspersed with typical collagen fibres (Fig. 2.15) [1]. This is usually associated with an increase in fibrocytes. The commonest cell type in untreated coeliac disease is the *plasma cell*. These cells are often found in clusters and may completely dominate the low-power field of examination at the EM level (Fig. 2.16). The most characteristic feature of the plasma cells is their cisternal dilatation [21, 22],

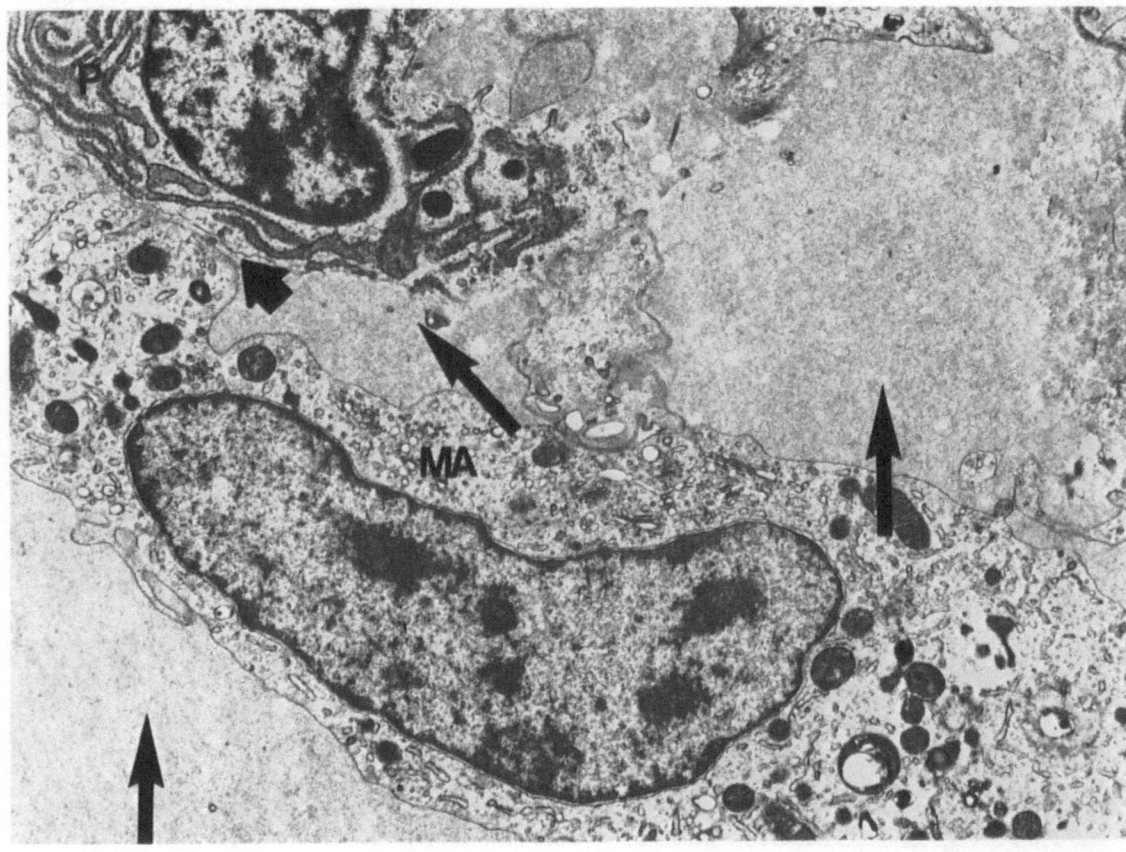

Fig. 2.14. Untreated coeliac disease: separation of connective tissue by spaces (*arrows*) which contain fine floccular material. The cells of the lamina propria appear sparser, though contact is maintained (*thick arrow*). The material within the spaces appears homogeneous and may be composed of fine fibrils or oedema fluid or both. *MA*, macrophage; *P*, plasma cell. (× 8400)

Fig. 2.15. Untreated coeliac disease: dense bundles of collagen fibres (*CO*) surround a lymphocyte (*LY*) in the ▷
lamina propria. The fibres, though not appearing electron dense, are identified as collagen by the size of their diameter. *N*, nucleus of lymphocyte. (× 16 860)

Fig. 2.16. Untreated coeliac disease: several plasma cells (*P*) identified by the chromatin pattern (*CR*) of their ▷
nuclei (*N*) or by the cisternal arrangement (*CY*) within their cytoplasm. The cisternae are usually widely dilated, probably indicating increased activity (immunoglobulin production), but some resemble young plasma cells (*arrow*) in which the tight cisternal pattern and the abundance of other cytoplasmic organelles suggest relative immaturity. *PO*, polymorphonuclear leucocyte. (× 8170).

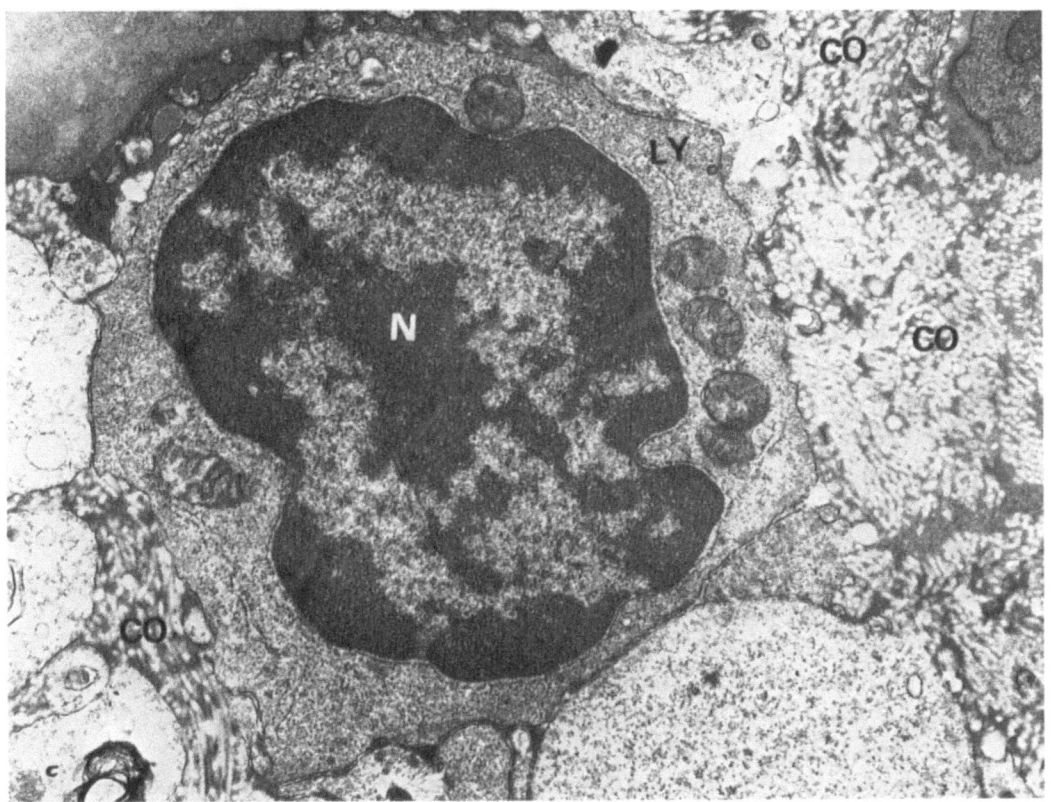

Fig. 2.15. △   Fig. 2.16. ▽

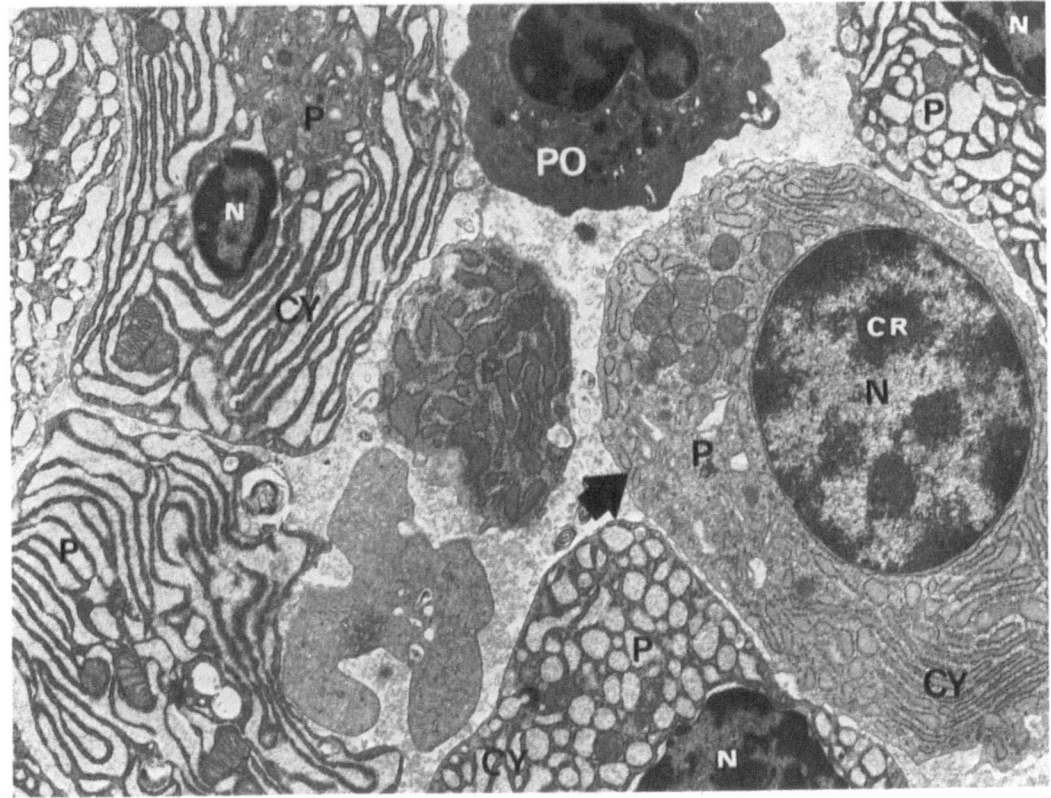

though this varies from cell to cell. The cytoplasm is often completely taken up with cisternae filled with a dense homogeneous substance, the immuno-globulin. Any increase in length of RER of the cisternae is known to be an indication of increased protein synthesis [8], confirmed by morphometry at the EM level [9]. Few mitochondria, smooth ER, Golgi vesicles or free-lying ribosomes are evident. The nucleus is placed excentrically within the cell.

The external membrane of the plasma cell often shows breaks in continuity so that cisternae are found lying free in the surrounding connective tissue medium [22]. Though rupture of the plasma cell membrane is a frequent finding in untreated coeliac disease, it may be due to an artefact arising from excessive fragility or it may signify overactivity of the cell itself. It should be noted that although this overactivity appears to be an integral feature of untreated coeliac disease it is not associated with lysis of the cell itself, since the nucleus of the plasma cells appears normal, lysosomes are absent and the mitochondrial membranes are intact. Increased numbers of mucosal plasma cells producing IgA, IgM, IgG and IgE have been reported in untreated coeliac disease [12, 14, 19], including the production of specific antigluten antibodies [4, 7]. The lamina propria lymphocytes are less conspicuous than the plasma cells. They can be seen in various stages of development but the large cell types, with clumps of nuclear chromatin and increase in cytoplasmic RER, pre-dominate [10] (Fig. 2.15). Their number is very variable and has only recently been critically studied at EM level in relation to the plasma cells [10].

Similar considerations apply to the *macrophage* counts in untreated coeliac disease, which could be more easily identified by histochemical techniques. Numerous macrophages with greater or lesser phagolysosomal activity may be seen with the EM (Fig. 2.14). Compared to the normal mucosa the impression is gained that the macrophages are increased in number and in phagolysosomal activity, though not to the extent found in mucosae in parasitic infestations, inflammatory bowel disease or multiple sclerosis. They appear, however, more numerous and active than in protein calorie malnutrition (see Chap. 4). Macrophages may be seen in intimate relation to both lymphocytes and plasma cells or along the side of small blood vessels. Invariably they are seen immediately below the basal laminae of enterocytes.

Great controversy surrounds the number of mucosal *mast cells* and the state of their granules. It has been claimed that with the light microscope and appropriate staining techniques fewer mast cells are seen in untreated coeliac disease compared to those after treatment [13], suggesting either degranulation or actual decrease in numbers. With the EM the impression is gained that there is no decrease in numbers but that many of the mast cells are partially or totally degranulated (Fig. 2.17). The role of mast cells in untreated coeliac disease is

Fig. 2.17. Untreated coeliac disease: a mast cell (*MC*) with a central nucleus (*N*) and a few granules (*GR*) in   ▷
the surrounding cytoplasm. Empty vacuoles (*Va*) and partially degranulated vacuoles (*arrows*) are seen close
to the surface membrane of the mast cell (compare with Fig. 1.46). (× 11 529)

Fig. 2.18. Untreated coeliac disease: an occasional polymorphonuclear leucocyte (*PO*) with multilobar nuclei   ▷
(*N*) and numerous small phagolysosomes (*L*) is seen in the lamina propria. Note plasma cells (*P*) showing
dilated cisternae. (× 4380)

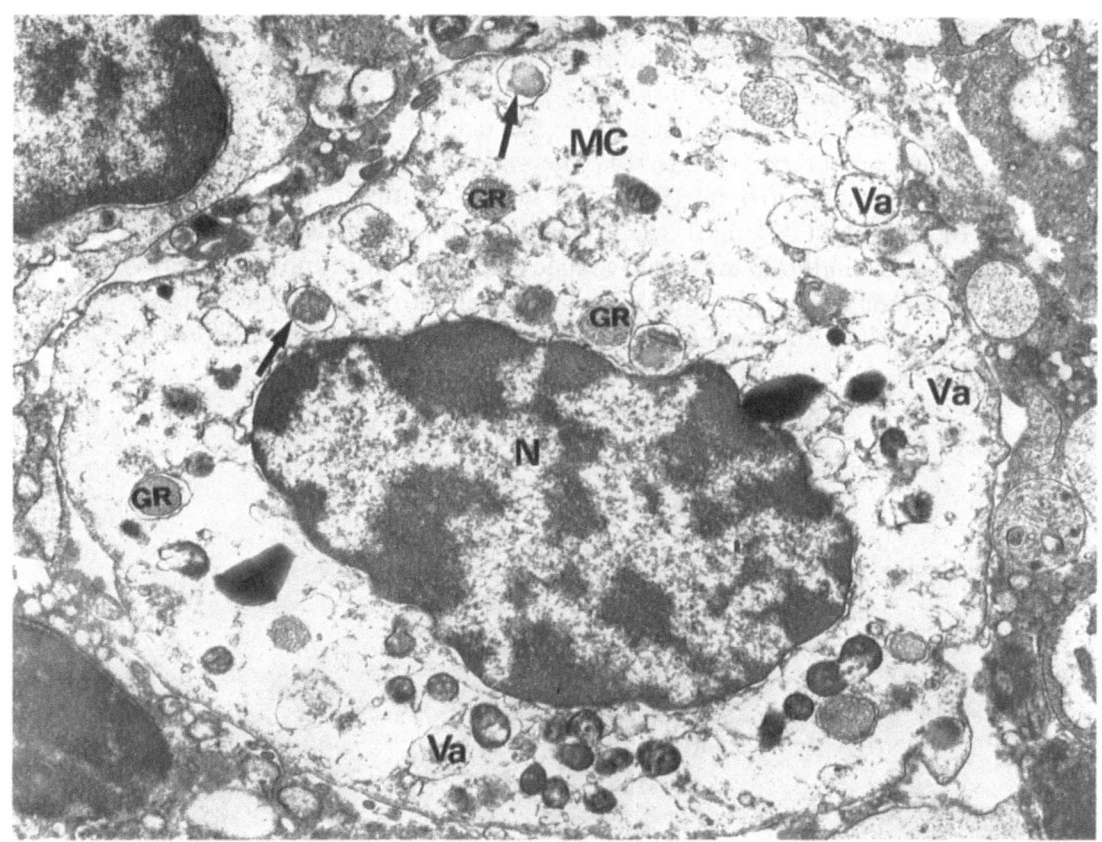

Fig. 2.17. △   Fig. 2.18. ▽

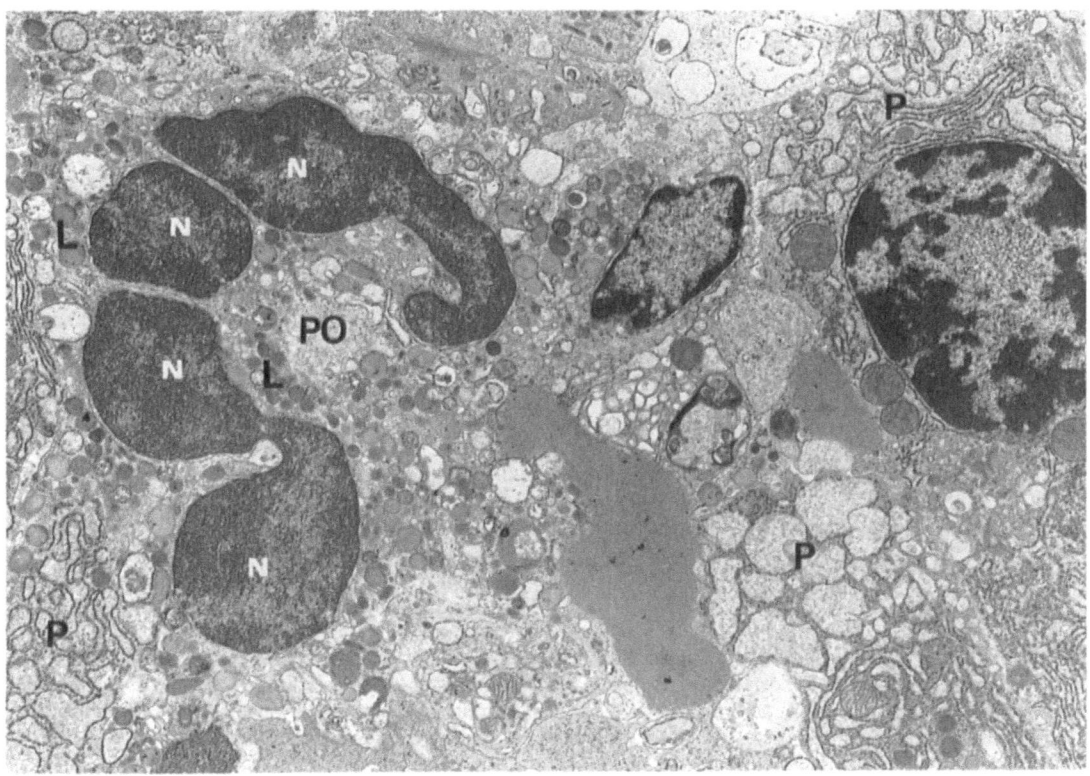

not understood, but they may play an important part in the pathogenesis of this disease. Eosinophils are often more plentiful in childhood than in adult untreated coeliac disease. *Polymorphonuclear leucocytes* may be seen in the lamina propria of untreated coeliac disease, particularly in children, but they are usually few in number (Fig. 2.18). The *endothelial cells* of small blood vessels may show hypertrophy (Fig. 2.19) with or without increase in the thickness of their basal lamina (Fig. 2.20). This is, however, a variable feature in both adult and childhood untreated coeliac disease. Little is know about any changes in the small nerve plexuses of the mucosa in untreated coeliac disease, though no structural abnormalities or decrease in numbers have been reported with the EM.

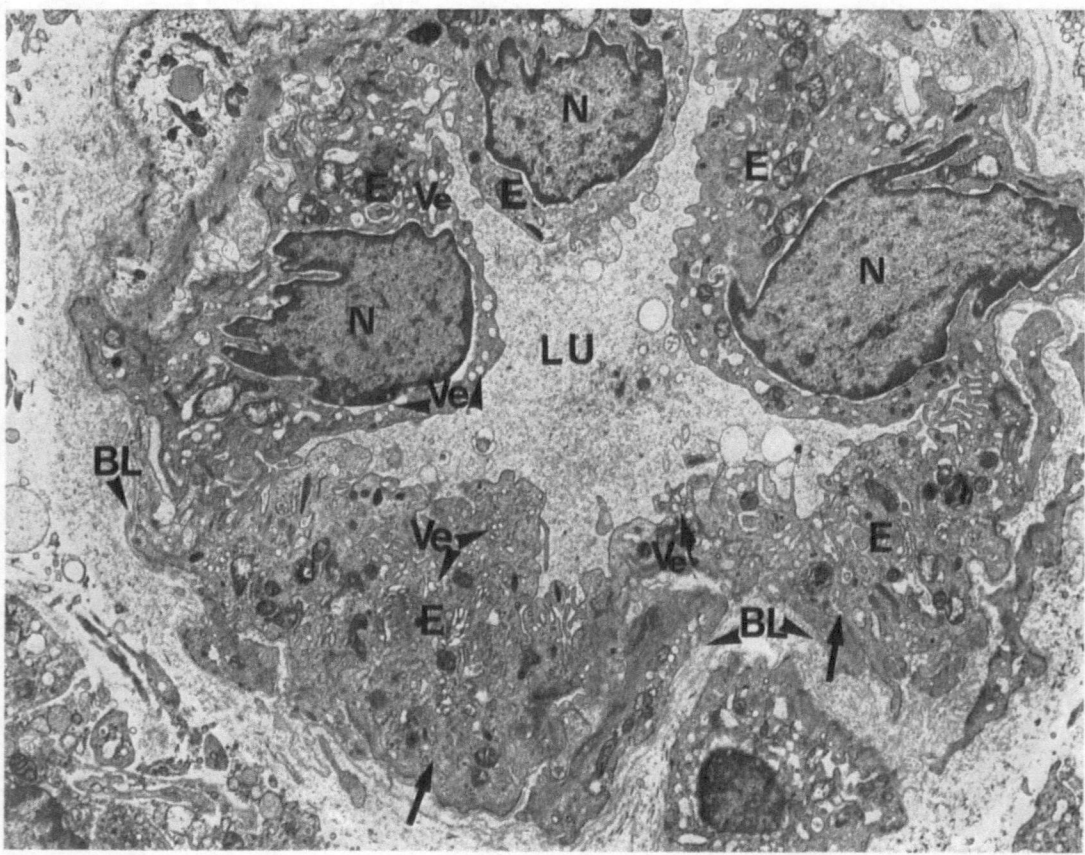

Fig. 2.19. Untreated coeliac disease: a small blood vessel in which the lumen (*LU*) is surrounded by several endothelial cells (*E*) seen at their nuclear level (*N*) or as cytoplasmic processes (*arrows*). The cytoplasmic organelles are hypertrophied and contain numerous cytoplasmic vesicles (*Ve*), mitochondria, Golgi complexes and small phagolysosomes. The basal laminae of the endothelium (*BL*) is not hypertrophied. (× 7310)

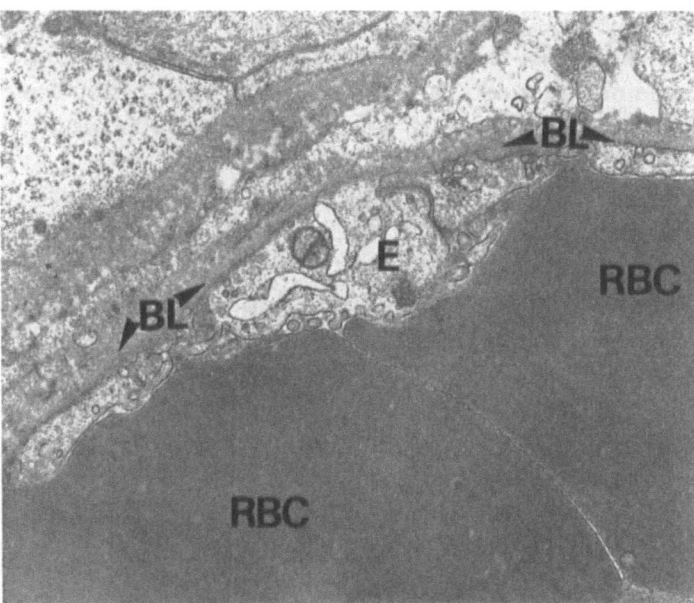

Fig. 2.20. Untreated coeliac disease: part of a small blood vessel showing hypertrophy of the basal lamina (*BL*) of the endothelial cells (*E*). *RBC*, red blood cell in lumen of vessel. (× 8643)

Comparison of adult and childhood coeliac disease

No significant differences in the ultrastructural appearances in untreated coeliac disease have been observed between adults and children. This is partly due to the variability of fine structural changes. Light microscopic appearances also appear to be identical between adults and children. After treatment with a gluten-free diet the mucosa reverts to histological normality with reappearance of the villi, shortening of the crypts and decrease in theliolymphocytes and lamina propria cellularity (Fig. 2.1b). This reversion to normal (or near normal) is variable both in time and extent, and may depend on the age of the patient and how strictly a gluten-free diet is adhered to. Although morphometric comparison between histological improvement in adults and children after treatment may be meaningless because of individual variability, histological impressions favour the view that villous regeneration is more complete in children. Subjective fine structural observations suggest that in the untreated coeliac child the enterocytes are more immature, the lamina propria connective tissue fibrils are denser and both lymphocytes and plasma cells are more numerous. The possible increase in eosinophils and polymorphs in childhood coeliac disease has already been mentioned. Any increases in macrophages and mast cells are even more difficult to evaluate.

Gluten challenge in treated children with normal mucosa (27 patients)

The ultrastructure of the mucosa was studied in each child on a gluten-free diet before gluten challenge, and 2, 5, 7, 11, 15, 24, 48, 72 and 96 h after a single dose of 20 g gluten, cooked or uncooked, given either by mouth or delivered by naso-duodenal tube [20, 24]. Each patient had between one and three biopsies.

Throughout the periods tested, no histological deterioration was evident when pre- and post-challenge biopsies were compared, and the enterocytes also remained ultrastructurally normal. Between 2 and 7 h after challenge there was oedema in the lamina propria with the appearance of eosinophils in the interepithelial spaces (Fig. 2.21) and lamina propria, and an increase in lamina propria mast cells (Fig. 2.22), some partially granulated, others degranulated. Plasma cells appeared moderately active but not increased. Between 11 and 24 h several changes occurred in the lamina propria: there was thickening of the basal lamina of enterocytes (Fig. 2.23) and increase in density of the fine

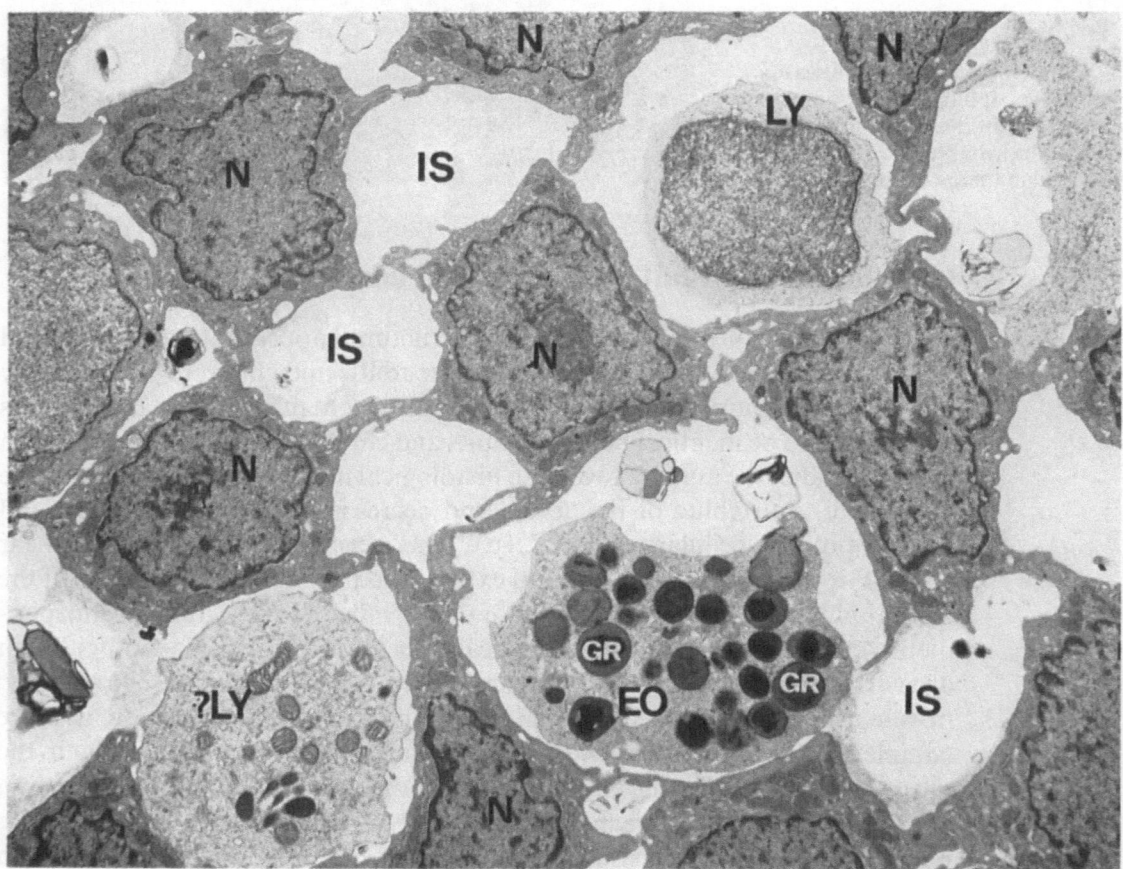

Fig. 2.21. Gluten challenge: widely dilated intercellular spaces (*IS*) between enterocytes shown at their nuclear level (*N*). These spaces appear empty or are filled with infiltrating cells, identified either as lymphocyte (*LY*) or eosinophil (*EO*), the latter showing typical granules (*GR*) in the cytoplasm. The identity of a third interepithelial cell (*?LY*) cannot be established. Biopsy taken between 2 and 7 h after gluten. (× 6200)

Fig. 2.22. Gluten challenge: two mast cells (*MC*) in the lamina propria seen at their nuclear level (*N*). In the   ▷ cytoplasm there are some granules present (*arrows*) but many vacuoles (*Va*) are either partly degranulated or totally empty. Biopsy taken between 2 and 7 h after gluten. (× 10 143)

Fig. 2.23. Gluten challenge: the basal lamina (*BL*) of enterocytes (*EN*) appears as a wide layer composed of   ▷ fine fibrous tissues. No distinct linear layer external to the basal membrane of the enterocytes (*arrow*) can be identified (compare with Fig. 1.12). *P*, plasma cell with nucleus (*N*). Biopsy taken between 11 and 24 h after gluten. (× 10 750)

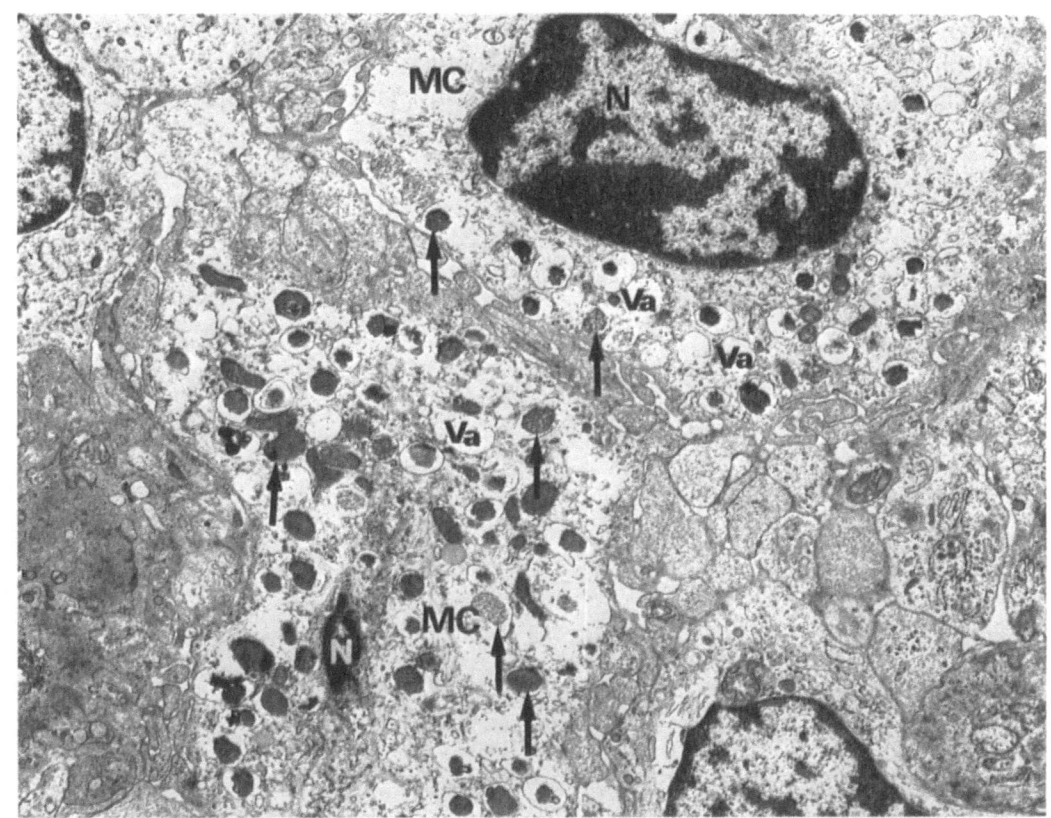

Fig. 2.22. △   Fig. 2.23. ▽

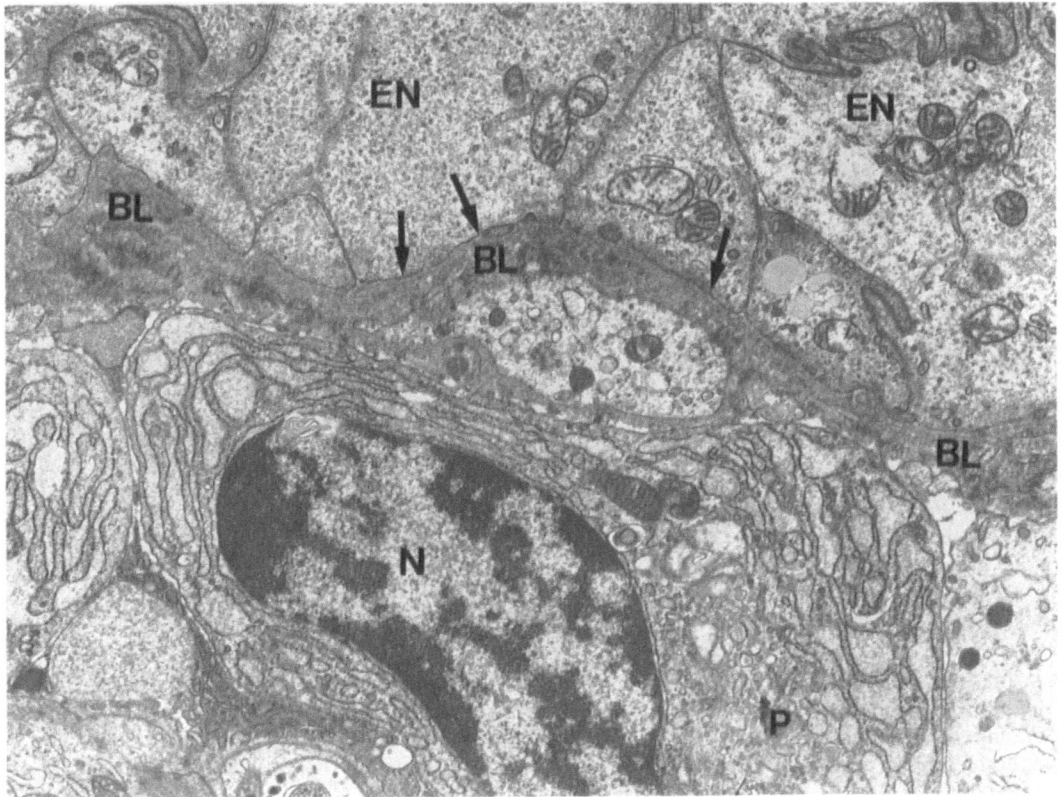

fibrils of the connective tissue. The basal laminae of the endothelial cells lining small blood vessels (Fig. 2.24) were also thickened and the endothelial cells themselves appeared swollen, with numerous pinocytotic vesicles (Fig. 2.25).

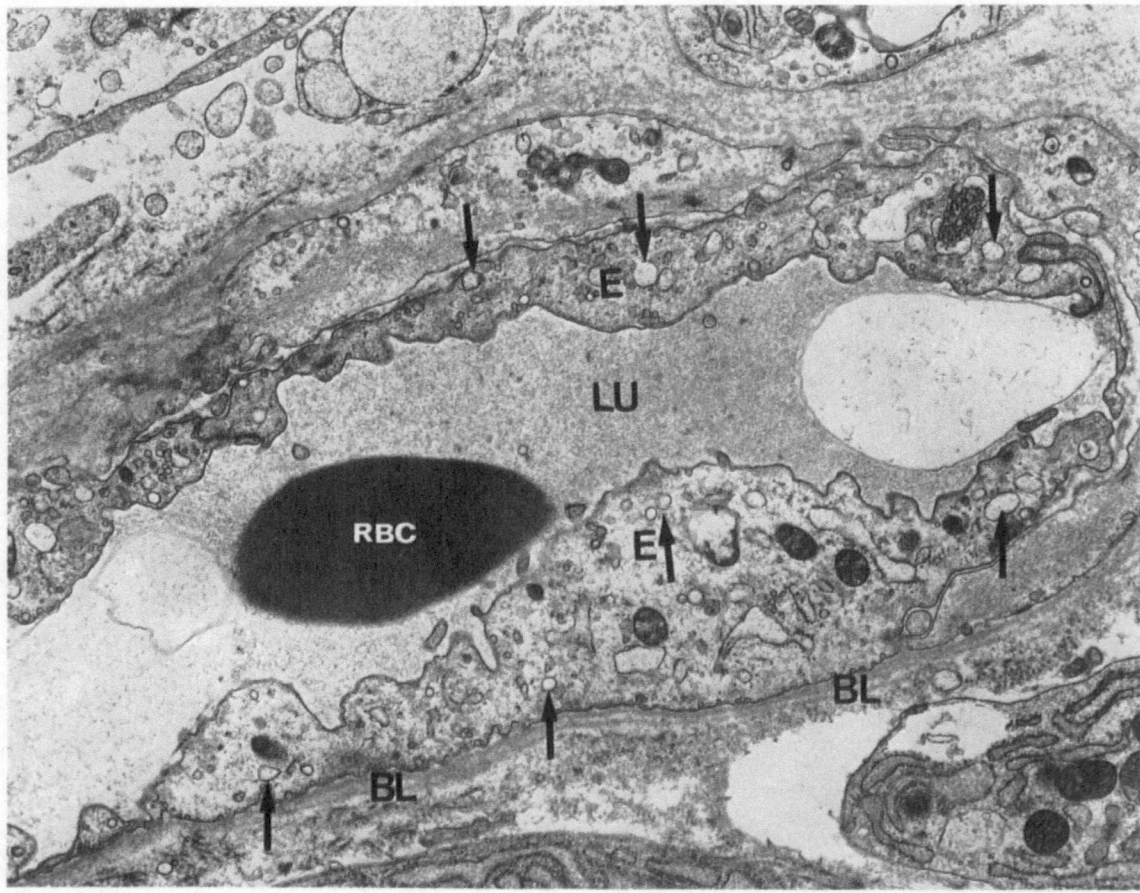

Fig. 2.24. Gluten challenge: the endothelium of a small blood vessel surrounding the lumen (*LU*), which contains a single red blood cell (*RBC*). There is early hypertrophy of the endothelial processes (*E*), which contain many vesicular bodies in their cytoplasm (*arrows*). The basal lamina (*BL*) surrounding the endothelium shows thickening and blends with the fibrous tissue external to it. Biopsy taken 11 h after gluten. (×11 490)

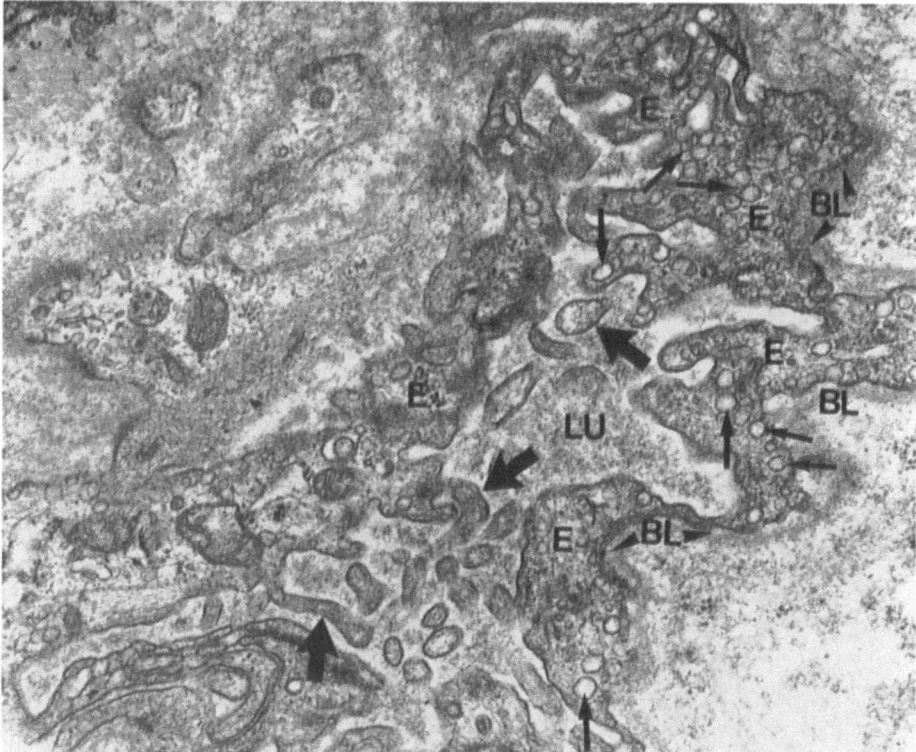

Fig. 2.25. Gluten challenge: processes of endothelial cells (*E*) surrounding the lumen (*LU*) of a small blood vessel and showing cytoplasmic hypertrophy with numerous marginal folds (*thick arrows*) and micropinocytotic vesicles (*arrows*) situated either within or attached to the outer cell membrane. The basal lamina (*BL*) of the endothelial cells is thickened and indistinct from the surrounding fibrous tissue. Biopsy taken 24 h after gluten. (× 30 500)

The lumen of the vessels was often narrowed due to this swelling. Occasional polymorphs were observed within the lamina propria. Cisternal dilatation within plasma cells, indicating increased cell activity, was more pronounced than earlier (Figs. 2.26, 2.27). Macrophages could be seen but there was no striking increase in their number or activity. After 48 h there was further increase in density of the connective tissue fibrils (Fig. 2.28) and the appearance of collagen fibres became a conspicuous feature in the lamina propria. The basal laminae of the epithelium (Fig. 2.28) and endothelium

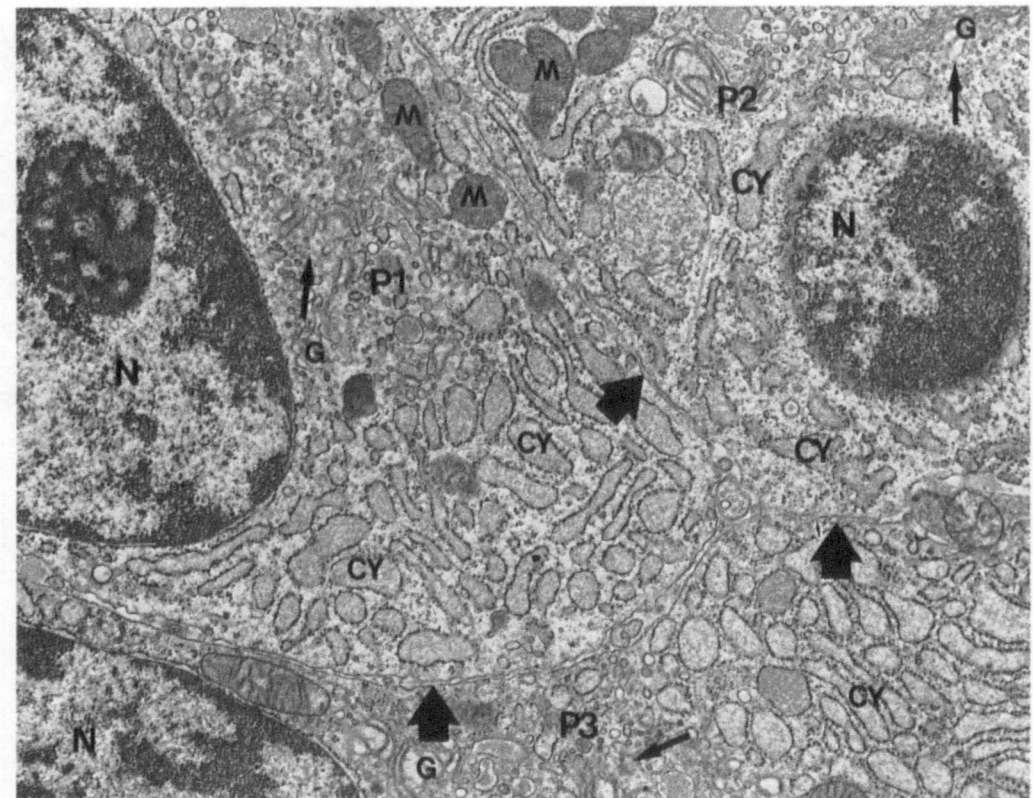

Fig. 2.26. △   Fig. 2.27. ▽

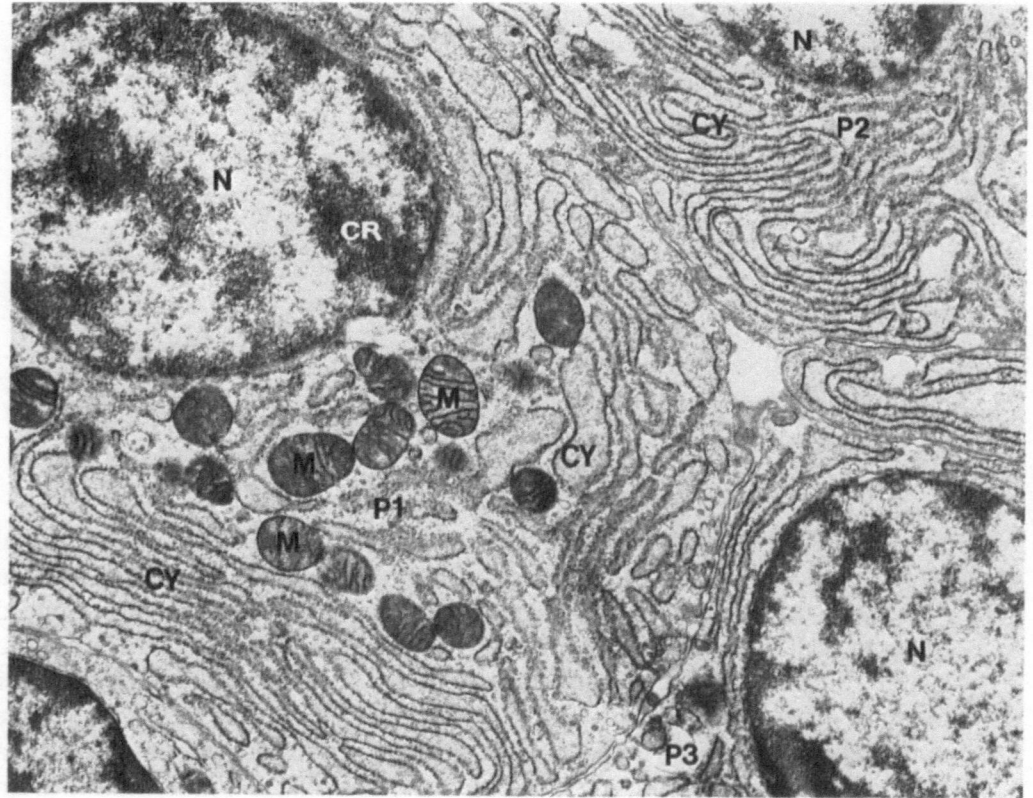

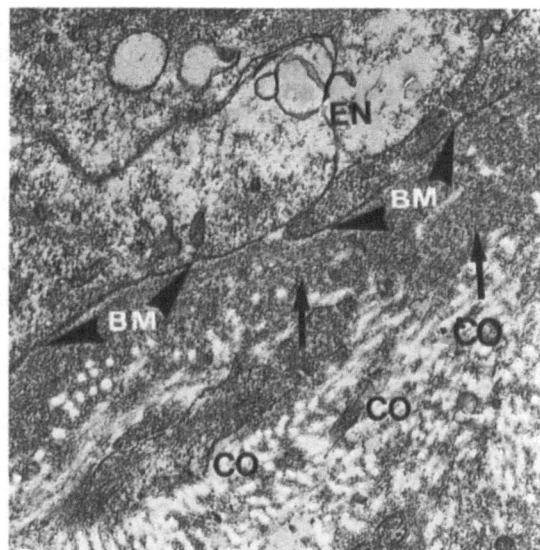

Fig. 2.28. Gluten challenge: increase in connective tissue fibrils (*arrows*) and collagen fibres (*CO*) in the lamina propria below the basal membrane (*BM*) of an enterocyte (*EN*). The basal lamina of the enterocyte is not distinguishable. Biopsy taken 48 h after gluten. (× 17 750)

◁ **Fig. 2.26.** Gluten challenge: three plasma cells (*P1, 2, 3*) shown at their nuclear level (*N*). The cell membranes (*arrows*) are in close apposition. Cytoplasmic cisternae (*CY*) are moderately dilated and contain dense material (immunoglobulin). All cells show perinuclear areas of cytoplasm (*thin arrows*) containing other organelles, such as ER, RER, Golgi (*G*) and mitochondria (*M*), indicating that they are young plasma cells. Biopsy taken 15 h after gluten. (× 25 490)

◁ **Fig. 2.27.** Gluten challenge: three plasma cells (*P1, 2, 3*) at their nuclear level (*N*) in close apposition to each other. Their cytoplasm contains elongated maze-like dilated cisternae (*CY*) which, with the exception of a few mitochondria (*M*), completely fill the cytoplasmic spaces. The plasma cell nuclei contains less chromatin (*CR*). Their appearance suggests greater maturity compared to those seen in Fig. 2.26. Biopsy taken 24 h after gluten. (× 29 230)

(Fig. 2.29) appeared thicker and denser and endothelial hypertrophy was again evident (Fig. 2.29). Numerous active plasma cells were seen, some with rupture of the membranes and escape of cytoplasmic cisternae. Increased numbers of lymphocytes, macrophages and mast cells were also seen. Eosinophils were identified, as were occasional polymorphs. The overall impression was that of increased cytopathological activity predominantly within the lamina propria, involving the connective tissue fibrils and collagen fibres, the endothelial cells and the infiltrating cells; of the latter, eosinophils, polymorphs and mast cells were increased in the early phases after challenge and plasma cells, lymphocytes and macrophages in the later stages.

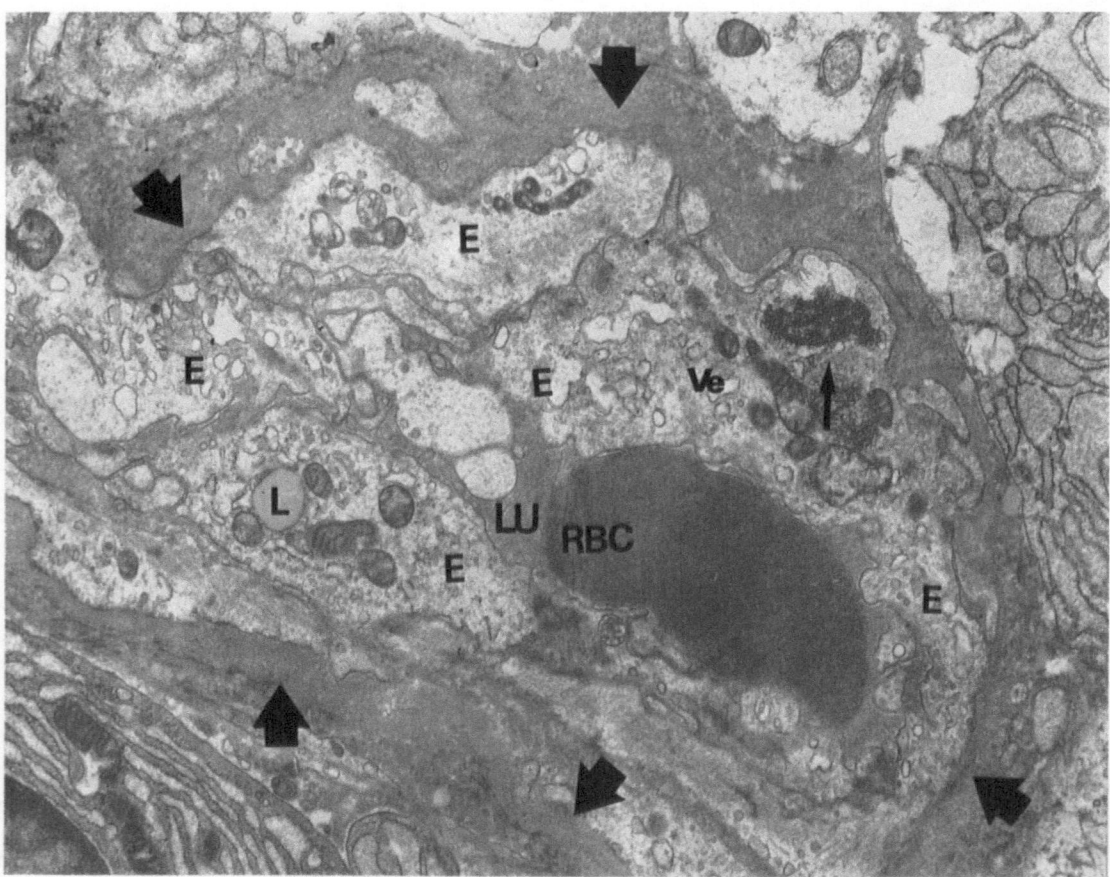

Fig. 2.29. Gluten challenge: a small blood vessel in which the lumen (*LU*) contains a single red blood cell (*RBC*) and is almost occluded by the hypertrophy of the endoplasmic processes of the endothelium (*E*). The cytoplasm of these processes contains numerous organelles, including small vesicles (*Ve*), lysosomes (*L*) and phagocytosed material (*arrow*). The basal lamina of the endothelium is obscured by a thick fibrous band (*thick arrows*) which surrounds the blood vessel. Biopsy taken 96 h after gluten. (×11 954)

Gluten challenge in children with partial repair of the mucosa (12 patients)

In the absence of strict dietary control the mucosa may be in a state of partial repair, showing histologically shorter villi, cuboidal enterocytes, elongated crypts and a moderate excess of theliolymphocytes and infiltrating cells (PVA) (Fig. 2.30). If this mucosa is challenged with gluten, a further flattening of the enterocytes and a rapid increase in the theliolymphocytes and infiltrating cells including polymorphs may be seen within 48 h, progressing to a subtotal villous atrophy within 96 h (Fig. 2.31). On EM, signs of enterocyte damage

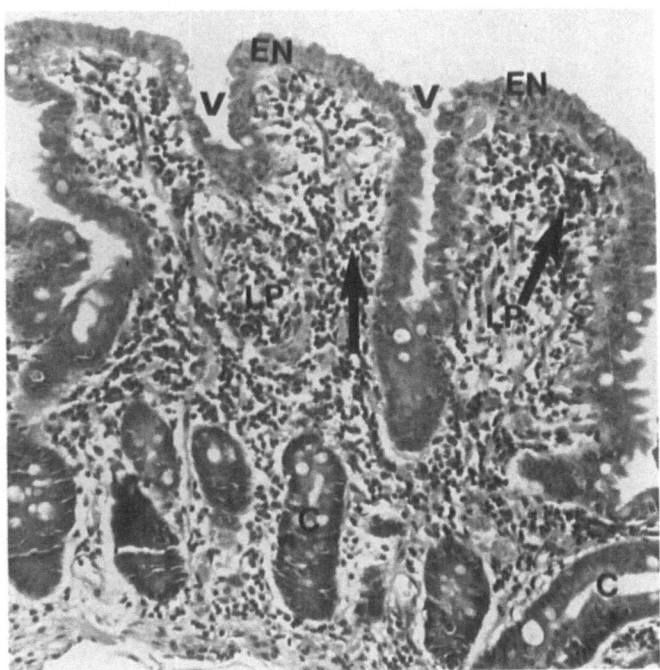

Fig. 2.30. Light microscopy of jejunal mucosa in the absence of strict dietary control of the gluten-free diet. The villi (*V*) are short and broad, the enterocytes (*EN*) appear cuboidal. Theliolymphocytes are increased. There is an excess of inflammatory cells (*arrows*) within the lamina propria (*LP*). The crypts (*C*) are elongated. (× 180)

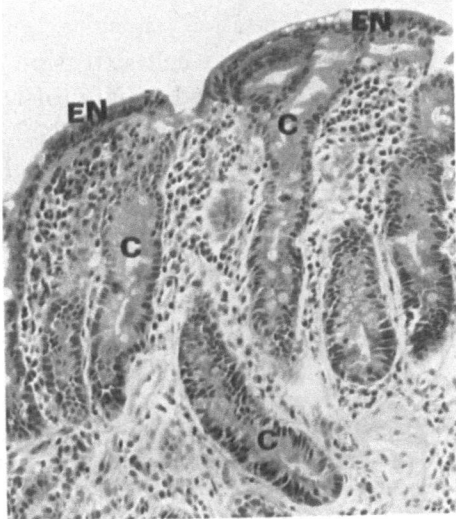

Fig. 2.31. Light microscopy of the mucosa from the same patient 96 h after gluten challenge. The surface of the mucosa appears flat with severe reduction in enterocyte height (*EN*), increase in theliolymphocytes and crypt hypertrophy (*C*). (× 150)

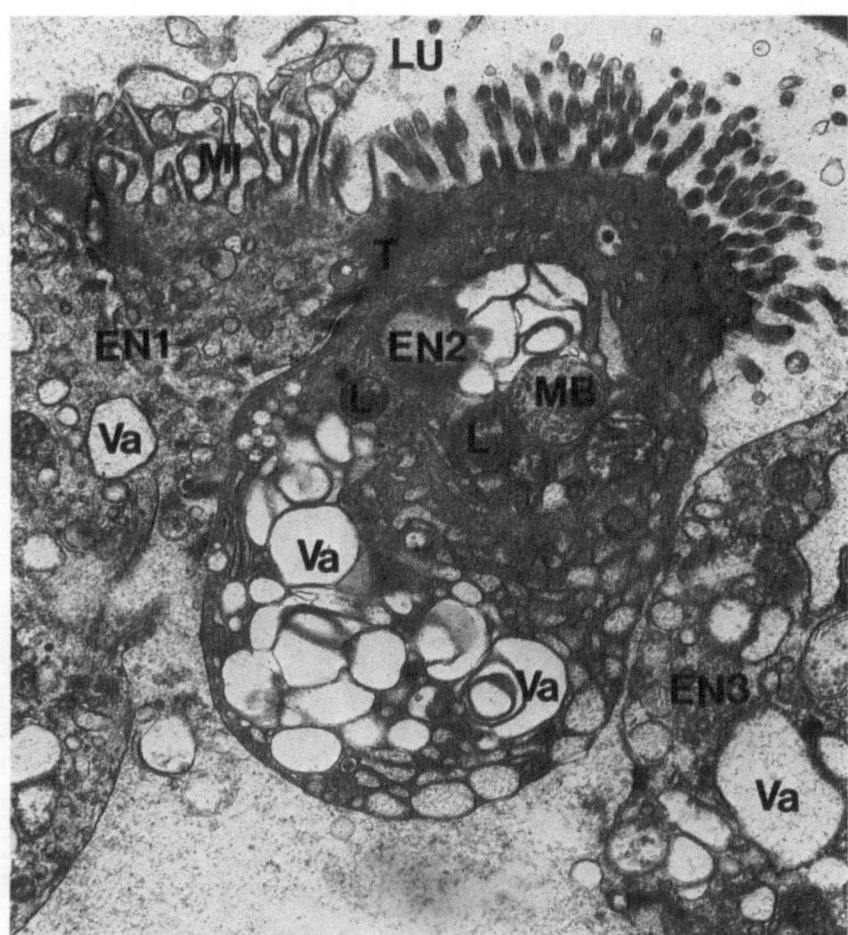

Fig. 2.32. Three enterocytes (*EN1, 2, 3*) facing the lumen of the bowel (*LU*) are seen in a degenerative state. A tight junction (*T*) between EN1 and EN2 is still observed on the left but is severed from cell EN3. The microvilli (*MI*) of cell EN1 are severely abnormal. All enterocytes show excessive vacuolation (*Va*) and EN2 shows excess lysosomes (*L*) and multivesicular bodies (*MB*). Biopsy from the same patient as in Fig. 2.31. (× 12 060)

such as excessive cell extrusion (Fig. 2.32), microvillous shortening and branching, increased activity of lysosomes, excessive vacuolation and mitochondrial damage (Figs. 2.33, 2.34) are seen. Theliolymphocytes may be particularly numerous (Fig. 2.35). In the lamina propria fewer plasma cells and more lymphocytes may be observed at 48 h after challenge (Fig. 2.36) than at 24 h. This may be due to rapid stimulation of lymphocytes to form new plasma cells.

Fig. 2.33. Low magnification electron micrograph showing several enterocytes (*EN*) in oblique section. They ▷ contain large vacuoles (*Va*) filled with apparently residual fatty material. The Golgi complexes (*G*) show widely dilated vesicles. Theliolymphocytes (*TL*) are seen in the interepithelial spaces. *N*, nuclei of enterocytes. Biopsy taken several days after gluten challenge. (× 9910)

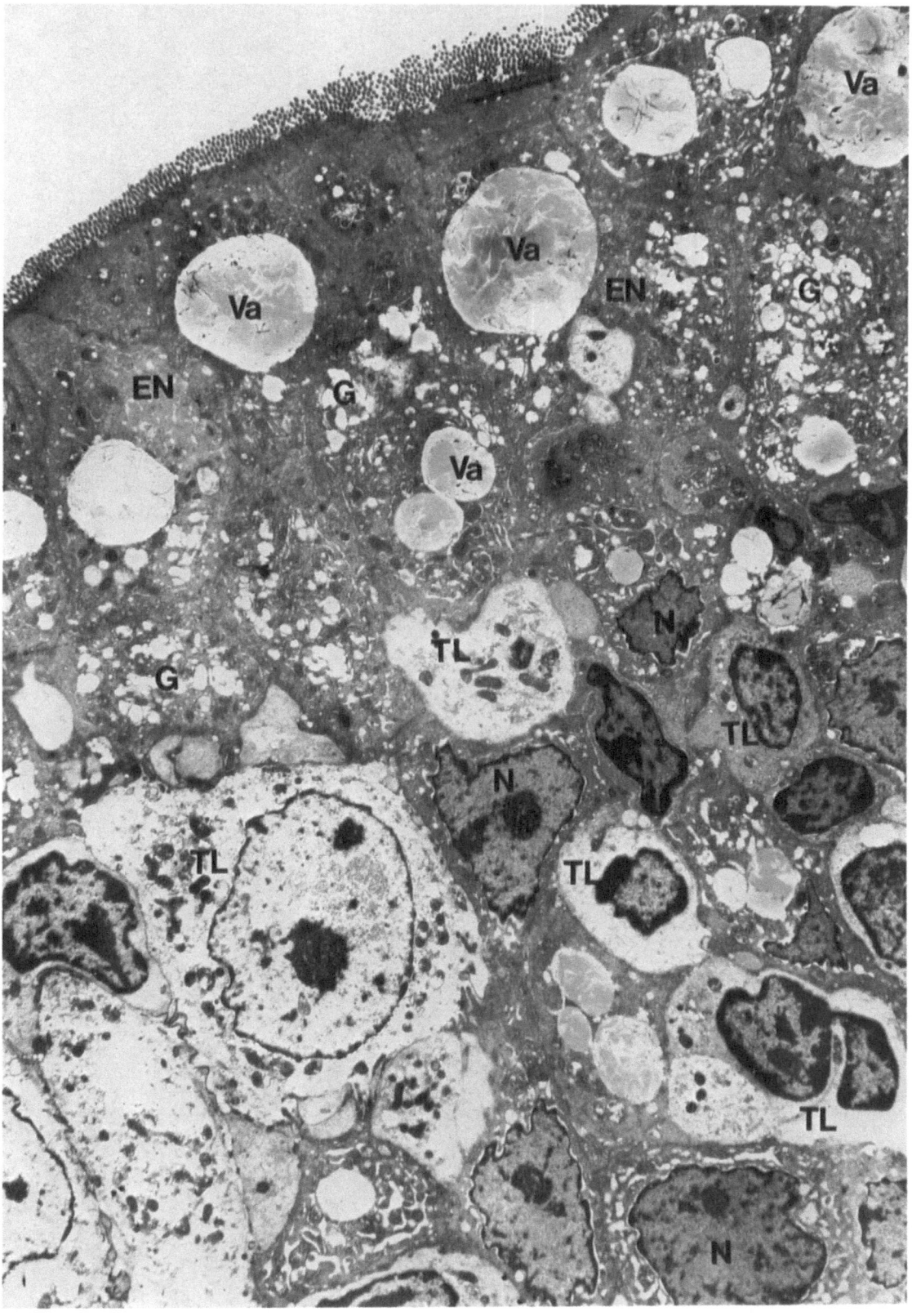

Fig. 2.33.

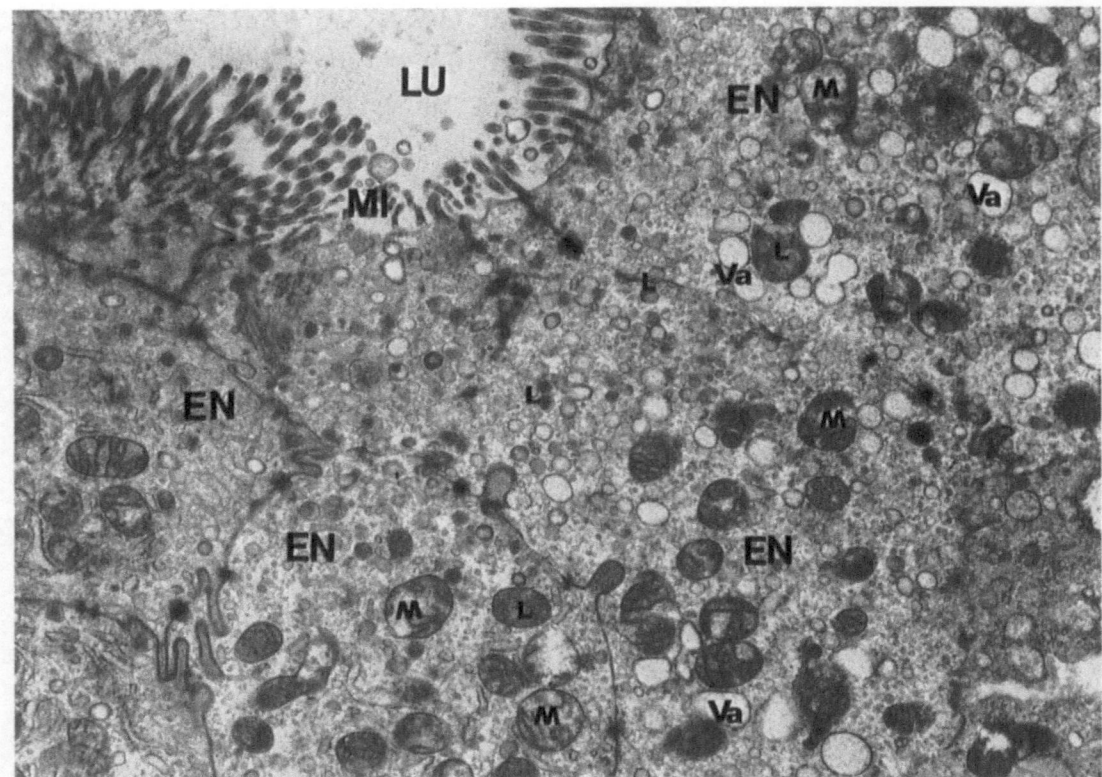

Fig. 2.34. △   **Fig. 2.35.** ▽

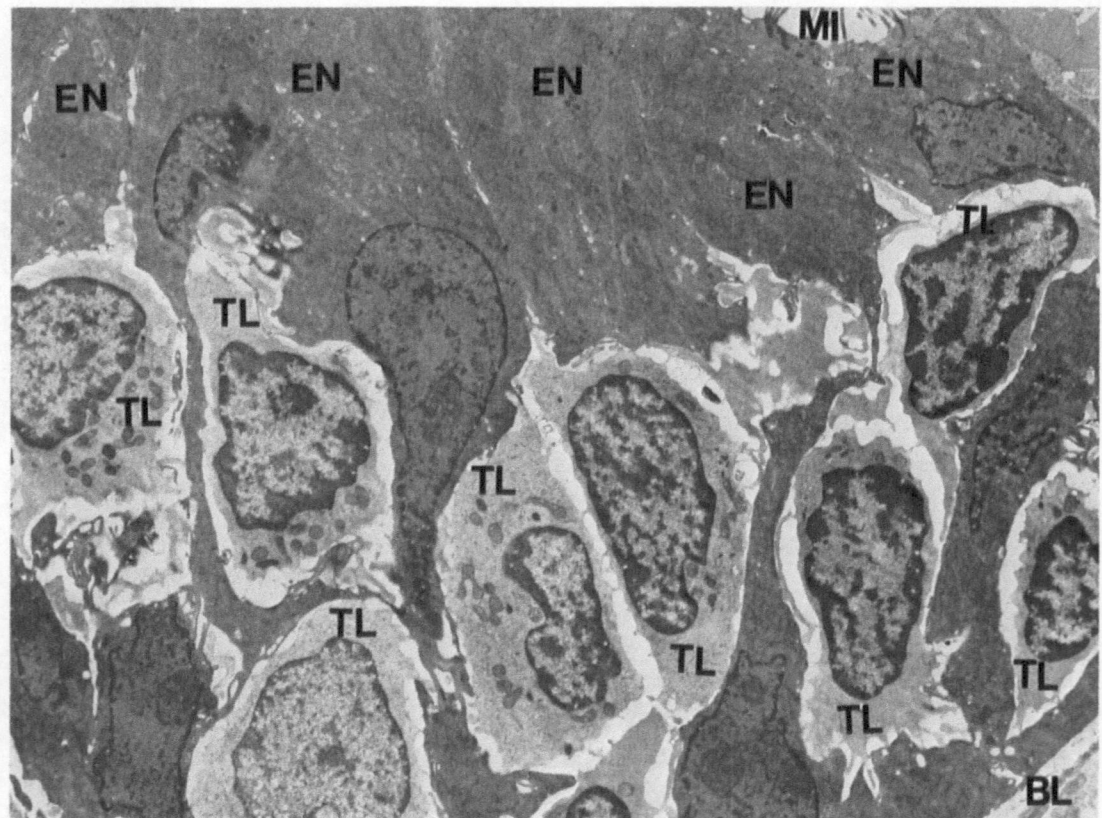

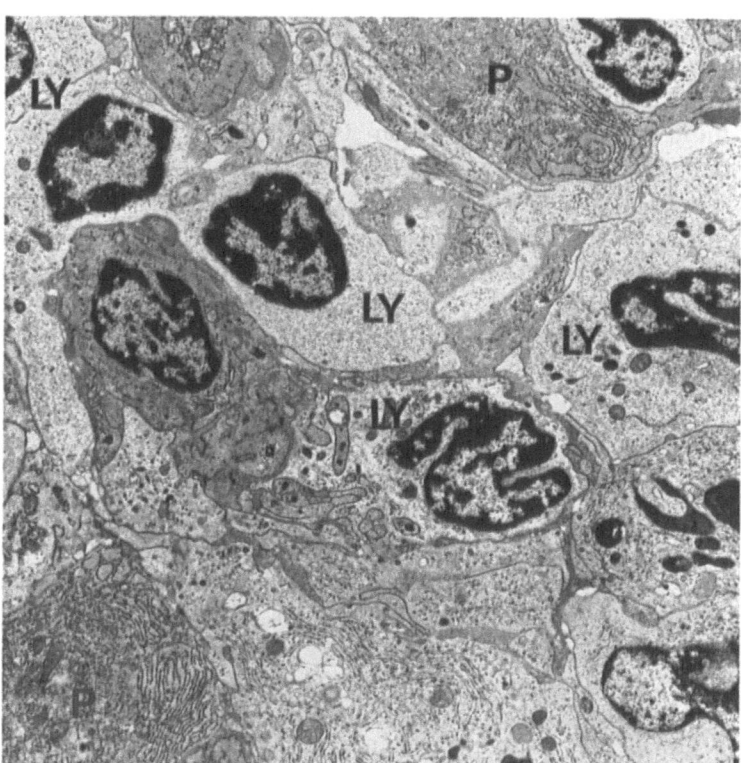

Fig. 2.36. The lamina propria is packed with small lymphocytes (*LY*) and fewer, as well as less active plasma cells (*P*). Biopsy taken 48 h after gluten challenge. (×1535)

The correlation of structure and function in coeliac disease

Untreated coeliac disease

It is important to re-emphasise that the histological and fine-structural features of untreated coeliac disease are identical in adults and children but may vary in degree. Quantitative immunological studies of the jejunal mucosa showing an increase in all major immunoglobulin classes correlate with the increased number of plasma cells seen histologically and with the dilatation of plasma cell cisternae observed ultrastructurally. The deposition of immune complexes in the lamina propria [5] which bind C3 complement may indicate a cytotoxic reaction (type 3 hypersensitivity) which may be directed against the epithelial component. The morphological expression of this may be crypt cell hyperplasia with emergence of a faulty generation of definitive absorbing cells, resulting in fewer and less viable cells (whence short or absent villi).

◁ **Fig. 2.34.** Several enterocytes (*EN*) facing the lumen of the bowel (*LU*) The cytoplasmic changes are relatively minor and show abnormality of the microvilli (*MI*), cytoplasmic vacuolation (*Va*) and numerous small and large lysosomes (*L*). The mitochondria (*M*) appear swollen and show abnormalities of their cristae. Biopsy taken several days after gluten challenge. (×7780)

◁ **Fig. 2.35.** Theliolymphocytes (*TL*) invading the intercellular spaces of enterocytes (*EN*). The ratio of *TL* to *EN* is between 1:1 and 1:2. *MI*, microvilli; *BL*, basal lamina. Biopsy taken several days after gluten challenge. (×4670)

Ultrastructural evidence is found in the emerging enterocytes lining the surface of the mucosa which appear immature and vacuolated, with swelling of mitochondria and an increase in lysosomes. The microvillous abnormalities of these enterocytes and their typical branching are not representative of degenerating microvilli, which usually appear bulbous or swollen, but resemble those found in normal crypt epithelium. Alternatively the appearance of the abnormal enterocytes may be the result of a cytotoxic factor (type 2 hypersensitivity) acting directly on their surface membranes, and the immaturity of these cells may be explained as an effort by the crypt cells to replace the damaged surface cells more rapidly than normal, much as immature red blood cells appear in the circulation in severe anaemia [6].

Gluten challenge after treatment with a gluten-free diet

Just as elimination of dietary gluten causes improvement in the jejunal mucosa, so re-introduction of gluten to the diet results in the return of mucosal histological abnormalities identical with those seen in untreated coeliac disease. Diagnostic gluten challenges are an accepted method in the management of the coeliac patient [17], but the time required to reproduce histological abnormalities is uncertain. It varies from patient to patient, may be more rapid in children than in adults and depends on the degree of histological normality achieved before challenge. In the author's experience histopathological changes of the mucosa of well-treated adults or children were not seen within 48 h after an oral dose of 20 g gluten. Higher doses have, however, been reported to cause early severe mucosal damage and exfoliation of the epithelium [18]. After 48 h variable mucosal abnormalities have been reported in both adults and children [11]. It is evident that sequential biopsies in the early hours after the gluten challenge should provide the most informative ultrastructural observations of aetiopathological value, but these have not been undertaken in adults as yet. In children our studies [20], although necessarily subjective, may provide a basis for further fine-structural observations.

Immunopathological observations suggest that a reaginic reaction may take place within the lamina propria in the early hours after gluten challenge. This has only been studied in children in a few instances (unpublished data) when a moderate increase in IgE-staining cells could be demonstrated. Ultrastructurally this coincides in time with oedema, an increase in eosinophils and the presence of degranulated mast cells. Later events, roughly from 11 h after gluten challenge onwards, show immunological and cytological evidence of a local Arthus reaction. This is suggested by the demonstration of immune complexes in the basal laminae of epithelia and endothelia [5,23] and ultrastructurally by increased density of the connective tissue fibrils, hypertrophy of endothelial cells and the appearance of polymorphs, followed in time sequence by further connective tissue reactions such as deposition of collagen fibres. The rapid increase in plasma cells predominantly in IgA and IgM production has been confirmed by immunofluorescence studies [23]. Theliolymphocytes are also increased after challenge but, as already mentioned, their significance in the cytopathogenetic events is not clear. The overall cytological changes after gluten challenge, observed mainly in the lamina propria and associated with distinct immunological reactions, emphasise again the importance of immunological factors in the aetiology of coeliac disease, for further details of which the reader is referred to the chapter on coeliac disease by Asquith and Haeney [2].

References

1. Araya M, Walker-Smith JA (1975) Specificity of ultrastructural changes in small intestinal epithelium in early childhood. Arch Dis Child 50:844–855
2. Asquith P, Haeney MR (1979) Coeliac disease. In: Asquith P (ed) Immunology of the gastro-intestinal tract. Churchill Livingstone, Edinburgh, London, New York, pp 66–94
3. Booth CC (1974) Definition of adult coeliac disease. In: Hekkens WTh, Hekkens JM, Peña AS (eds) Coeliac disease. Proceedings of the second international coeliac symposium. Stenfert Kroese, Leiden, pp 17–22
4. Brandtzaeg P, Baklien K (1976) Immunohistochemical studies of the formation and epithelial transport of immunoglobulins in normal and diseased human intestinal mucosa. Scand J Gastroenterol 2, suppl. 36:5–45
5. Doe WF, Henry K, Booth CC (1974) Complement in coeliac disease. In: Hekkens WTh, Hekkens JM, Peña AS (eds) Proceedings of the second international coeliac symposium. Stenfert Kroese, Leiden, pp 189–196
6. Doniach I, Shiner M (1960) Histopathology of the stomach in pernicious anaemia and jejunum in steatorrhoea. Br J Radiol 33:238–242
7. Falchuk ZM, Gebhard RL, Sessoms C, Strober W (1974) An in-vitro model of gluten-sensitive enteropathy. Effect of gliadin on intestinal epithelial cells of patients with gluten-sensitive enteropathy in organ culture. J Clin Invest 53:487–500
8. Ghadially FN (1977) Ultrastructural pathology of the cell. Butterworths, London, pp 222–254
9. Guix M, Skinner JM, Whitehead R (1979) Ultrastructural analysis of plasma cells in coeliac patients. Gut 20:504–508
10. Guix M, Skinner JM, Whitehead R (1979) Morphometric electron and light microscopic analysis of lymphoid cells in coeliac disease. Scand J Gastroenterol 14:261–265
11. Jos J, Rey J, Frezal J (1969) Effets précoces de la réintroduction du gluten sur la muqueuse intestinale dans al maladie coelique en rémission. Arch Fr Pediatr 26:849–859
12. Kilby A, Walker-Smith JA, Wood CBS (1976) Studies on the immunoglobulin containing cells and intraepithelial lymphocytes in the small intestinal mucosa of infants with the post-gastroenteritis syndrome. Austr Paediatr J 12:241
13. Kingston D, Pearson J, Shiner M (1979) The mast cell in gastrointestinal allergy. In: Pepys J, Edwards AM (eds) The mast cell, its role in health and disease. Pitman Medical, London, pp 394–405
14. Maffei HVL, Kingston D, Hill ID, Shiner M (1979) Histological changes and the immune response within the jejunal mucosa in children under and over 2 years. Pediatr Res 13:733–736
15. Marsh MN (1975) Studies of intestinal lymphoid tissue. 1. Electron microscopic evidence of 'blast transformation' in epithelial lymphocytes of mouse small intestinal mucosa. Gut 16:665–674
16. Mavromichalis J, Brueton MJ, McNeish AS, Anderson CM (1976) Evaluation of the intraepithelial lymphocyte count in the jejunum in childhood enteropathies. Gut 17:600–603
17. Meeuwisse GW (1970) Diagnostic criteria in coeliac disease. Acta Paediatr Scand 59:461–463
18. Rubin CE, Brandborg LL, Phelps PC et al. (1960) Studies of coeliac disease. II. The apparent irreversibility of the proximal intestinal pathology in coeliac disease. Gastroenterology 38:517–535
19. Savilahti E (1972) Intestinal immunoglobulins in children with coeliac disease. Gut 13:958–964
20. Shiner M (1973) Ultrastructural changes suggestive of immune reactions in the jejunal mucosa of coeliac children following gluten challenge. Gut 14:1–12

21. Shiner M (1974) Electron microscope appearances of jejunum in coeliac disease. In: Cooke WT, Asquith P (eds) Clinics in gastroenterology, vol.3, no.1. Saunders, Philadelphia, London, Toronto, pp 33–54
22. Shiner M (1974) Cell distribution in the jejunal mucosa in coeliac disease. In: Hekkens WTh, Hekkens JM, Peña AS (eds) Coeliac disease. Proceedings of the second international coeliac symposium. Stenfert Kroese, Leiden, pp 121–137
23. Shiner M, Ballard J (1972) Antigen–antibody reactions in jejunal mucosa in childhood coeliac disease after gluten challenge. Lancet i: 1202–1205
24. Shiner M, Shmerling DH (1972) The immunopathology of coeliac disease. Digestion 5: 69–88
25. Toner PG, Carr KE, Al Yassin TM (1980) The gastrointestinal tract. Small intestine. In: Johannessen JV (ed) Electron microscopy in human medicine, vol. 7, Digestive system. McGraw-Hill, London, pp 144–145
26. Trier JS, Browning PH (1970) Epithelial-cell renewal in cultured duodenal biopsies in coeliac sprue. N Engl J Med 283: 1245–1250
27. Walker-Smith J (ed) (1979). Coeliac disease. In: Diseases of the small intestine in childhood. 2nd edn. Pitman Medical, London, pp 91–138

Select bibliography

Biempica L, Toccalino H, O'Donnell JC (1968) Cytochemical and ultrastructural studies of the intestinal mucosa of children with celiac disease. Am J Pathol 52: 795–823

Booth CC, Peters TJ, Doe WF, (1977) Immunopathology of coeliac disease. Ciba Found Symp 46: 329–346

Boshkov SP (1981) Ultrastructural changes in the small intestine mucosa in patients with primary malabsorption syndromes. Z Gesamte Inn Med 36 [Suppl]: 204–206

Canepa M, Buffa D (1969) Ultrastructural studies on jejunal mucosa in 'idiopathic sprue' before and during treatment with gluten free diet. Verh Dtsch Ges Pathol 53: 181–185

Dissanayake AS, Jerrome DW, Offord RE, Truelove SC, Whitehead R (1974) Identifying toxic fractions of wheat gluten and their effect on the jejunal mucosa in coeliac disease. Gut 15: 931–946

Dodero M, Celle G, Canepa M, Michetti P (1970) Some ultramicroscopic aspects of Lieberkühn's intestinal crypts during sprue-celiac disease before and during gluten-free diet. Minerva Gastroenterol 16: 131–135

Gasbarrini G (1969) Electron microscopic contribution to the knowledge of the etiopathogenesis and diagnosis of various diseases of the small intestine with malabsorption syndromes. Bull Sci Med (Bologna) 141: 425–434

Gasbarrini G, Miglio F, Serra MA, Bernardi M (1974) Immunological studies of the jejunal mucosa in normal subjects and adult celiac patients. Digestion 10: 122–128

Guix M, Skinner JM, Whitehead R (1979) Morphometric electron and light microscopic analysis of lymphoid cells in coeliac disease. Scand J Gastroenterol 14: 261–265

Guix M, Skinner JM, Whitehead R (1979) Ultrastructural analysis of plasma cells in coeliac disease. Gut 20: 504–508

Jos J, Labbé F (1976) Ultrastructural localisation of IgA globulins in normal and coeliac intestinal mucosa using immunoenzymatic methods. Biomedicine 24: 425–434

Jos J, Lenoir G, Ritis G, Rey J (1975) In-vitro pathogenetic studies of coeliac disease. Effects of protein digests on coeliac intestinal biopsy speciments maintained in culture for 48 hours. Scand J Gastroenterol 10: 121–128

Jos J, Labbé F, Geny B, Griscelli C (1979) Immunoelectron-microscope localization of immunoglobulin A and secretory component in jejunal mucosa from children with coeliac disease. Scand J Immunol 9: 441–450

Labbé F, Labbé JP, Jos J (1976) Use of peroxidase-labelled antibodies for ultrastructural localisation of immunoglobulins in normal and coeliac intestinal mucosa. In: Feldman G et al. (eds) Proceedings of the first international symposium on immunoenzymatic techniques. Elsevier, Amsterdam, New York, p 135

Labo G, Gasbarrini G, Migli F, Bernardi M (1978) Thelio- and propriolymphocyte count in normal subjects and in primary and secondary enteropathy. GEN 32: 403–417

Lojda Z (1974) Cytochemistry of enterocytes and of other cells in the mucous membrane of the small intestine. Biomembranes 4A: 43–122

Madara JL, Trier JS (1980) Structural abnormalities of jejunal epithelial cell membranes in celiac sprue. Lab Invest 43:254–261

Marche C, Laumonier R, Metayer J (1972) Villous atrophy. Histological, histochemical and ultrastructural aspects. Ann Gastroenterol Hepatol (Paris) 8:387–405

Mylotte M, Egan-Mitchell B, Fottrell PF, McNicholl B, McCarthy CF (1974) Family studies in coeliac disease. Q J Med 43:359–369

Otto HF (1973) The interepithelial lymphocytes of the intestinum. Morphological observations and immunologic aspects of intestinal enteropathy. Curr Op Pathol 57:81–121

Peters TJ, Doe WF, Heath JR, Mitchell JD (1973) Lysosomal acid hydrolase activity in intestinal biopsies from control subjects and patients with coeliac disease. Gut 14:430

Polak JM, Pearse AG, Van Noorden S, Bloom SR, Rossiter MA (1973) Secretin cells in coeliac disease. Gut 14:870–874

Rubin W, Ross LL, Sleisenger MH, Weser E (1966) An electron microscope study of adult coeliac disease. Lab Invest 15:1720–1747

Rusconi R, Galluzzo C, Roggero P, Porro CB (1978) Morphological and ultrastructural aspects of intestinal mucosa in coeliac disease. Minerva Pediatr 30:7–14

Rusconi R, Roggero P, Galluzzo C, Careddu P (1979) Lateral junctions and intercellular spaces. Ultrastructural morphological evaluation of the intestinal epithelium in normal subjects and patients with gluten intolerance. Minerva Pediatr 31:759–764

Chapter 3

Cow's Milk Protein Intolerance (CMPI)

This syndrome, seen in children during the first and second years of life, may be defined as an intolerance to and malabsorption of a protein component in cow's milk, resulting in diarrhoea, weight loss and generally failure to thrive. Although it has been shown that beta-lactoglobulin is the most 'allergenic' [1,14] protein in cow's milk, it is not the only protein to which intolerance may be developed [3]. The syndrome is clinically recognised when withdrawal of cow's milk causes improvement and re-introduction results in deterioration [3,15].

Tolerance to cow's milk is usually, though not invariably, acquired after the second year of life. Intolerance may be part of an atopic (allergic) condition [2] or may be secondary to viral or bacterial infection of the gastrointestinal tract [16]. Histologically the mucosa varies from normal appearances to some degree of villous atrophy (Fig. 3.1), but sometimes a subtotal villous atrophy is seen, indistinguishable from that of untreated coeliac disease [13]. An increase in infiltrating cells within the lamina propria is commonly observed. Damage to

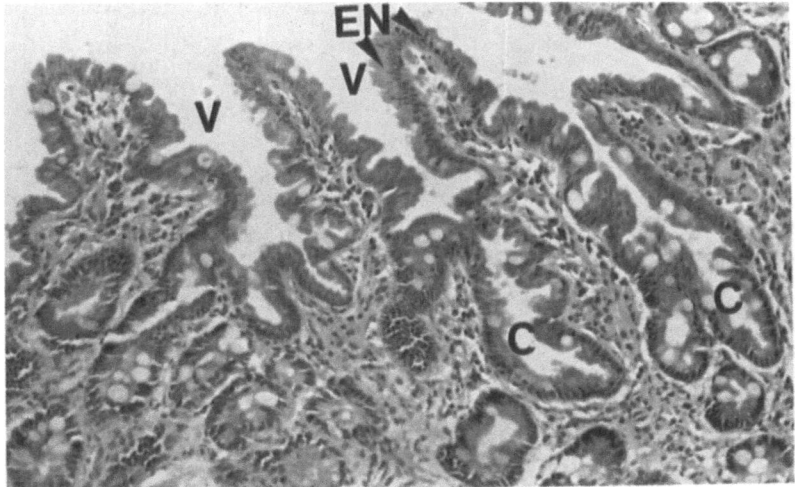

Fig. 3.1. Light microscopy of the jejunal mucosa from a patient with cow's milk protein intolerance (CMPI). The villi (*V*) are shorter than normal and the crypts (*C*) of Lieberkühn are elongated and tortuous. The enterocytes (*EN*) are usually normal in height and theliolymphocytes are within normal range. The inflammatory cells of the lamina propria are usually increased and occasional polymorphonuclear leucocytes may be present. (× 150)

the enterocytes may lead to secondary lactose malabsorption, also a feature of coeliac disease. Repair of the mucosal damage after cow's milk elimination may be slow, particularly after infection, and therefore rapid clinical improvement should not be expected. Equally, after a period of dietary treatment the re-introduction of cow's milk may not cause immediate clinical relapse, even though histological changes can already be demonstrated [11]. For these reasons the clinical evaluation of cow's milk protein intolerance is not always easy and the study of the reaction of jejunal mucosa immunologically, histologically and ultrastructurally before and after milk challenge has helped to provide a firm basis for the recognition of this syndrome [13, 15].

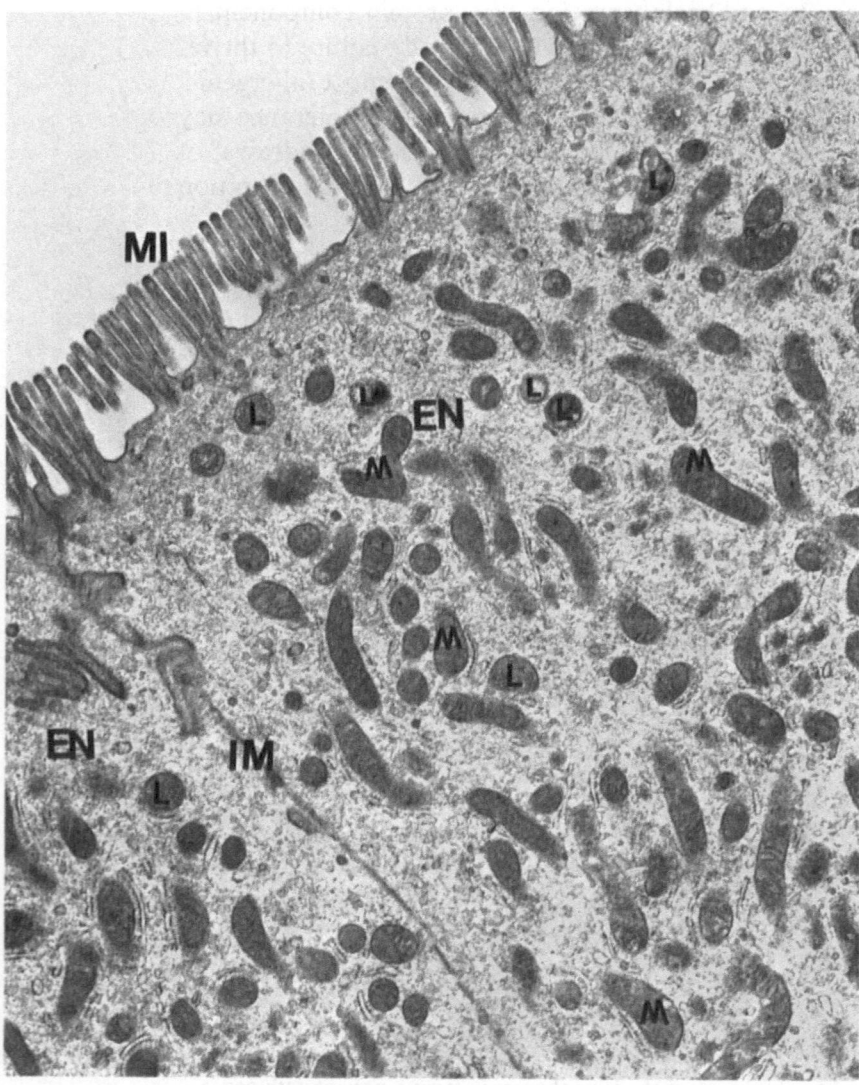

Fig. 3.2. Upper parts of enterocytes (*EN*) in CMPI showing branching of the microvilli (*MI*) and some increase in intracytoplasmic lysosomes (*L*) and multivesicular bodies. The other cytoplasmic organelles are normal and the general appearance is that of mature absorbing type epithelium. *M*, mitochondria; *IM*, intercellular membranes. (× 13 700)

Untreated

The ultrastructural appearance of the mucosa in CMPI is non-specific. The enterocytes lining the usually short villi appear mature, but may show short branched or irregular microvilli [4] and an increase in intracytoplasmic lysosomes (Fig. 3.2). Intraepithelial lymphocytes may be increased but are usually fewer than in untreated coeliac disease. The basal laminae are not thickened. The lamina propria may be oedematous or show some increase in connective tissue fibrils. The plasma cells (Fig. 3.3), though numerous, appear to contain fewer dilated cisternae than in coeliac disease. The ratio of lymphocytes to plasma cells appears normal. Macrophages are plentiful and active. Often an increased number of eosinophils and mast cells as well as an occasional polymorph are seen. As in coeliac disease, elimination of cow's milk from the diet causes complete reversion of the ultrastructural appearances to normal, but the time required for this change is variable and individual.

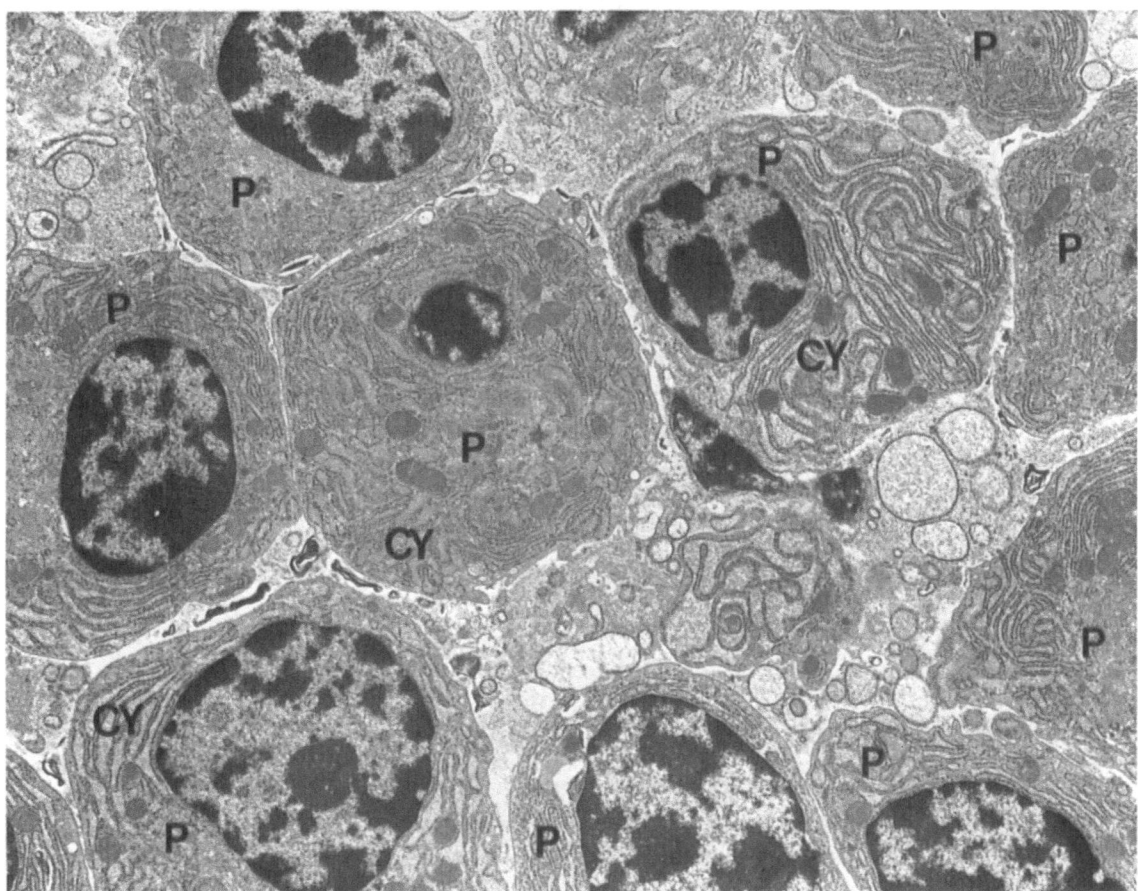

Fig. 3.3. The lamina propria contains increased numbers of plasma cells (*P*) in CMPI but, compared to those seen in coeliac disease, their cytoplasmic cisternae (*CY*) are only moderately dilated. ($\times$ 4750)

Cow's milk challenge

Challenges with cow's milk are usually undertaken after 3 months of milk exclusion, at which time the histology and ultrastructure of the small intestinal mucosa should appear normal. A dose of 1.0–3.0 ml milk is given orally and may be repeated in the absence of symptoms.

Histology and immunology

As in coeliac disease, jejunal biopsy should always be done immediately before the challenge so that histological and immunological (and ultrastuctural) comparison of the mucosa can be made before and after milk challenge. Post-challenge biopsies can either be performed at the time of clinical relapse [6] or routinely at a chosen time [5, 11, 12]. These authors were able to demonstrate histological changes consisting of shortening of villi and increase in inflammatory cell infiltration. This was accompanied by increase in IgA and IgM plasma cells as demonstrated by immunofluorescence staining [10]. Our own studies [11, 12] were designed to show the earlier changes within the jejunal mucosa after milk challenge. Two groups of patients were studied: those with clinical relapse within a few hours after challenge and those without symptoms at a chosen time of repeat biopsy. In the first group jejunal biopsy 6 h after a single dose of cow's milk showed no histological abnormalities. However, an increase in mucosal IgE plasma cells could be demonstrated by immunofluorescence. At 11 h the post-challenge mucosa showed short, broad villi with decreased enterocyte height and increase in inflammatory cells, including polymorphonuclear infiltration. Simultaneous immunofluorescence showed increases in IgE and IgA plasma cells, indicating that pathological and immune reactions had taken place within the jejunal mucosa at the time of clinical relapse. The second group (seven patients) did not show any symptoms after single or repeat milk challenges and were re-biopsied 20–24 h after the first dose. In four of the seven patients the jejunal mucosa showed shortening or loss of villi with irregular short enterocytes and increase in theliolymphocytes and inflammatory cell infiltration, including polymorphs (Fig. 3.4). Increases in IgE, IgA and IgM plasma cells were found with fluorescence techniques. Milk exclusion was immediately instituted. The other three patients, with no obvious histological change up to 24 h, were continued on a milk regimen but relapsed 5–7 days later.

Ultrastructural observations

At 6 h after milk challenge few ultrastructural changes can be seen. The enterocytes are not affected, the microvilli are normal and the basal laminae show the usual fine fibrillar structure. In the lamina propria there is some oedema but no obvious increase in plasma cell activity. Granulated mast cells can be seen (Fig. 3.5). At 11 h after milk challenge the enterocytes show some increase in lysosomes but are generally of normal appearance. Plasma cells

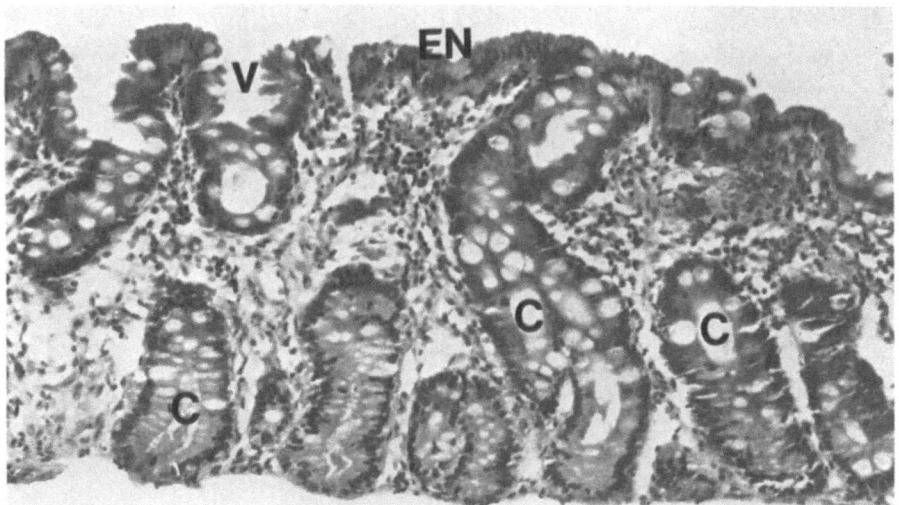

Fig. 3.4. Light microscopy of the jejunal mucosa in an 8-month-old patient with CMPI 21 h after cow's milk challenge. The villi (*V*) are severely reduced in height and the enterocytes (*EN*) appear flattened in some areas. The crypts (*C*) are elongated and the inflammatory infiltrate in the lamina propria is increased. Polymorphonuclear leucocytes are invariably seen below the level of the enterocytes. (× 200)

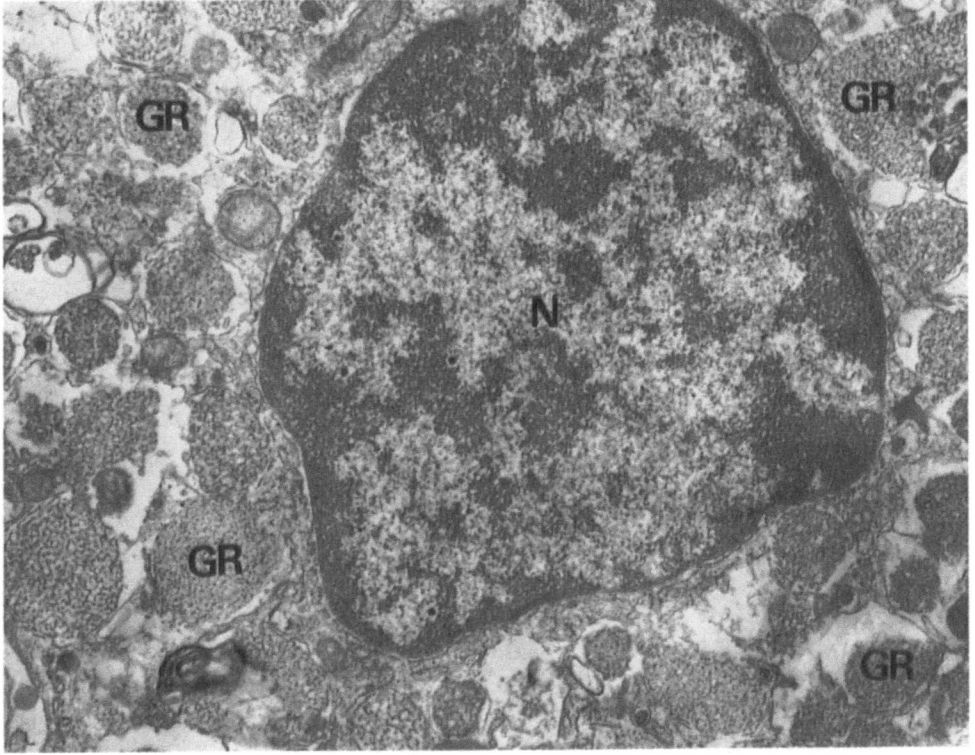

3.5. Part of a mast cell with a central nucleus (*N*) and round, granulated cytoplasmic bodies (*GR*). Six hours after cow's milk challenge. (× 21 632)

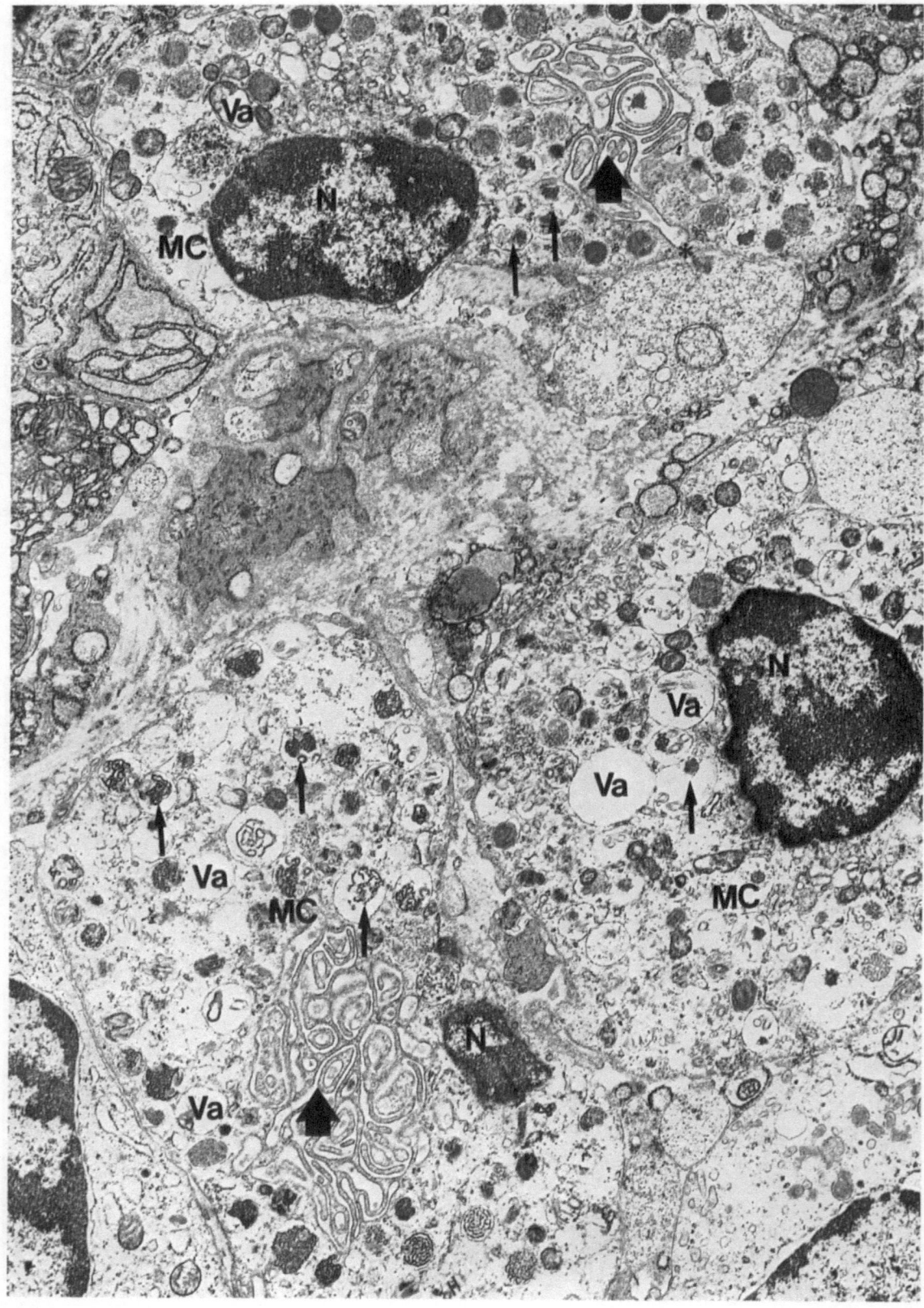

Fig. 3.6.

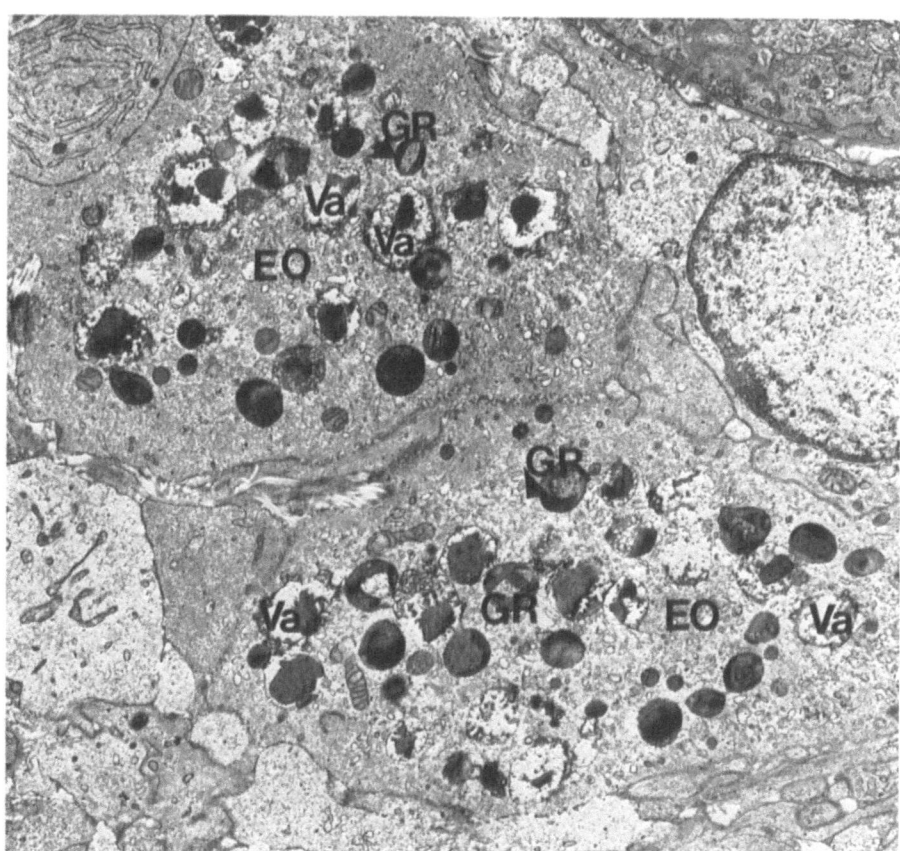

Fig. 3.7. Eosinophil (*EO*) in the lamina propria. Most of the cytoplasmic granules (*GR*) are seen as degranulated vacuoles (*Va*) containing small amounts of dense material. Eleven hours after cow's milk challenge. (× 13 400)

begin to look more active, with dilated cisternae. The most noticeable feature is an increase in mast cells, which can be seen in clusters of two or three, showing degranulation and often labyrinth formation (Fig. 3.6). Eosinophils can also be readily seen, often with deformed or degenerate cytoplasmic granules (Fig. 3.7). At 20–24 h after milk challenge changes within the enterocytes (Fig. 3.8) can be observed and in this respect CMPI differs from coeliac disease. The microvilli may show bulbous dilatation at their tips and the cytoplasm may become vacuolated with increase in lysosomes, swelling of mitochondria and irregularity of the cell nucleus. Similar enterocyte changes have been observed by others [4, 5, 15]. Detachment of one or more enterocytes from

◁ **Fig. 3.6.** Three mast cells (*MC*) in the lamina propria showing gross degranulation of many of the cytoplasmic bodies. Large empty vacuoles (*Va*) are seen. Others show partial degranulation (*arrows*). Two of the mast cells contain intracytoplasmic channels (labyrinths) lined by ER (*thick arrows*), which may extend to and fuse with the cell membrane (*asterisk*). These channels are thought to indicate active degranulation within mast cells. *N*, nucleus of mast cells. Eleven hours after cow's milk challenge. (× 9250)

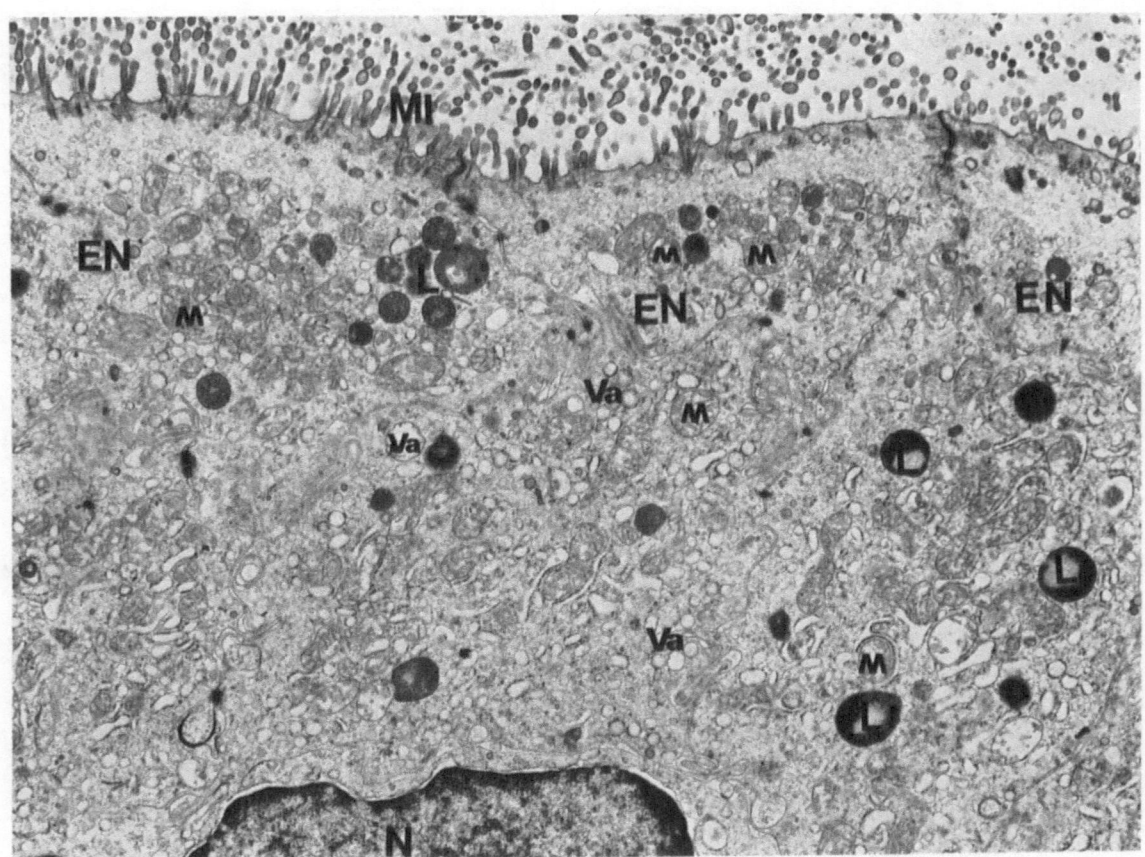

Fig. 3.8. Upper parts of enterocytes (*EN*) showing damage of the microvilli (*MI*), increase in cytoplasmic lysosomes (*L*), swelling of the mitochondria (*M*) and increase in small vacuoles (*Va*). The enterocyte appears short and shows the upper part of its nucleus (*N*). Twenty-four hours after cow's milk challenge. (× 6470)

adjacent cells and consequent extrusion into the bowel lumen may be observed (Fig. 3.9). Polymorphs may be numerous in the intercellular spaces of the enterocytes (Fig. 3.10) and theliolymphocytes may also be seen in increased numbers (Fig. 3.11). In the lamina propria there is increase in fibrous tissue and collagen (Fig. 3.11) or oedema with infiltration of inflammatory cells (Fig. 3.12) consisting of plasma cells, eosinophils, polymorphs and mast cells, some granulated, others degranulated. The endothelial cells of small blood vessels appear normal (Fig. 3.12). Macrophages appear to be active but not overfilled with phagocytosed material.

The most noticeable features on ultrastructural examination are therefore enterocyte damage and inflammatory cell density with increase of plasma cells, polymorphs, eosinophils and mast cells.

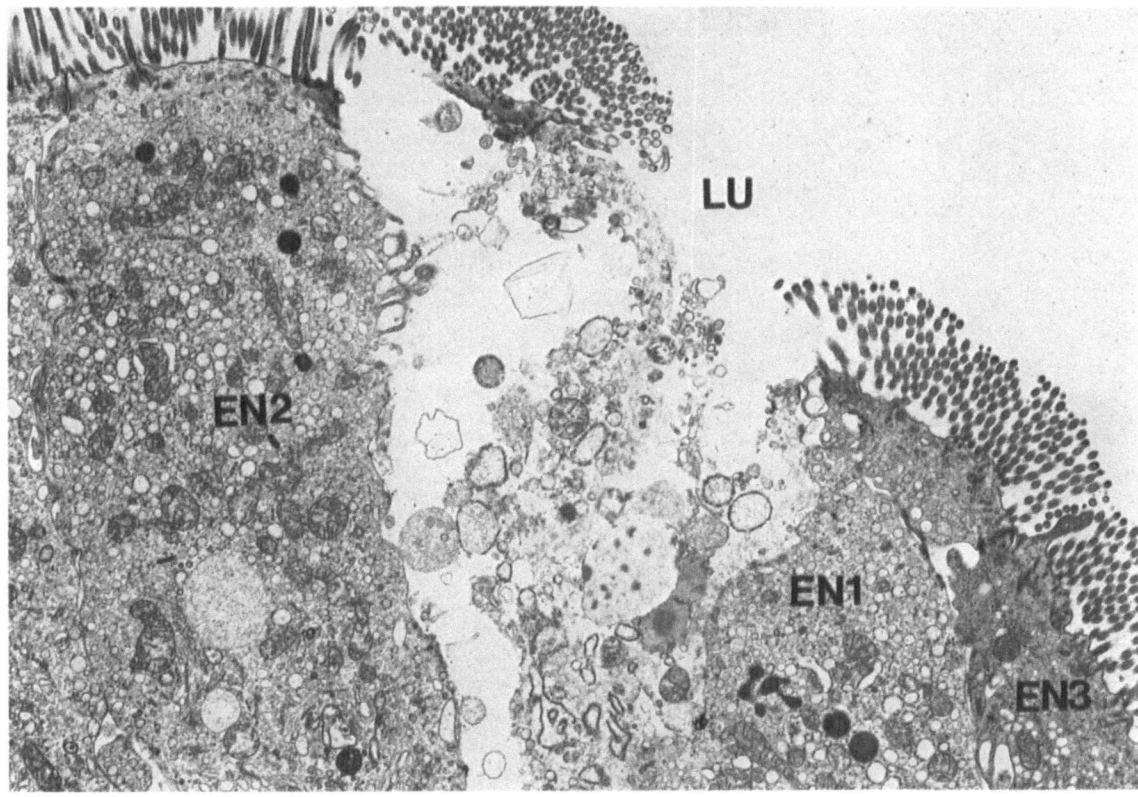

Fig. 3.9. Lysis of an enterocyte (*EN1*) bordered by two viable cells *EN2* and *EN3*. The contents of the lysed cell are discharged into the bowel lumen (*LU*). Twenty-four hours after cow's milk challenge. (× 7500)

Overleaf (pages 106–107):

Fig. 3.10. Polymorphonuclear cells (*PO*) amongst enterocytes (*EN*) seen in oblique section and showing micro- ▷
villi (*MI*) in the upper left corner. *N*, nucleus of enterocytes. The nuclei of the polymorphs appear smaller and darker than those of the enterocytes. Twenty hours after cow's milk challenge. (× 8130)

Fig. 3.11. Oblique section through lower parts of several enterocytes with nuclei (*N*) showing three thelio- ▷
lymphocytes (*TL*). The lamina propria below the basal lamina (*BL*) shows thickening of the connective tissue fibrils (*arrows*), which appear to blend with the basal lamina. Collagen fibres (*CO*) are seen immediately below this area. Twenty-four hours after cow's milk challenge. (× 5300)

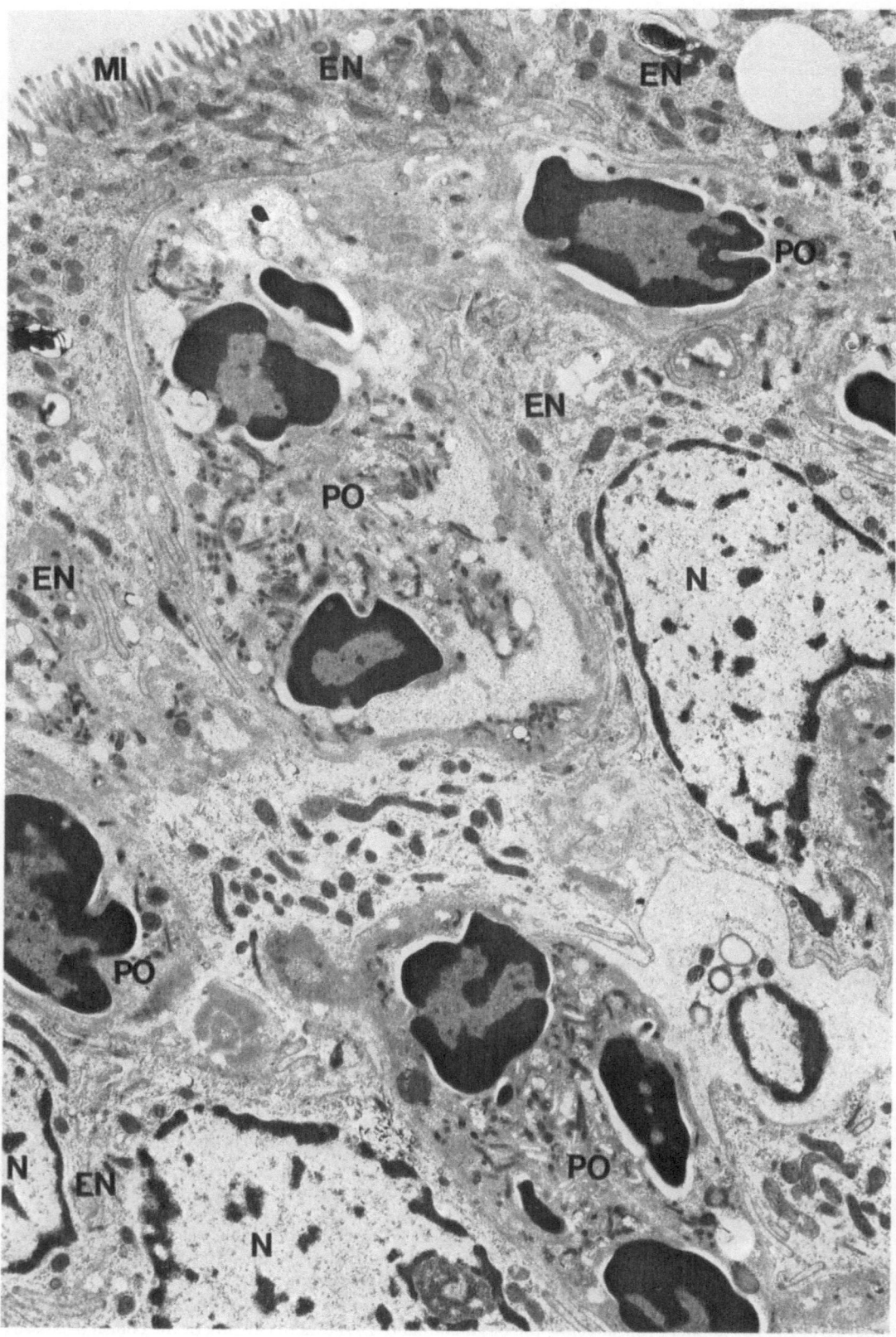

Fig. 3.10.

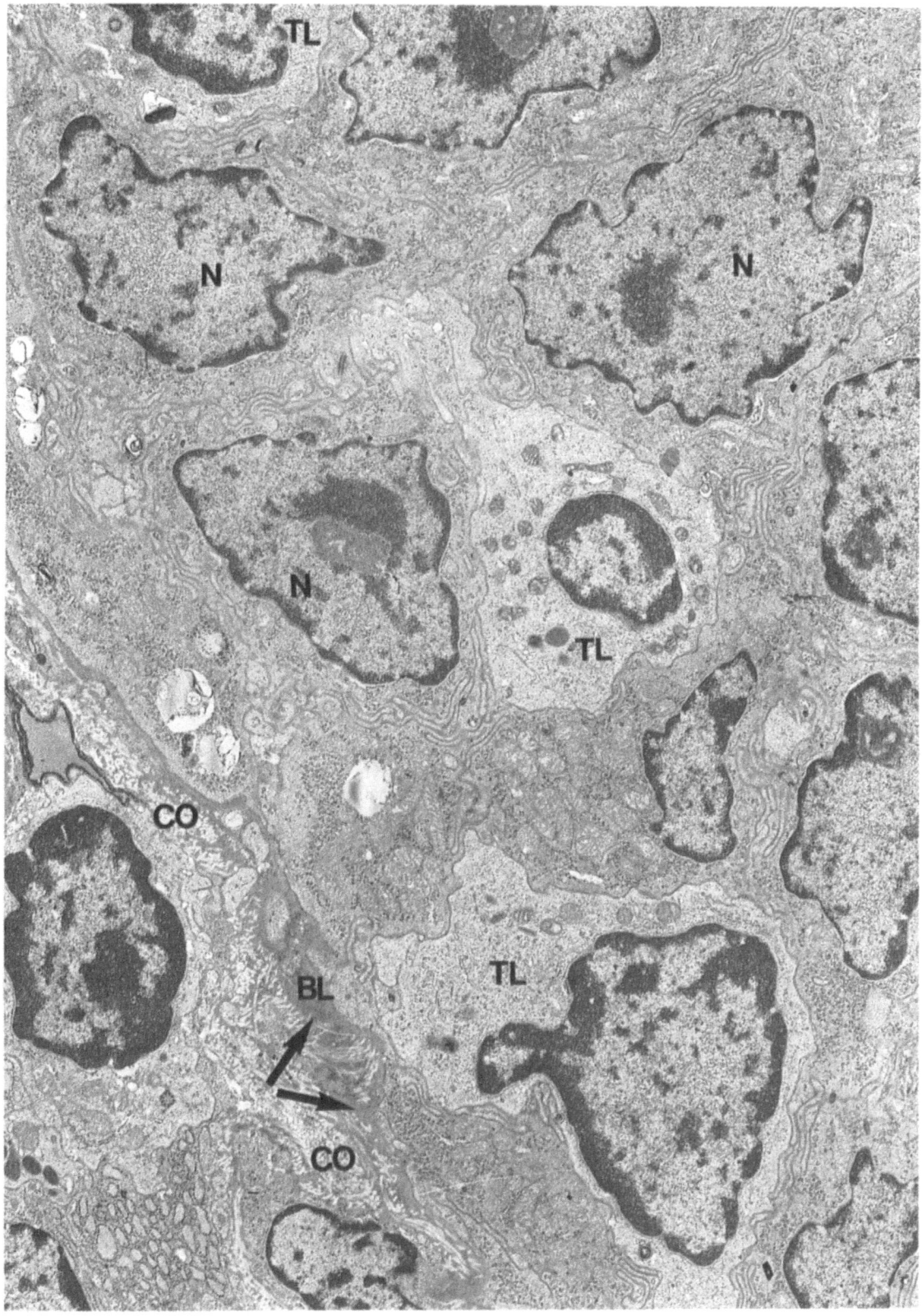

Fig. 3.11.

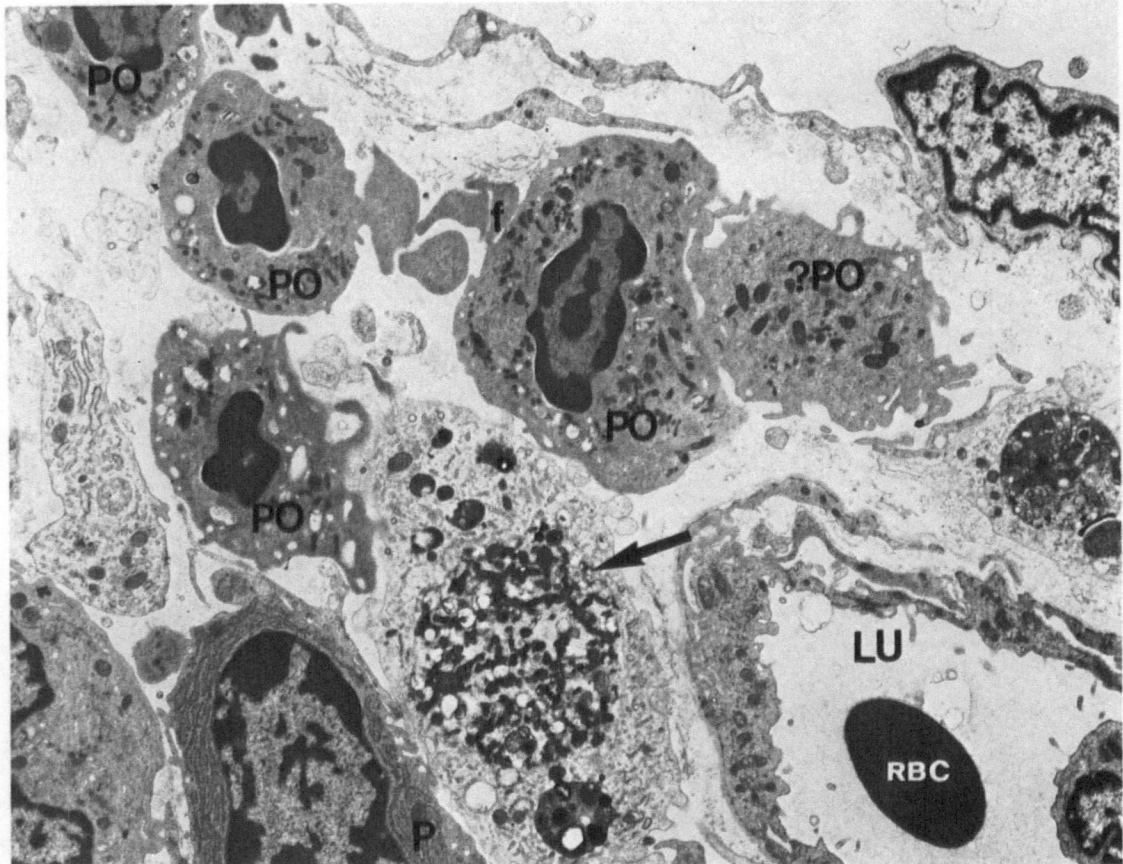

Fig. 3.12. Various inflammatory cells within the lamina propria including at least four polymorphonuclear cells (*PO*), a plasma cell (*P*) and an unidentified cell with apparent nuclear lysis (*arrow*). *LU*, lumen of small blood vessel with *RBC*. Twenty-three hours after cow's milk challenge. (× 5000)

Clinical, morphological and immunological correlation

Too few studies have been undertaken to distinguish the morphological or immunological changes within the mucosa of primary CMPI from those of secondary (postinfective) CMPI. Even on clinical grounds it is not always possible to rule out viral or bacterial infection which might have preceded cow's milk intolerance. What appears certain is that morphological damage may occur within the jejunal mucosa after milk challenge without coincident clinical manifestations. Though in some patients this damage may appear early (within 24 h), in other patients it may be delayed. Thus in three out of seven patients studied to date in whom the jejunal mucosa appeared normal at 24 h after milk challenge and who were continued on cow's milk, clinical relapse was seen within a week of the onset of the challenge (unpublished observations). Jejunal biopsies aimed to show any delayed morphological damage were not carried out.

From coincident immunological studies it appears that plasma cells were activated. The early increase in IgE plasma cells may be part of a reaginic reaction within the mucosa which may be followed by a (delayed) Arthus reaction (appearance of increased plasma cells, eosinophils and polymorphs) and, possibly with the activation of complement [7], lead to cytotoxic destruction of enterocytes. Though increased activity of IgE plasma cells and mast cell increase with degranulation have been demonstrated in the early hours after milk challenge[12], this needs confirmation. Although of great importance to the understanding of reaginic reactions within the jejunal mucosa, both cell types are difficult to study and improved methods are urgently awaited, since morphometry of mast cells is inaccurate in the presence of degranulation and the existence of IgE plasma cells in the human intestinal mucosa has only recently been demonstrated by immunocytochemical techniques [8]. The demonstration of reaginic reactions within the human mucosa after cow's milk challenge awaits further immunocytochemical studies. The recent demonstration of IgA and IgE plasma cells within the jejunal mucosa reacting specifically against beta-lactoglobulins, and their increase in patients with CMPI [9], is further proof of local immune reactions in this syndrome.

References

1. Freier S, Kletter B, Gery I, Lebenthal E, Geifman M (1969) Intolerance of milk protein. J Pediatr 75:623–631
2. Gerrard JW, MacKenzie JWA, Goluboff N, Garson JZ, Maningas CS (1973) Cow's milk allergy: prevalence and manifestations in an unselected series of newborns. Acta Paediatr Scand [Suppl] 234:1–21
3. Goldman AS, Anderson DW, Sellers W et al. (1963) Milk allergy. I. Oral challenge with milk and isolated milk proteins in allergic children. Pediatrics 32:425–443
4. Iancu T, Elian E (1976) The intestinal microvillus. Ultrastructural variability in coeliac disease and cow's milk intolerance. Acta Paediatr Scand 65:65–73
5. Kuitunen P, Rapola, J, Savilahti E, Visakorpi JK (1973) Response of the jejunal mucosa to cow's milk in the malabsorption syndrome with cow's milk intolerance. Acta Paediatr Scand 62:585–595
6. Kuitunen P, Visakorpi JK, Savilahti E, Pelkonen P (1975) Malabsorption syndrome with cow's milk intolerance: clinical findings and course in the light of 54 cases. Arch Dis Child 50:351–356
7. Matthews TS, Soothill JF (1970) Complement activation after milk feeding in children with cow's milk allergy. Lancet ii:893–895
8. Patterson S, Roebuck P, Platts-Mills TAE et al. (1981) IgE plasma cells in human jejunum demonstrated by immune electron microscopy. Clin Exp Immunol 46:301–304
9. Pearson JR Kingston D, Shiner M (1981) Specific antibody production to milk proteins in the jejunal mucosa of children with cow's milk protein intolerance. Gut 22:A421
10. Savilahti E (1973) Immunochemical study of the malabsorption syndrome with cow's milk intolerance. Gut 14:491–501
11. Shiner M. Ballard J, Brook CGD, Herman S (1975) Intestinal biopsy in the diagnosis of cow's milk protein intolerance without acute symptoms. Lancet ii:1060–1063
12. Shiner M, Ballard J, Smith M (1975) The small intestinal mucosa in cow's milk allergy. Lancet i:136–140
13. Visakorpi JK (1979) Milk allergy and the gastrointestinal tract in children. In: Asquith P (ed) Immunology of the gastrointestinal tract. Churchill Livingstone, Edinburgh, London, New York, pp 183–194
14. Visakorpi JK, Immonen P (1967) Intolerance to cow's milk and wheat gluten in the primary malabsorption syndrome in infancy. Acta Paediatr Scand 56:49–56
15. Walker-Smith J (1979) Cow's milk protein intolerance. In: Diseases of the small intestine in childhood. Pitman Medical, London, pp 143–158
16. Walker-Smith J (1979) Cow's milk protein intolerance: In: Diseases of the small intestine in childhood, 2nd edn. Pitman Medical, London, p 145

Chapter 4

Protein-Energy Malnutrition (P-EM)

Histology

Several authors [2,3,4,5,11,13] have described the morphological jejunal mucosal appearances in P-EM (marasmus, kwashiorkor) of children in underdeveloped countries. These vary from near normal to a subtotal villous atrophy, although the most common histological picture is a partial villous atrophy (Fig. 4.1a). This is usually accompanied by lengthening of crypts, and by increases in theliolymphocytes and in cellular infiltration of the lamina propria. It is likely that the mucosal appearances depend on whether the clinical picture is predominantly marasmus (total malnutrition) or kwashiorkor (mainly

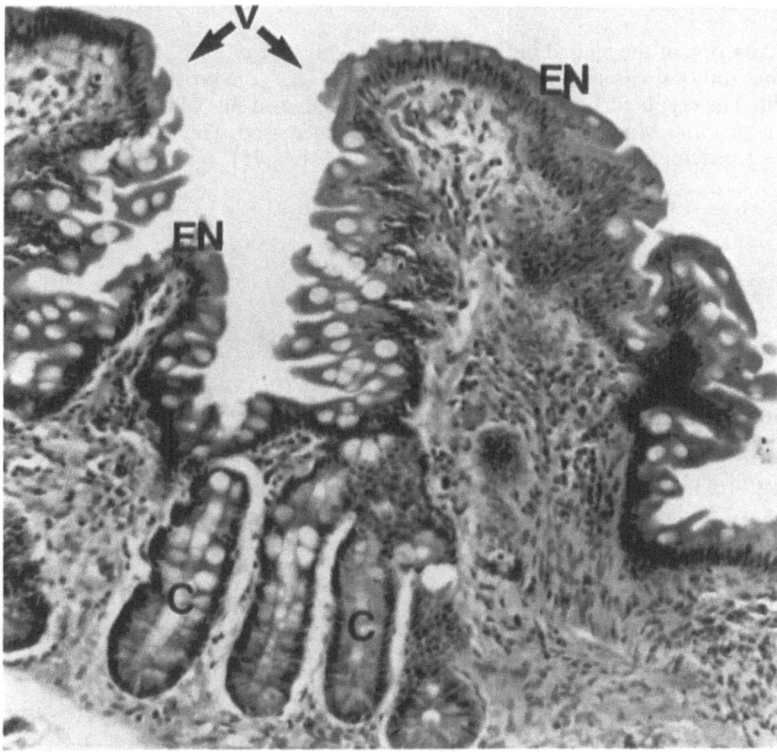

Fig. 4.1a. Light microscopy of the jejunal mucosa in a child with marasmus. (H & E × 180)

protein deprivation), on the presence of other common factors such as parasitic infestations and viral and bacterial overgrowth, and on the chronicity and severity of malnutrition at the time of investigation. We and others [8, 10, 11] have found the most severe villous atrophy in children with P-EM presenting clinically with severe kwashiorkor (Fig. 4.1b). The mucosal appearances were indistinguishable from those of coeliac disease in severely affected children. The lamina propria showed increases in eosinophils and plasma cells.

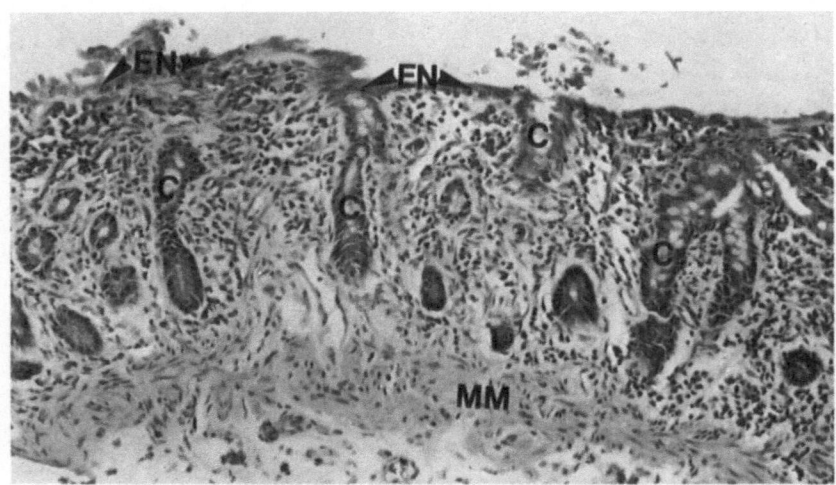

Fig. 4.1b. Light microscopy of the jejunal mucosa in a child with severe kwashiorkor showing subtotal villous atrophy. The enterocytes (*EN*) are grossly diminished in height. The crypts of Lieberkühn (*C*) appear lengthened but widely spaced in the lamina propria. Mucosal inflammatory cells are increased. The lamina propria shows oedema. *MM*, muscularis mucosae. (H & E × 75)

Ultrastructure

Few reports on the fine ultrastructure of the jejunal mucosa in P-EM have been published [4, 6, 8, 9, 10, 14]. The less severely involved mucosal ultrastructure described in the literature agrees with our own findings. The enterocytes appear short (Fig. 4.2) and may show mitochondrial damage and excess vacuolation (Fig. 4.3). In other enterocytes, cytoplasmic organelles may be normal but lysosomes may be increased (Fig. 4.4). Some microvilli may be long and densely spaced (Fig. 4.5) or they may be short and widely spaced [10] (Fig. 4.4), but branching is generally not marked. Lipid retention within enterocytes [8, 10] has been noted. A search for parasites (Figs. 4.5, 4.6, 4.7) overlying the microvilli or partly destroyed by intracytoplasmic hydrolases will often be

Fig. 4.2. Upper two-thirds of an enterocyte (*EN*) from the jejunal mucosal villi of a child with moderately ▷ severe protein-energy malnutrition (P-EM). Histology showed a PVA. The cell appears short and the large nucleus (*N*) takes up a considerable part of it. The microvilli (*MI*) are short and irregular. The cytoplasmic organelles appear normal and are those of a mature absorbing cell. *M*, mitochondria; *G*, Golgi; *L*, lysosomes; *MB*, multivesicular body. (× 30 000)

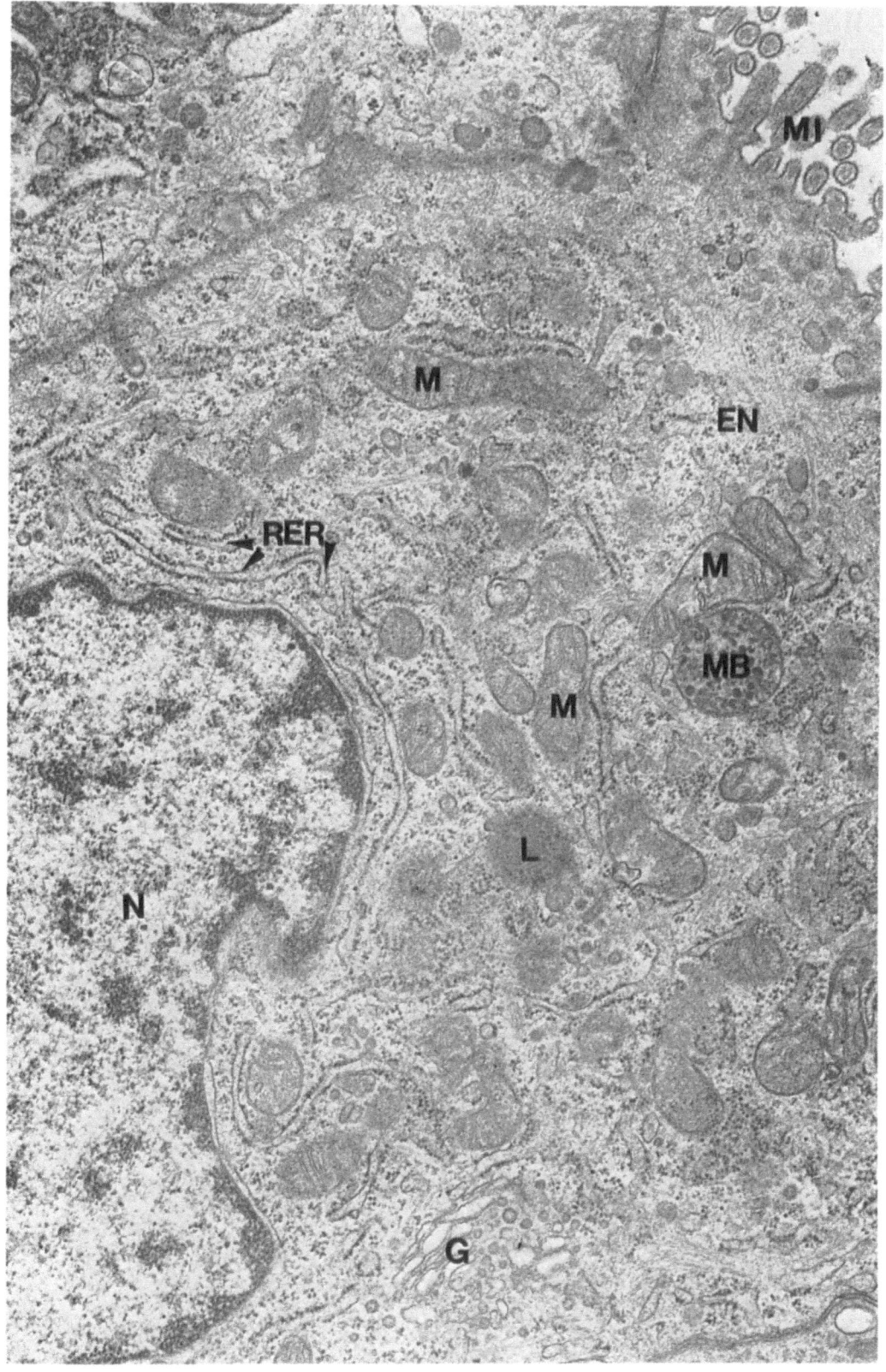

Fig. 4.2.

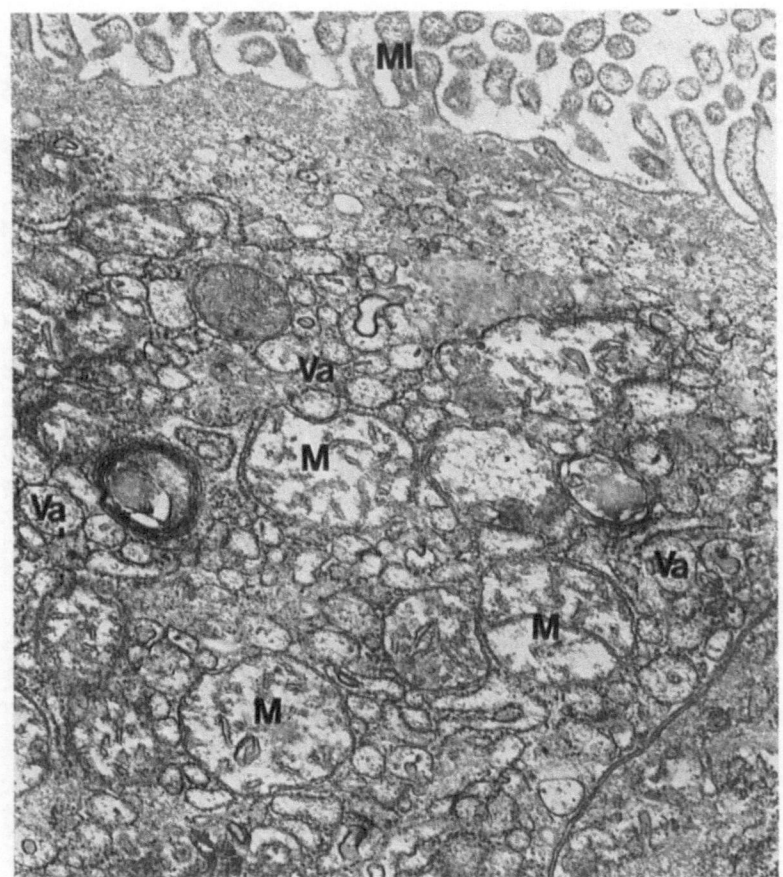

Fig. 4.3. △   **Fig. 4.4.** ▽

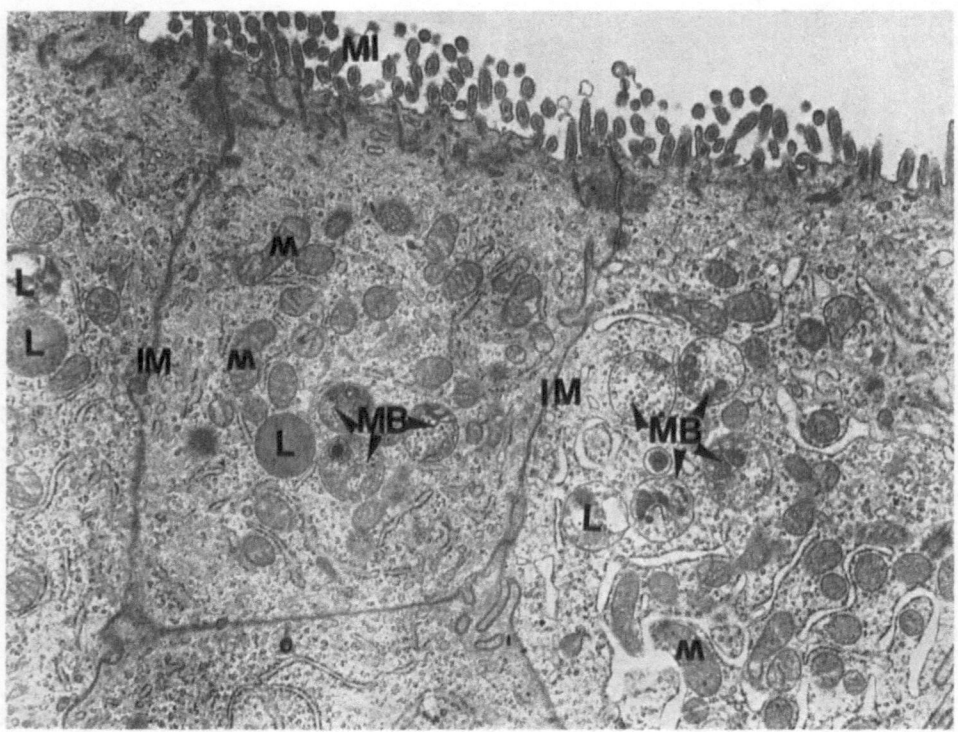

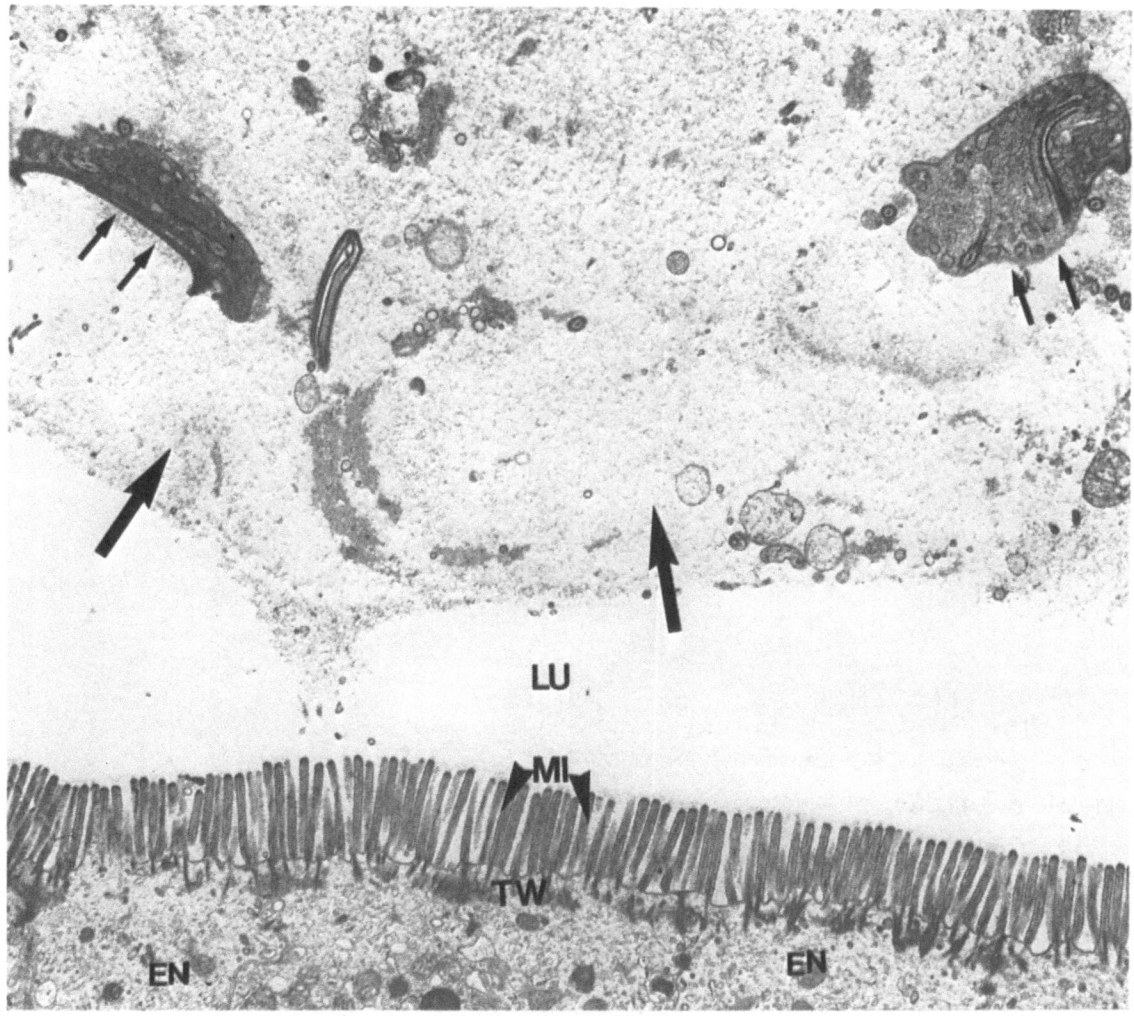

Fig. 4.5. Mucous layer (*thick arrows*) overlying the microvilli (*MI*) of several enterocytes (*EN*). The microvilli appear normal and their filaments enter the upper part of the cytoplasm to form a distinct terminal web (*TW*). In the mucous layer two protozoal bodies (*arrows*) are seen, of which one (*left*) has the characteristic features of *Giardia lamblia* and the other (*right*), though swollen, is probably also of the same type. *LU*, lumen of bowel. (× 12 214)

◁ **Fig. 4.3.** Upper half of an enterocyte from the villi of the same mucosa as Fig. 4.2, showing less organised cytoplasmic appearances with increase in vacuoles (*Va*) and swelling of many of the mitochondria (*M*). Note the irregular, short and bulbous microvilli (*MI*). (× 48 020)

◁ **Fig. 4.4.** Oblique section across several enterocytes from the villi of the same mucosa as in Figs. 4.2 and 4.3, showing increase in multivesicular bodies (*MB*) and also lysosomes (*L*). The mitochondria (*M*) appear normal but the microvilli (*MI*) are short and irregular. *IM*, intercellular membranes. (× 15 670)

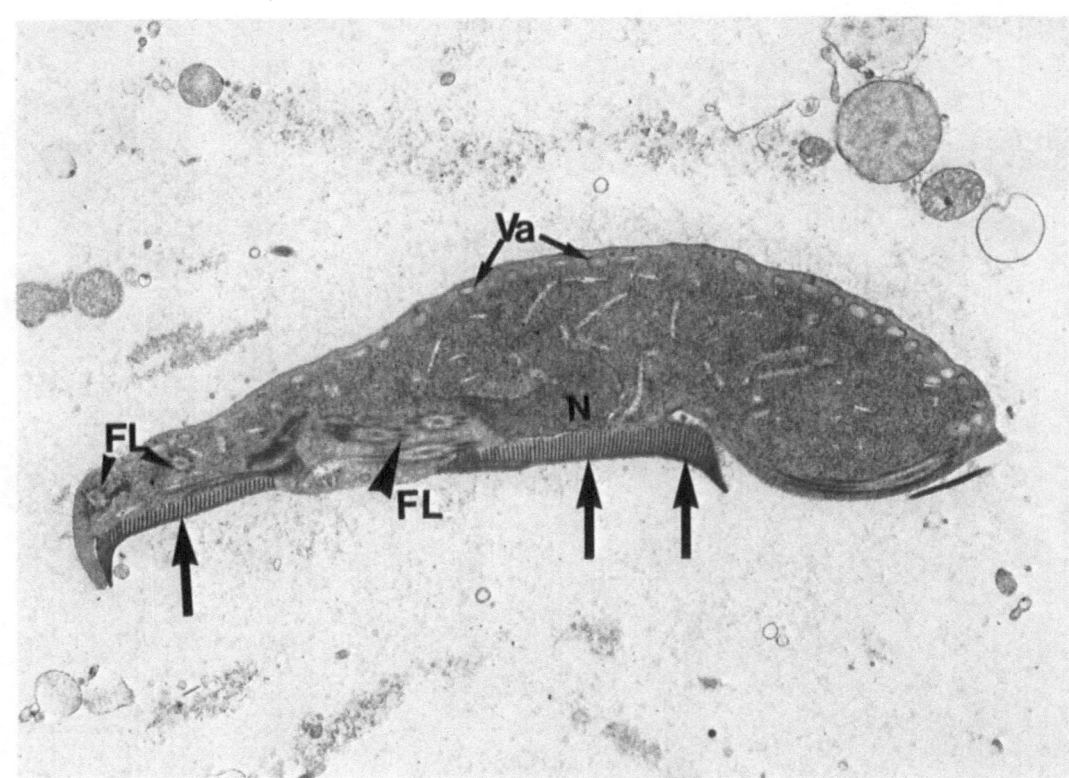

Fig. 4.6. △   **Fig. 4.7.** ▽

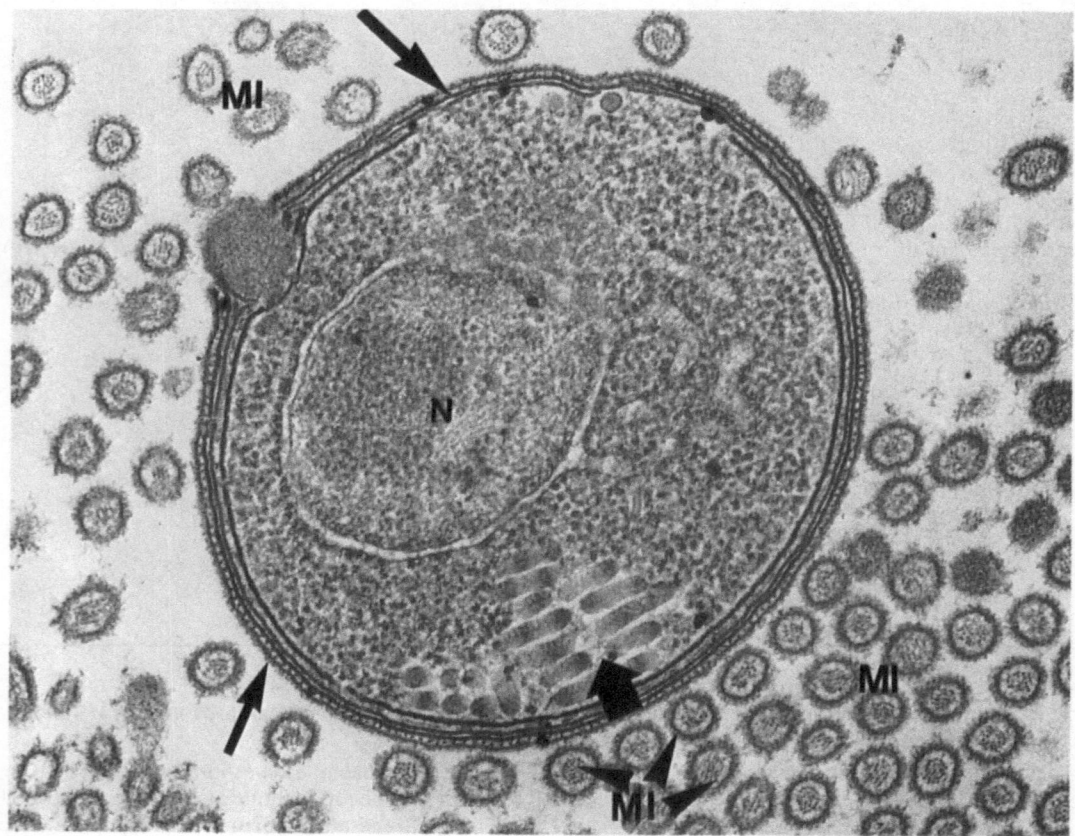

rewarded (Fig. 4.8). In one patient mycoplasma-like bodies (Fig. 4.9) were seen on the luminal side of the microvilli. The presence of parasites, cysts or other bodies is not necessarily associated with lysis of enterocytes in contact with these organisms. The basal laminae of the enterocytes may be thickened (Fig. 4.10) and blend with connective tissue fibrils which often give the lamina propria a denser than normal appearance. Collagen fibres may be evident. The small blood vessels and their endothelial cells and the distribution and appearances of lymphocytes and mast cells are normal. Eosinophils and macrophages are often numerous. Plasma cells are readily identified (Fig. 4.11)

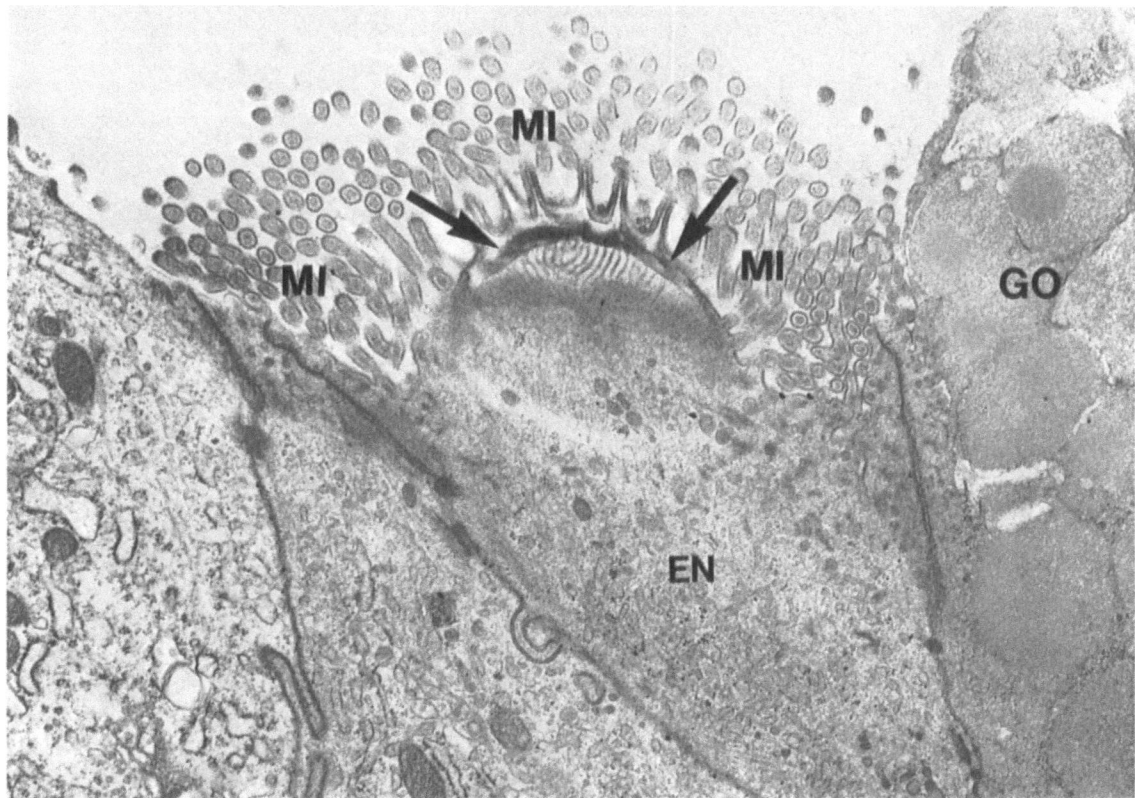

Fig. 4.8. Upper part of an enterocyte (*EN*) in P-EM showing lysis of a parasite (*arrows*) situated just beneath, and surrounded by, microvilli (*MI*). Note that neither the enterocyte nor the invading parasite possesses a clear limiting membrane. The microvilli appear normal as they surround the invading organism. *GO*, goblet cell. (× 16 850)

◁ **Fig. 4.6.** Higher magnification of a *Giardia lamblia* trophozoite. The body is elongated and wider at one end than the other. The cytoplasm contains a number of vacuoles (*Va*) on its dorsal surface immediately beneath the triple layered limiting membrane, and a striated structure (suction disc) on its ventral surface (*arrows*). Flagellae (*FL*) are seen in cross section arising from the main body. *N*, nucleus of trophozoite. (× 135 430)

◁ **Fig. 4.7.** *Giardia lamblia* in cross section. Note the multilayered capsule (*arrows*) which appears intact even though the parasite is in close contact with the microvilli (*MI*) (see in cross-section) of enterocytes. The cytoplasmic contents of the trophozoite contain granules (?ribosomes), membrane-lined channels and a zone of dense, elongated tubules at one end (*thick arrows*) staked in parallel. *N*, nucleus. (× 43 000)

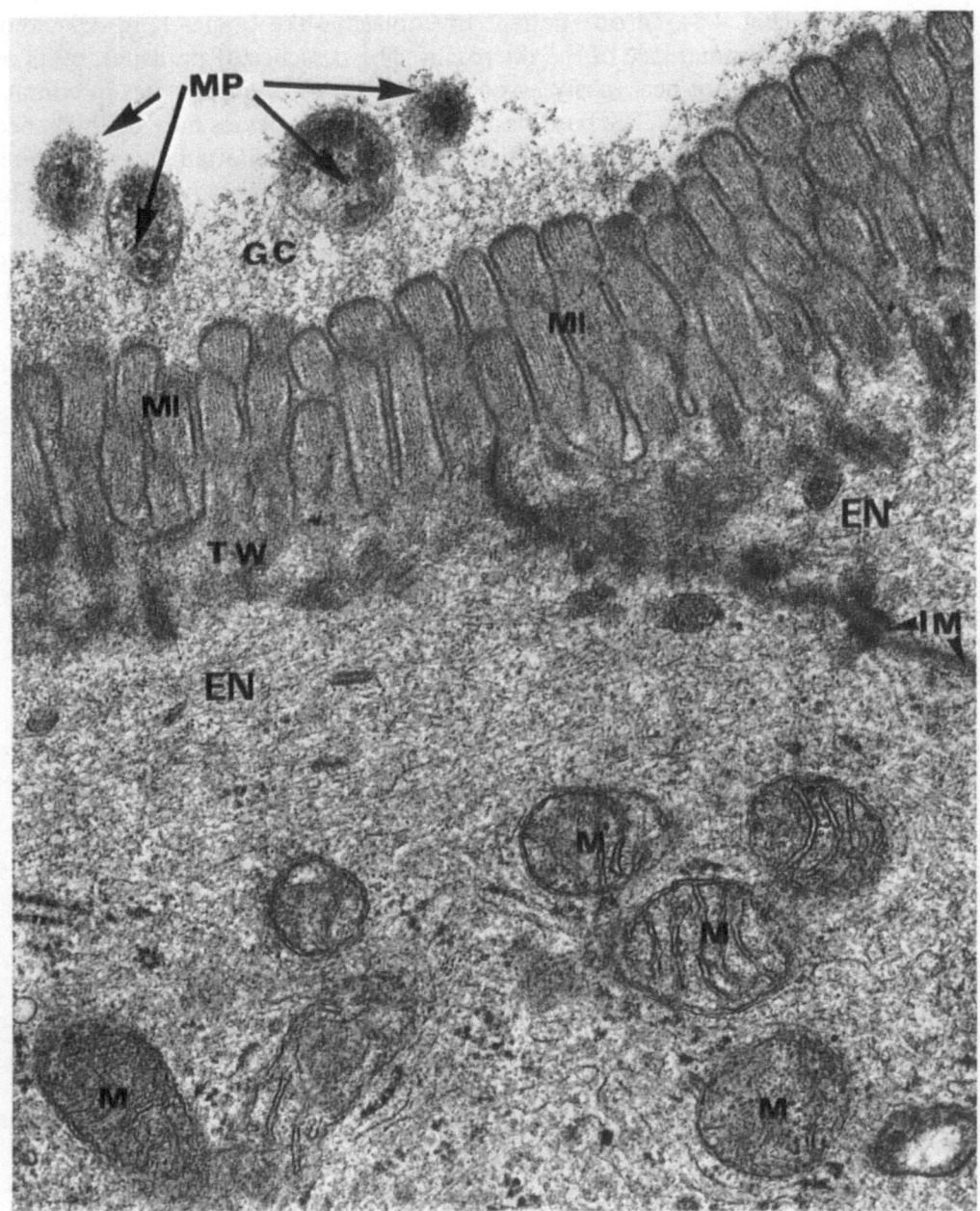

Fig. 4.9. Round, membrane-bound bodies (*MP*) in the region of the glycocalyx (*GC*) overlying the microvilli (*MI*) of enterocytes (*EN*). From the biopsy of a child with marasmus, without a respiratory infection. The size of the bodies is consistent with that of mycoplasma. *M*, mitochondria; *TW*, terminal web; *IM*, intercellular membranes. (× 75 970)

Fig. 4.10. Basal region of enterocyte (*EN*) showing thickening of the basal lamina (*BL*) and of the connective ▷ tissue fibrils with deposition of collagen fibres (*CO*). From the biopsy of a child with moderately severe marasmus. *N*, nucleus of fibrocyte (*FC*). (× 30 530)

Fig. 4.11. Plasma cells (*P*) are seen on the right, identified by their nuclear pattern (*N*) and cytoplasmic ▷ cisternae (*CY*). Though the cells appear to have reached maturity the cisternae are less dilated than normal and contain sparse material (immunoglobulin). *FC*, fibrocyte. A macrophage (*MA*) with its nucleus (*N*) and small phagolysosomes (*L*) is seen in the centre. Same biopsy as in Fig. 4.10. (× 9940)

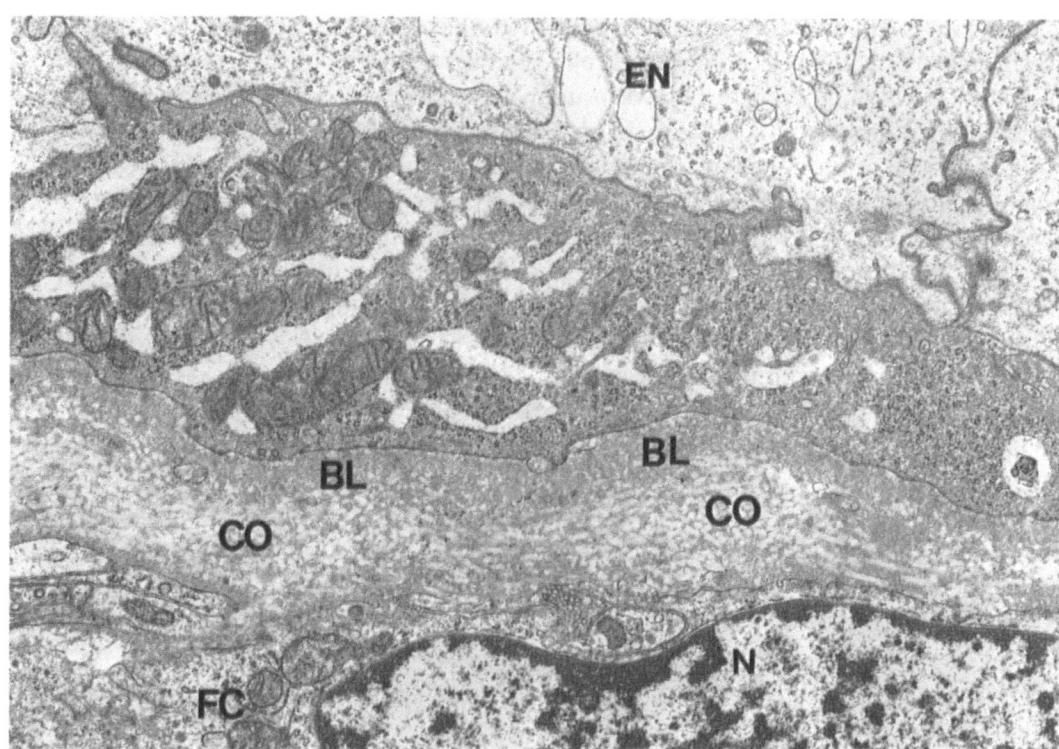

Fig. 4.10. △   Fig. 4.11. ▽

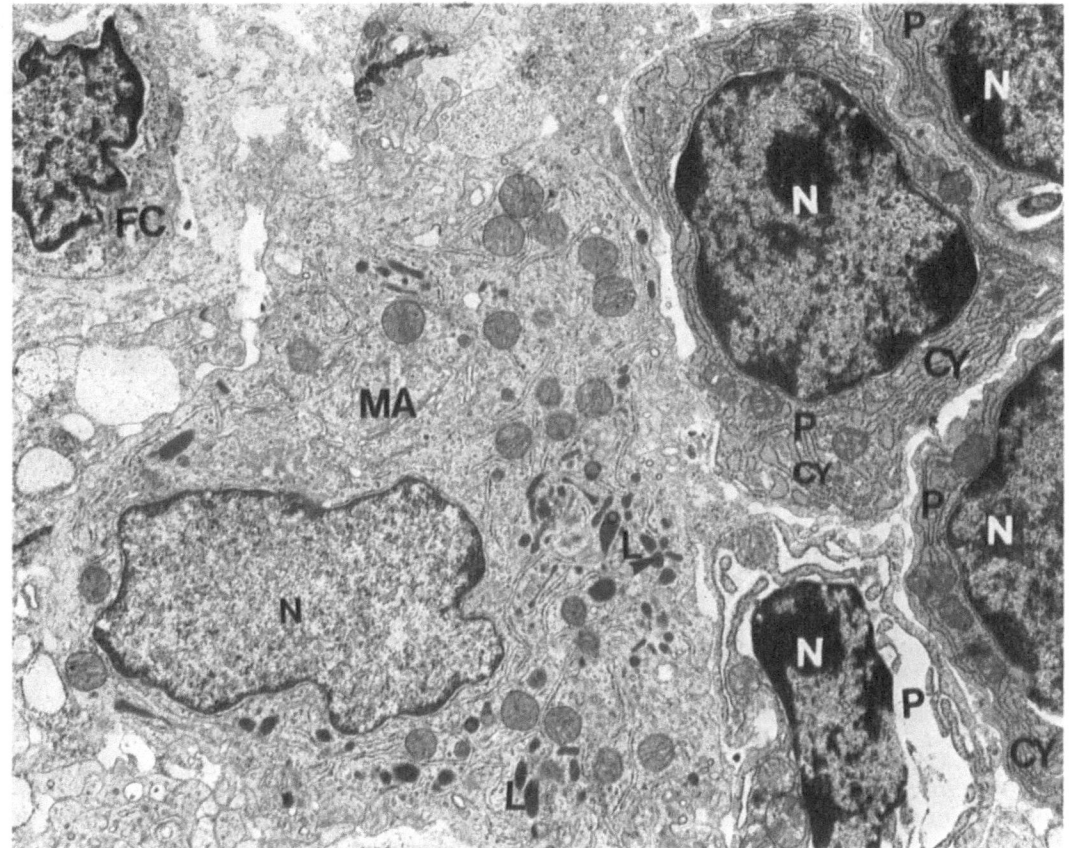

but the majority of cytoplasmic cisternae are collapsed and stacked in parallel fashion towards the periphery of the cell. The ultrastructure of the less severely affected mucosa, therefore, shows non-specific changes, such as short and often irregular microvilli, increase in epithelial lysosomes and thickening of the fibrous tissue component of the lamina propria. The histologically observed increase in plasma cells [10] is not paralleled by increased activity within their cytoplasmic cisternae, although the maturity of the plasma cell nuclei and the amount of cytoplasmic RER appears normal [10]. In contrast to the mildly affected mucosa of marasmus, the ultrastructure of the jejunal mucosa of three children with clinical manifestations of kwashiorkor and histological subtotal villous atrophy appeared severely altered [11]. The enterocytes showed short, sparse microvilli (Fig. 4.12). The cells appeared cuboidal and the nuclei large in

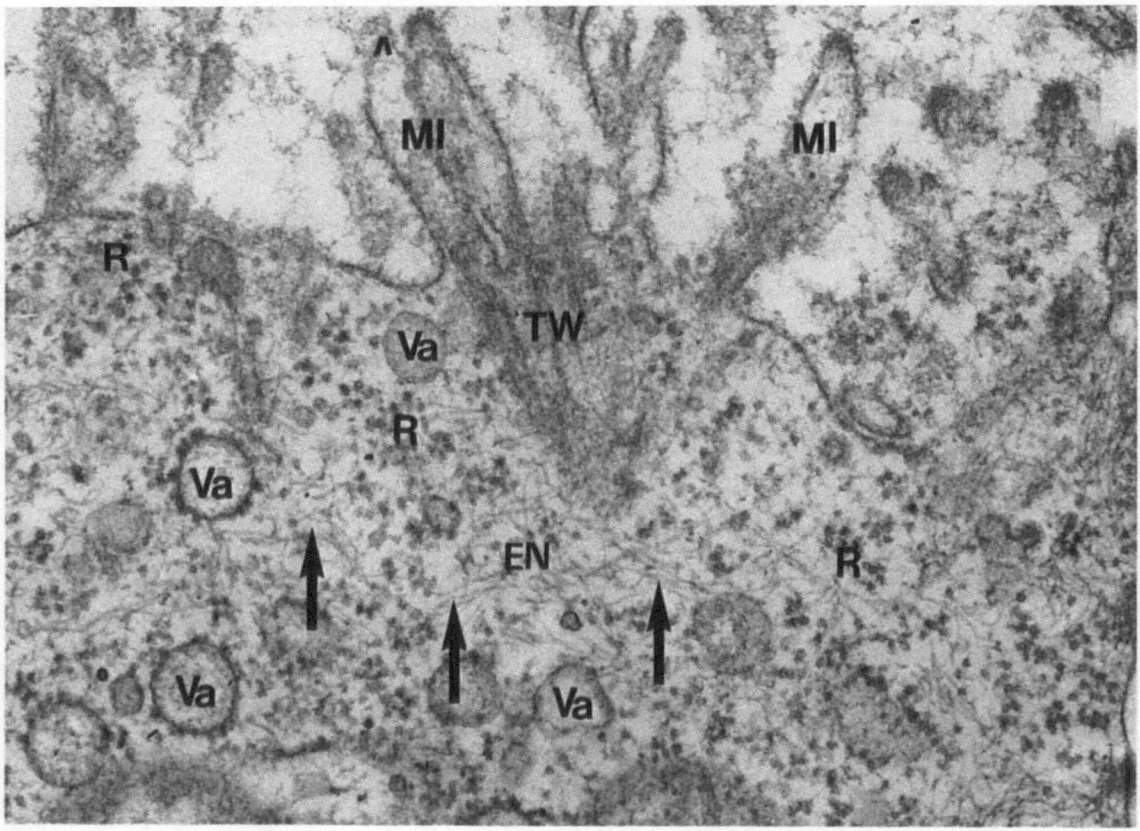

Fig. 4.12. Upper part of an enterocyte (*EN*) from the biopsy shown histologically in Fig. 4.1b. The microvilli (*MI*) are sparse, short and distended. The cell cytoplasm lacks normal density and its organelles consist mainly of free-lying ribosomes (*R*) and dilated vacuoles (*Va*), some lined by ER, others by RER. Fibres of the terminal web (*TW*) are sparse. Cytoplasmic fibrils and tubules are clearly seen (*arrows*). (× 50 500)

comparison to the cytoplasmic volume. Although often irregular in contour, nuclear degeneration was not evident. The cytoplasmic organelles were severely affected: the mitochondria appeared swollen with disruption of their cristae (Fig. 4.13), and an excess of vacuoles, lined by smooth or rough ER,

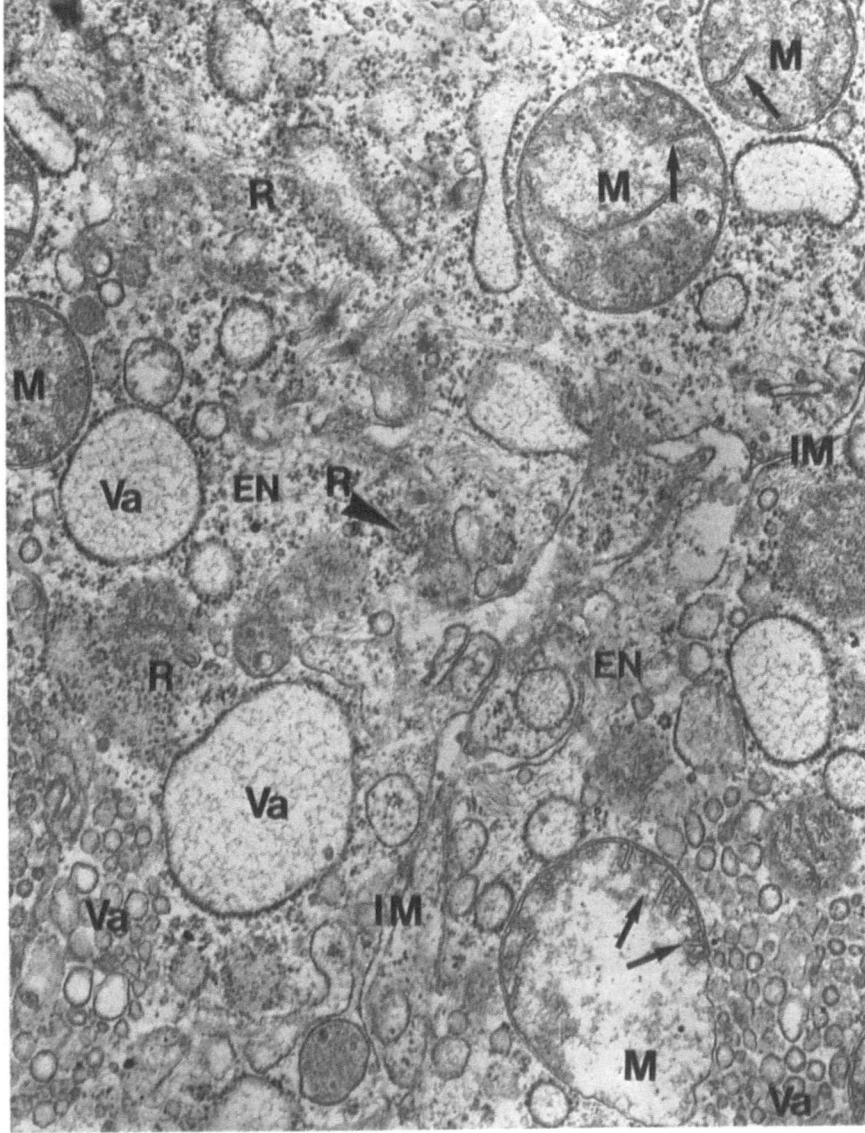

Fig. 4.13. Upper part of two enterocytes (*EN*) from the flat jejunal mucosa of a child with severe kwashiorkor. The cytoplasmic organelles show lack of organisation with swelling of the mitochondria (*M*) and disruption of the cristae (*arrows*). There is increased vacuolation (*Va*) affecting both ER- and RER-lined vesicles and numerous free-lying ribosomes and polysomes (*R*). *IM*, intercellular membrane. (× 60 000)

and ribosomes were seen. The Golgi complex showed dilated vesicles (Fig. 4.14). A most remarkable feature was the general lack of density of the cytoplasmic ground substance, which included the core of the microvilli, the terminal web, the mitochondrial ground substance and the basal lamina (Figs. 4.15, 4.16). Beyond the enterocytes the connective tissue fibrils of the lamina propria appeared equally sparse (Fig. 4.17). The endothelium of the small

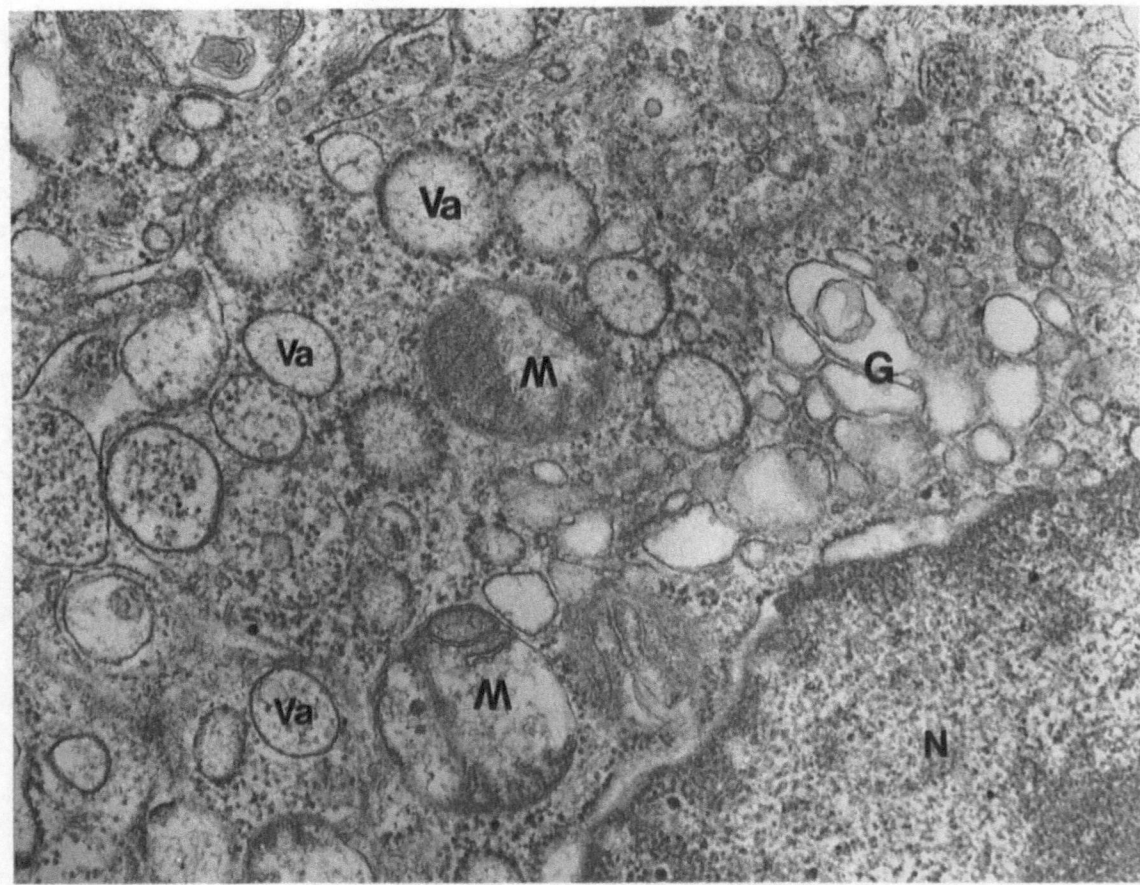

Fig. 4.14. Kwashiorkor: supranuclear portion of an enterocyte from the same mucosa as Fig. 4.13. showing the dilated vesicles of the Golgi complex (*G*) and similar changes of the mitochondria (*M*) and ER- and RER-lined vacuoles (*Va*) as in Fig. 4.13. *N*, nucleus. (× 55 310)

Fig. 4.15. Kwashiorkor: upper half of an enterocyte from the mucosa of a similar case, showing gross changes ▷ of the microvilli (*MI*), disorganised terminal web fibrils (*TW*), severe damage to the mitochondria (*M*) and increase in vacuoles (*Va*). The cytoplasmic background substance appears less electron dense than normal and contains numerous free-lying ribosomes (*R*), tubules and fibrils (*arrows*). (× 56 250)

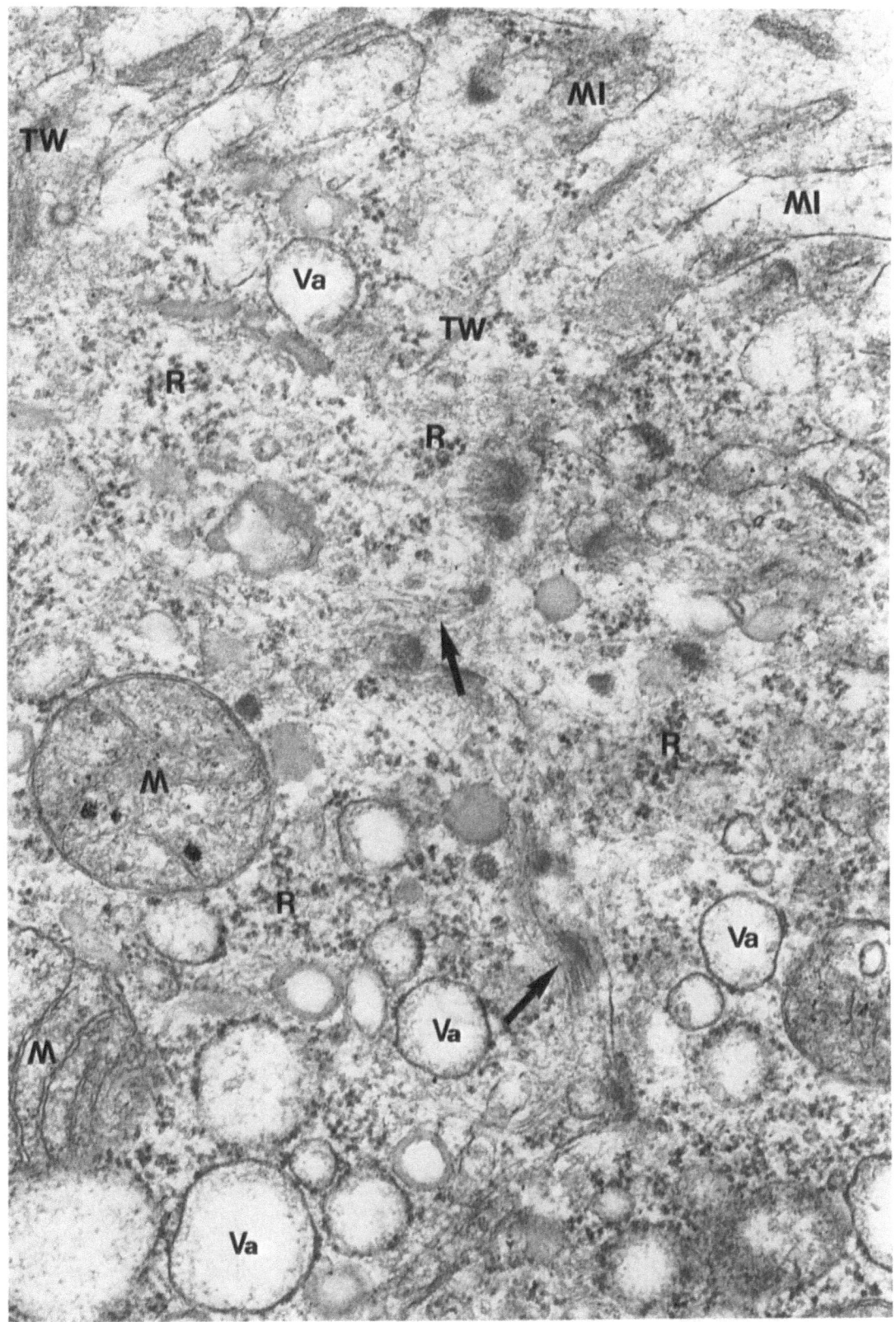

Fig. 4.15.

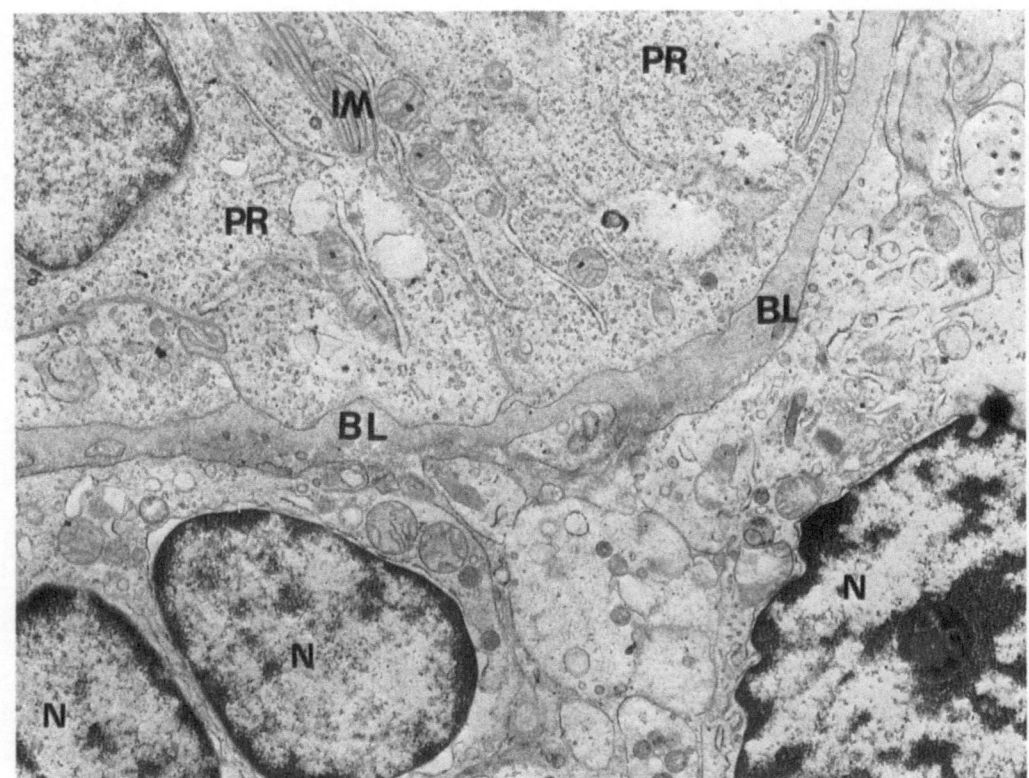

Fig. 4.16. △   Fig. 4.17. ▽

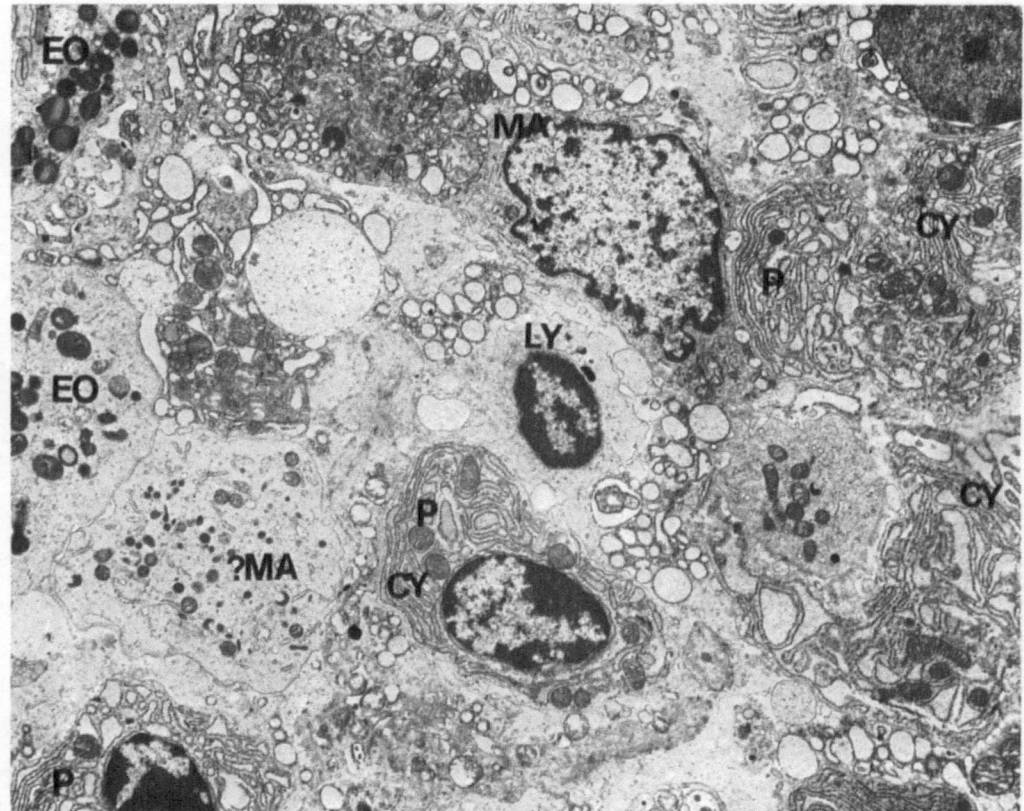

blood vessels appeared swollen (Fig. 4.18) and showed increased cytoplasmic translucency. Fibrocytes and macrophages appeared fewer than normal and a lack of phagolysosomal activity within the macrophages was observed (Figs. 4.17, 4.19). The plasma cells (Fig. 4.20) were mature but sparse in RER and cisternal activity. The fine structural appearances of the mucosa therefore suggested a lack of ground substance affecting most cell types and lack of activity within macrophages and plasma cells.

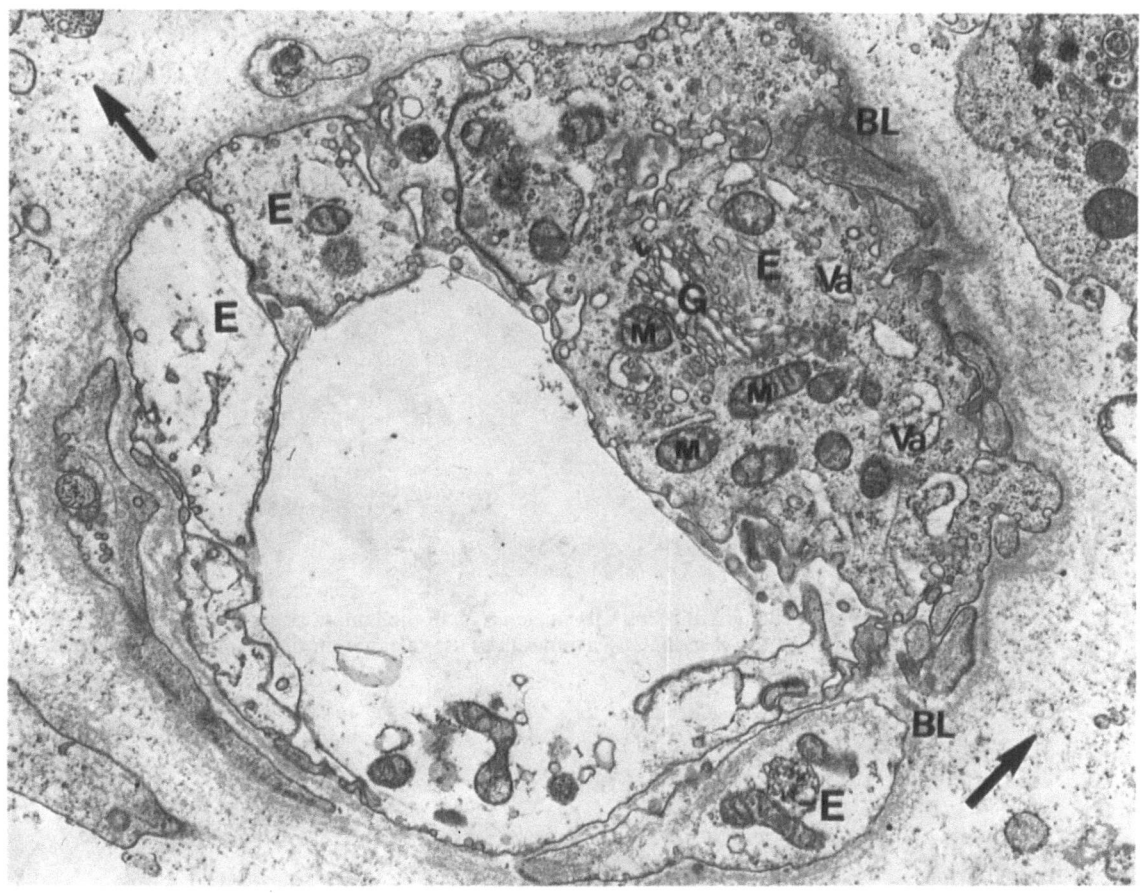

Fig. 4.18. Kwashiorkor: a small blood vessel in the lamina propria showing swelling of the endothelium (*E*) and increased translucency of the cytoplasmic substance. There is dilatation of RER-bound vacuoles (*Va*) but the Golgi complex (*G*) and the mitochondria (*M*) appear normal. A basal lamina (*BL*) surrounds the endothelium but beyond it the connective tissue fibrils are sparse (*arrows*). (× 15 750)

◁ **Fig. 4.16.** Kwashiorkor: the basal lamina (*BL*) of crypt epithelial cells appears as an ill-defined, finely granular area that lacks electron density. A distinct line representing the basal lamina cannot be seen. *PR*, precursor cells of the crypts; *IM*, intercellular membranes; *N*, nuclei of various lamina propria cells. (× 5440)

◁ **Fig. 4.17.** Kwashiorkor: various cell types of the lamina propria seen against a background that lacks electron density. Plasma cells (*P*), eosinophils (*EO*), macrophages (*MA*) and a lymphocyte (*LY*) are seen. Note the relative sparsity and lack of dilatation of the cisternae (*CY*) of the plasma cells. (× 6544)

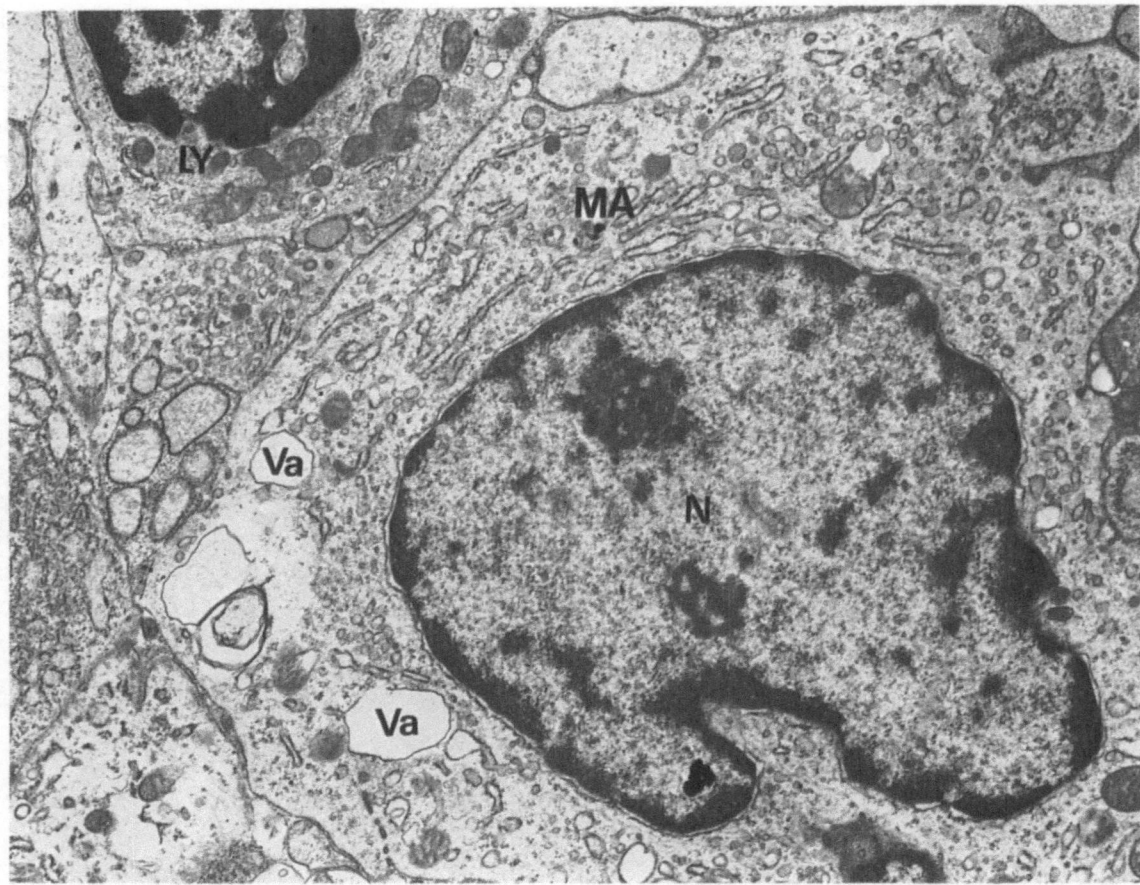

Fig. 4.19. Kwashiorkor: a macrophage (*MA*) with its nucleus (*N*) in the lamina propria showing a virtual absence of phagolysosomal bodies. A few dilated vacuoles (*Va*) are seen within the cytoplasm. *LY*, lymphocyte. (× 10 760)

Correlation of clinical and morphological data

It is possible that in the marasmic child, slowing of growth protects the patient from protein deficiency severe enough to affect every cell in the body. This would also be reflected in the adequate cell production and differentiation which leads to either a normal jejunal mucosa or a partial villous atrophy. The latter appearances may not be due to malnutrition itself but may be a reflection of the prevailing 'contaminated' environment. Surprisingly, plasma cell activity is not increased. Although immunological data of the jejunal mucosa are not available, T-cell deficiency, impairment of cell-mediated immunity and thymic atrophy have been reported in P-EM[7, 12] and it is possible that this may also affect the B-cells and macrophages of the lamina propria. Where the

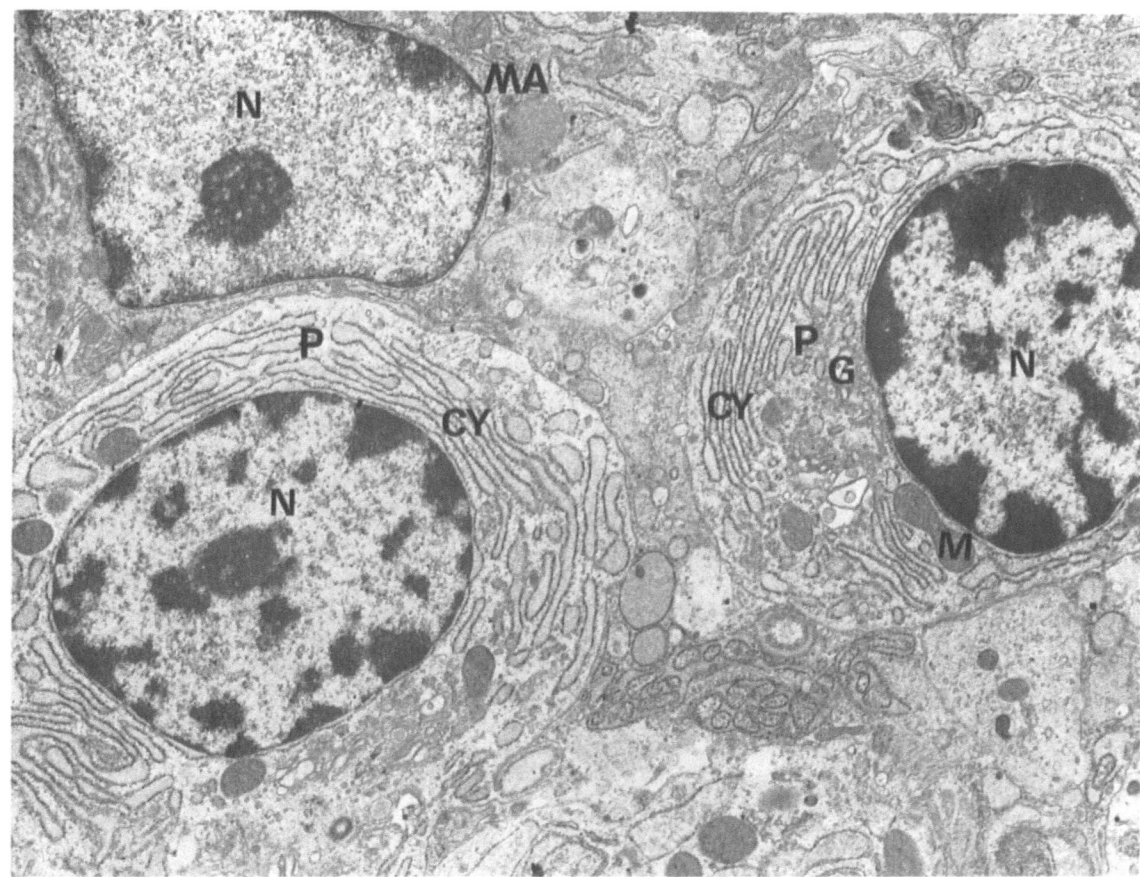

Fig. 4.20. Kwashiorkor: two plasma cells (*P*) and part of a macrophage (*MA*) in the lamina propria, showing normal nuclei (*N*). The cisternae (*CY*) within the plasma cell cytoplasm are collapsed and deficient in contents (immunoglobulin). The mitochondria (*M*) and Golgi complex (*G*) appear normal. (× 8830)

clinical picture is one of severe protein deficiency (kwashiorkor) the morphological appearances may be the result of inadequate cell formation at the crypts[3]. This is reflected by the lack of cells required to form normal villi and in the abnormality of the fine structure of the enterocytes lining the surface of the mucosa. Insufficient numbers of enterocytes are paralleled by their immaturity, shown by an excess of ribosomes. Intracytoplasmic ER and ground substance fibrils require protein for their formation and the lack of it may explain some of the structural abnormalities observed. In addition the cells of the immune system appear inactive and deficient. In the absence of immunological mucosal data it is only possible to point to the appearance of the macrophages and plasma cells as suggesting inadequate immune protection of the jejunal mucosa against entry of foreign material. This may set the scene for the frequency of giardial and other parasitic infestations [1].

References

1. Ament ME, Rubin CE (1972) Relation of giardiasis to abnormal intestinal immuno-deficiency syndromes. Gastroenterology 62:216–226
2. Barbezat GO, Bowie MD, Kaschula ROC, Hansen JDL (1967) Studies on the small intestinal mucosa of children with protein calorie malnutrition. S Afr Med J 41:1031–1036
3. Brunser O, Reid A, Monckeberg F, Maccioni A, Contreras I (1966) Jejunal biopsies in infant malnutrition with special reference to mitotic index. Pediatrics 38:605–612
4. Brunser O, Castillo C, Araya M (1976) Fine structure of the small intestinal mucosa in infantile marasmic malnutrition. Gastroenterology 70:495–507
5. Burman D (1965) The jejunal morphology in kwashiorkor. Arch Dis Child 40:526–531
6. Campos JV, Neto, UF, Particio FR et al. (1979) Jejunal mucosa in marasmic children. Clinical, pathological and fine structural evaluation of the effect of protein-energy malnutrition and environmental contamination. Am J Clin Nutr 32:1575–1591
7. Chandra RK (1972) Immunocompetence in under-nutrition. J Pediatr 81:1194–1200
8. Evans GW (1971) Structure and function of the jejunum in kwashiorkor. Nutr Rev 29:205–207
9. Mayoral LG, Triphathy K, Bolanos O et al. (1972) Intestinal functional and morphologic abnormalities in severely protein-malnourished adults. Am J Clin Nutr 25:1084–1091
10. Nassar AM, El Tantawy SA, Khalifa S, Abdel Fattah S, Abdel Hamid J (1980) Ultrastructural changes in the mucosa of the small intestine due to protein-calorie malnutrition. J Trop Pediatr 26:62–72
11. Shiner M, Redmond AO, Hansen JD (1973) The jejunal mucosa in protein-energy malnutrition. A clinical, histological and ultrastructural study. Exp Mol Pathol 19:61–78
12. Smythe PM, Schonland M, Brereton-Stiles GG et al. (1971) Thymolymphatic deficiency and depression of cell mediated immunity in protein-calorie malnutrition. Lancet ii:939–943
13. Stanfield JP, Hutt MSR, Tunnicliffe R (1965) Intestinal biopsy in kwashiorkor. Lancet ii:519–523
14. Theron JJ, Wittmann W, Prinsloo JG (1971) The fine structure of the jejunum in kwashiorkor. Exp Mol Pathol 14:184–199

Chapter 5

Miscellaneous

Malignancies

The malignancies most likely to affect the jejunal mucosa are the lymphomas or lymphosarcomas or more rarely the adenocarcinomas. They are usually diagnosed radiologically or at laparotomy and only very rarely by jejunal mucosal biopsy. Most malignancies of the jejunum in Western countries are circumscribed masses located in the middle or lower jejunum, and therefore not in the site normally biopsied by peroral technique. This contrasts with the so-called 'Mediterranean lymphomas' or IPSID (immunoproliferative small intestinal diseases) which are often diffuse, usually affect the duodenum and upper jejunum (but may also extend into the lower parts of the small intestine), and are therefore within reach of the endoscope or peroral jejunal biopsy technique. Again, limited information is available on the ultrastructural appearances of both types of lymphomas [11, 19, 20, 21, 22, 23, 24, 38]. We had the opportunity to study the ultrastructure of mucosal biopsy material in the following patients [21]:

1) one patient with Mediterranean lymphoma in whom the diffusely infiltrated duodenal and jejunal mucosa was biopsied under direct vision;

2) one patient with alpha-chain disease, a condition allied to Mediterranean lymphoma or IPSID in which the jejunal mucosa is uniformly affected though not necessarily malignant in the early stages;

3) six patients with 'Western' lymphoma involving either the ileum or mesenteric lymph nodes, in whom the 'uninvolved' upper jejunal mucosa was studied for possible identification of hyperactive, reactive or neoplastic inflammatory cells.

Fine structure of involved mucosa with IPSID

Histologically this patient's jejunal biopsy showed a subtotal villous atrophy with pleomorphic cellular infiltration, including abnormal histiocytes (Fig. 5.1), lymphocytes and plasma cells. The enterocytes appeared normal except for areas of increased cell lysis leading to superficial ulcerations. Ultrastructurally some histiocytes in the lamina propria showed large, irregular and/or multiple nuclei with prominent nucleoli and mitochondrial abnormalities (Figs. 5.2, 5.3). The plasma cell was more commonly found

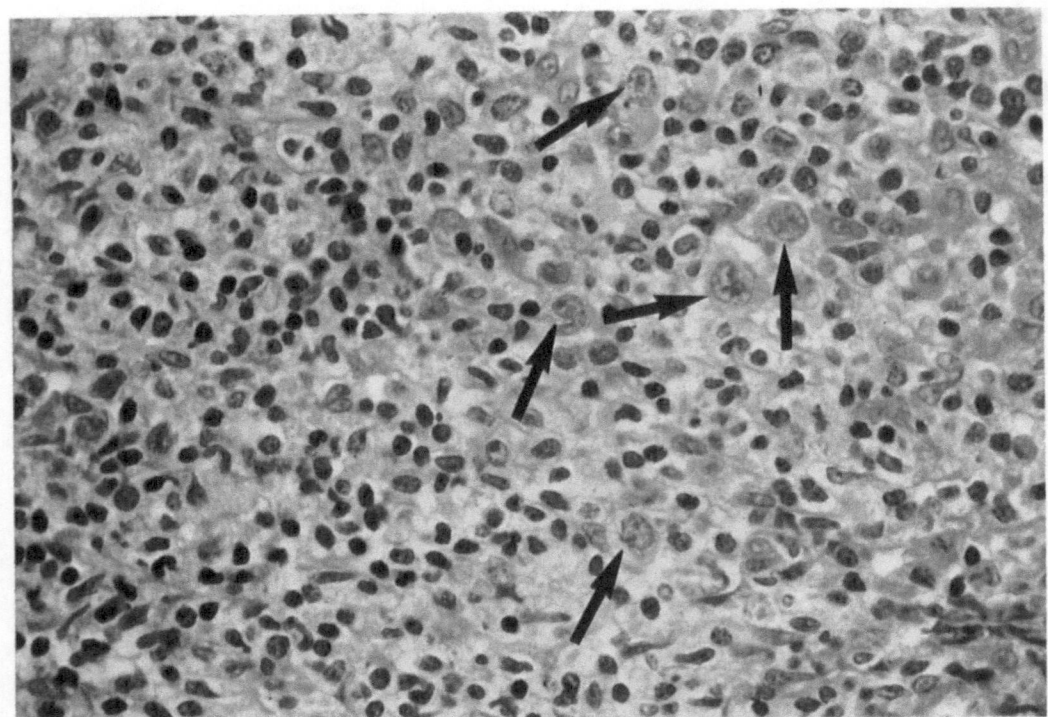

Fig. 5.1. △   **Fig. 5.2.** ▽

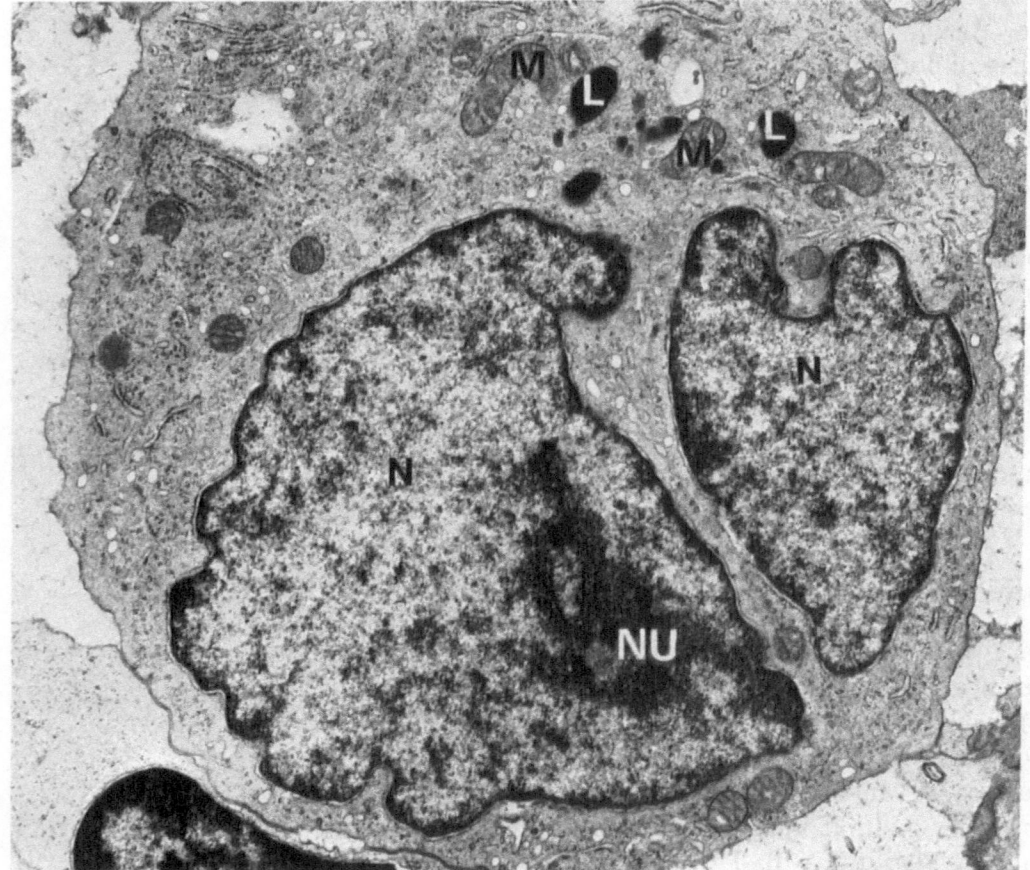

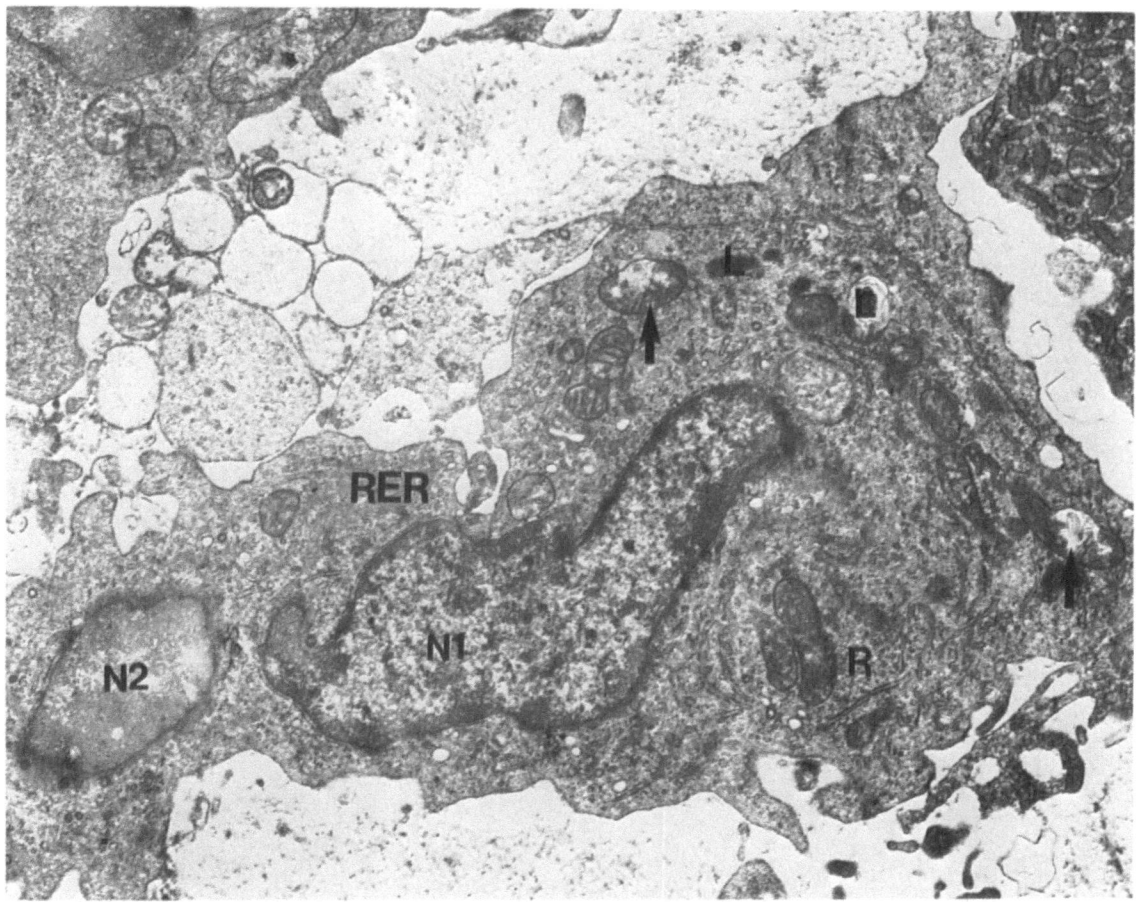

Fig. 5.3. Another histiocyte from the same mucosa as Fig. 5.2 showing pronounced abnormality of nuclear shape and the presence of two nuclei, *N1* and *N2*. The cytoplasm is rich in *RER* and ribosomes (*R*) but contains few lysosomes (*L*). Some of the mitochondrial cristae appear disrupted (*arrows*). (× 10 940)

to be abnormal, showing one or often multiple nuclei with irregular contours, indistinct nuclear chromatin pattern and more than one nucleolus (Figs. 5.4, 5.5). In the plasma cell cytoplasm the mitochondria were often swollen, disrupted or lysed, lysosomes were increased and the cisternae showed great irregularity. These abnormal histiocytes and plasma cells were diffusely distributed in the lamina propria and were interspersed with more normal appearing cells of the same type. Fibrocytes, macrophages and lymphocytes were numerous but showed no apparent cellular abnormalities.

◁ **Fig. 5.1.** Light microscopy of cells within the lamina propria from the jejunal biopsy of a patient with immunoproliferative small intestinal disease (IPSID). Cells with large irregular nuclei are seen (*arrows*). (× 400)

◁ **Fig. 5.2.** A histiocyte from the region of the lamina propria of a patient with immunoproliferative small intestinal disease (IPSID) showing two nuclei (*N*) with irregular contours and a large nucleolus (*NU*). The nucleus may be horseshoe-shaped and single, appearing as two separate parts. The cytoplasmic organelles show no abnormality. *M*, mitochondria; *L*, lysosomes. (× 8880)

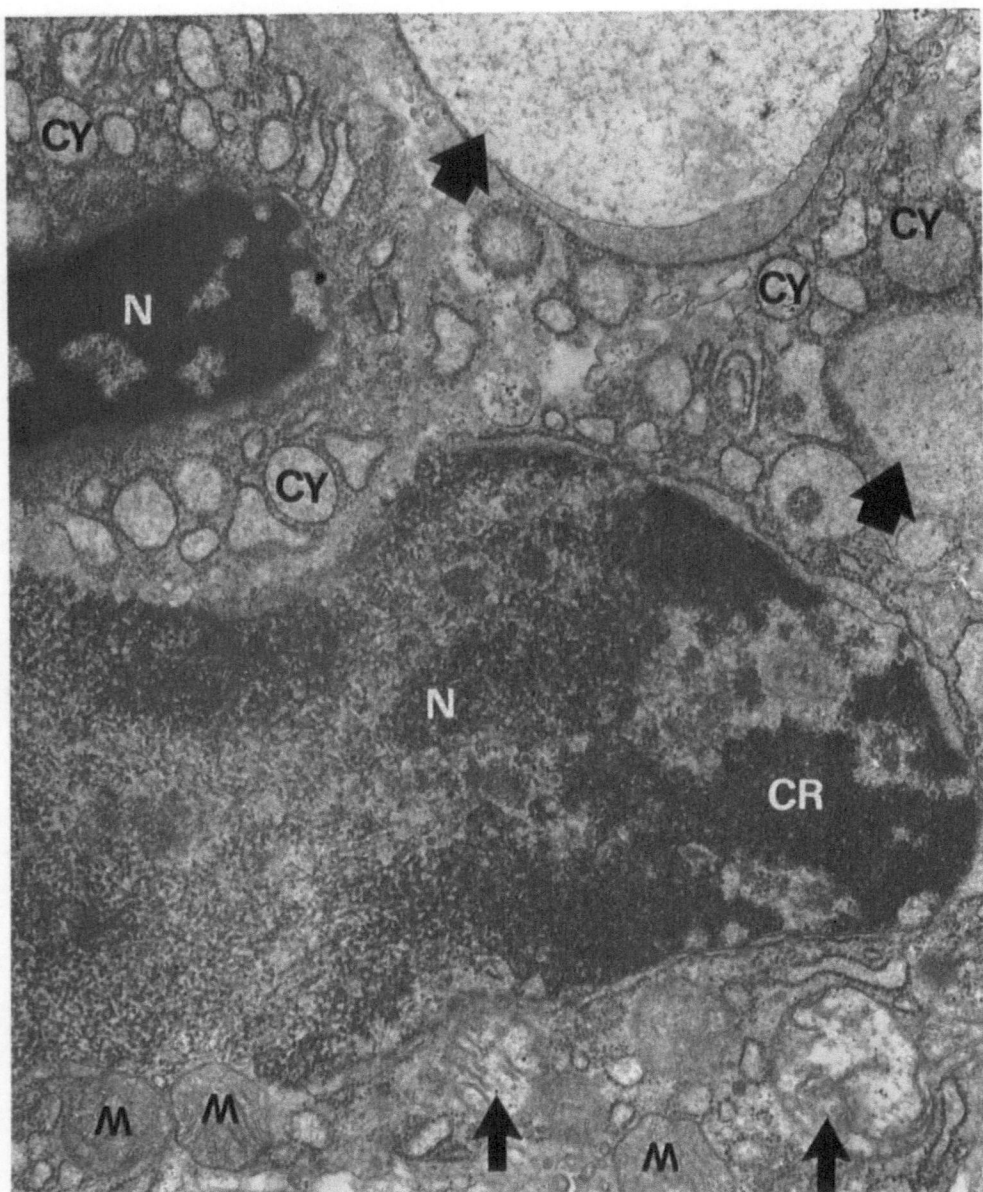

Fig. 5.4. Part of a plasma cell in the lamina propria in IPSID, identified by the chromatin (*CR*) pattern within the nuclei (*N*) and the presence of dilated cisternae (*CY*) containing immunoglobulin. Two separate nuclei are seen, the larger one showing marked abnormality of shape and distribution of the chromatin (*CR*). Within the cytoplasm the mitochondria (*M*) appear globular and some show disruption of the cristae (*arrow*). The distribution of the cisternae lacks regularity and some are grossly dilated (*thick arrows*). (× 15 600)

Fine structure of the mucosa in alpha-chain disease

The histology of this patient's jejunal biopsy showed a subtotal villous atrophy, normal enterocytes and a dense infiltration with apparently normal mature plasma cells (Fig. 5.6). Immunofluorescence techniques showed an absence of IgA light chains (kappa and lambda) within the plasma cells.

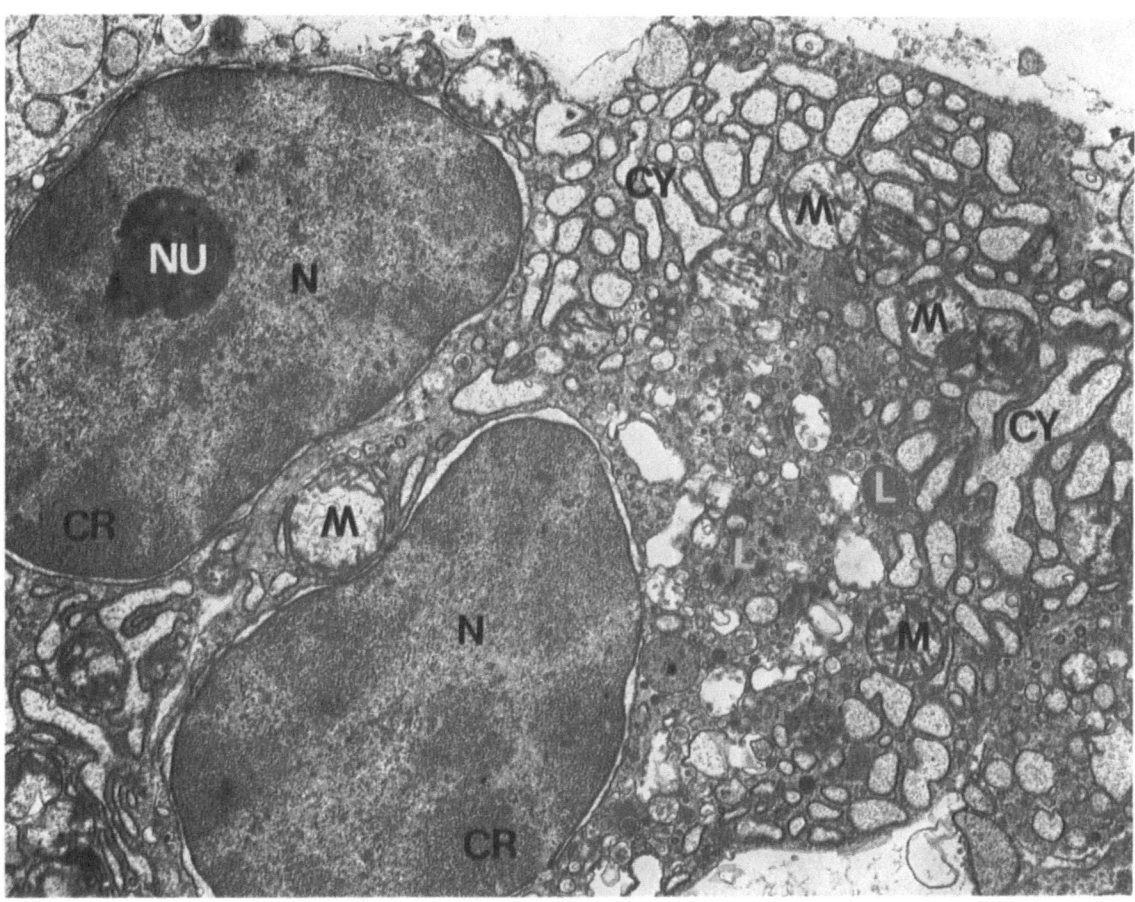

Fig. 5.5. Another plasma cell from the same mucosa showing two nuclei (*N*) with a large nucleolus in one (*NU*). The nuclear chromatin pattern (*CR*) is indistinct. The cytoplasmic cisternae (*CY*) are irregularly arranged and, though dilated, appear partly empty. There is gross abnormality of the mitochondria (*M*). Small and large lysosomes (*L*) are present. (× 13 016)

Fine-structural examination of the lamina propria plasma cells showed many hyperactive though normal-appearing plasma cells with single nuclei with regular contours and normal chromatin pattern, normal mitochondria and cytoplasmic cisternae arranged in an orderly fashion. There were, however, other plasma cells which resembled those seen in the patient with malignant IPSID. These cells were multinucleated (Fig. 5.7) and their cell membrane was often poorly delineated. Increase in cytoplasmic lysosomes and irregularity of the mitochondrial cristae and of cisternal arrangements were evident. The cisternae were sometimes filled with homogeneous material of increased electron density (Fig. 5.8). Rarely, distinct crystal formation was seen within the cisternal matrix [39] (Fig. 5.9 and inset). Similar crystals have been reported in the cisternae of plasma cells in plasmacytomas [9] and other lymphoproliferative disorders [37] and have been confirmed in alpha-chain disease (F. Tavarela Veloso, personal communication).

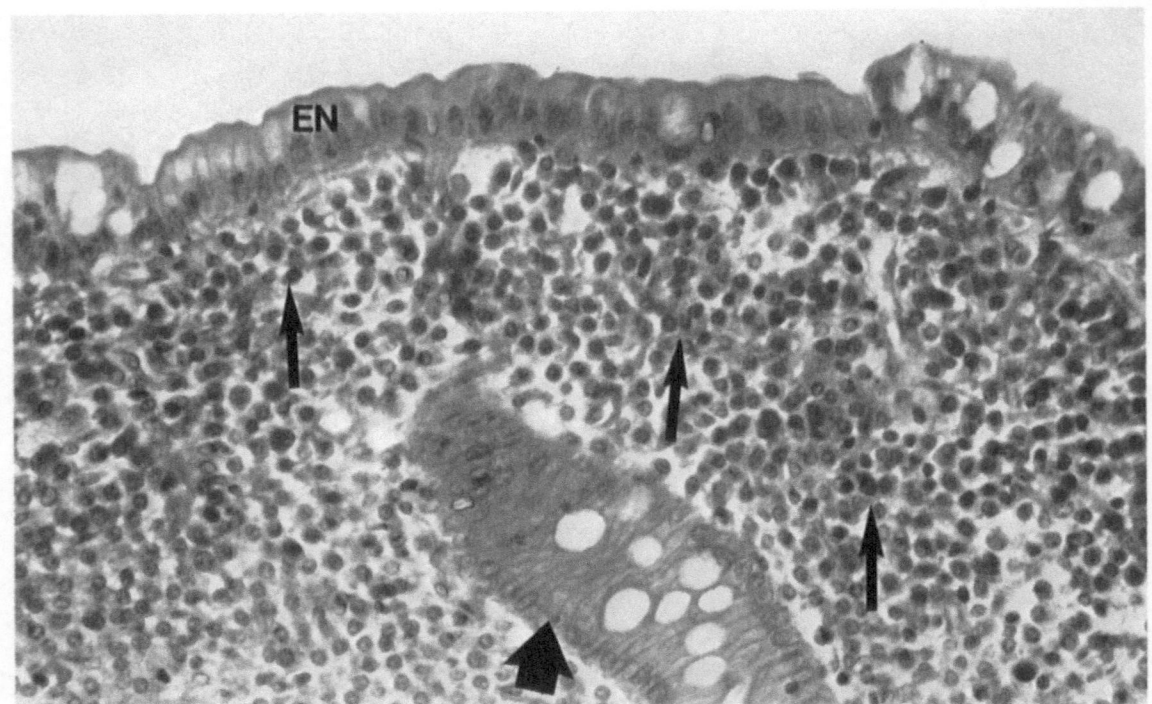

Fig. 5.6. △   **Fig. 5.7.** ▽

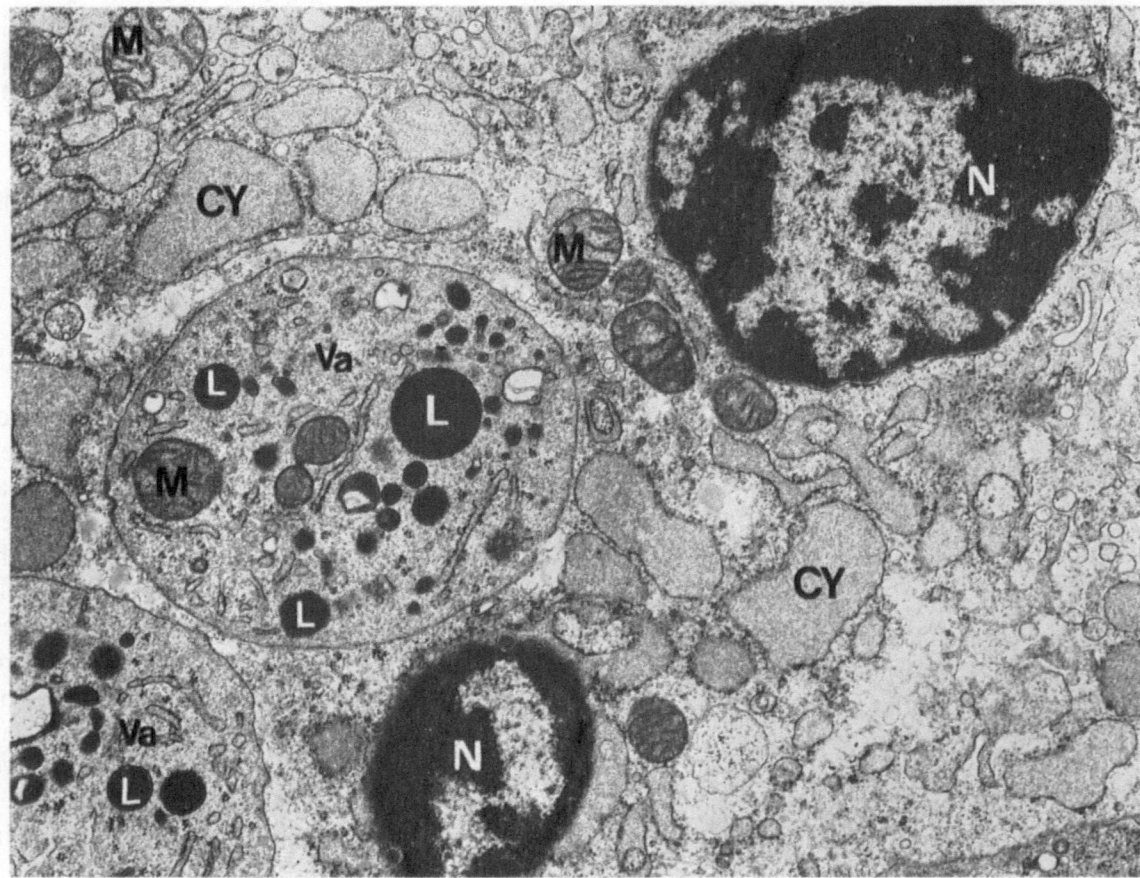

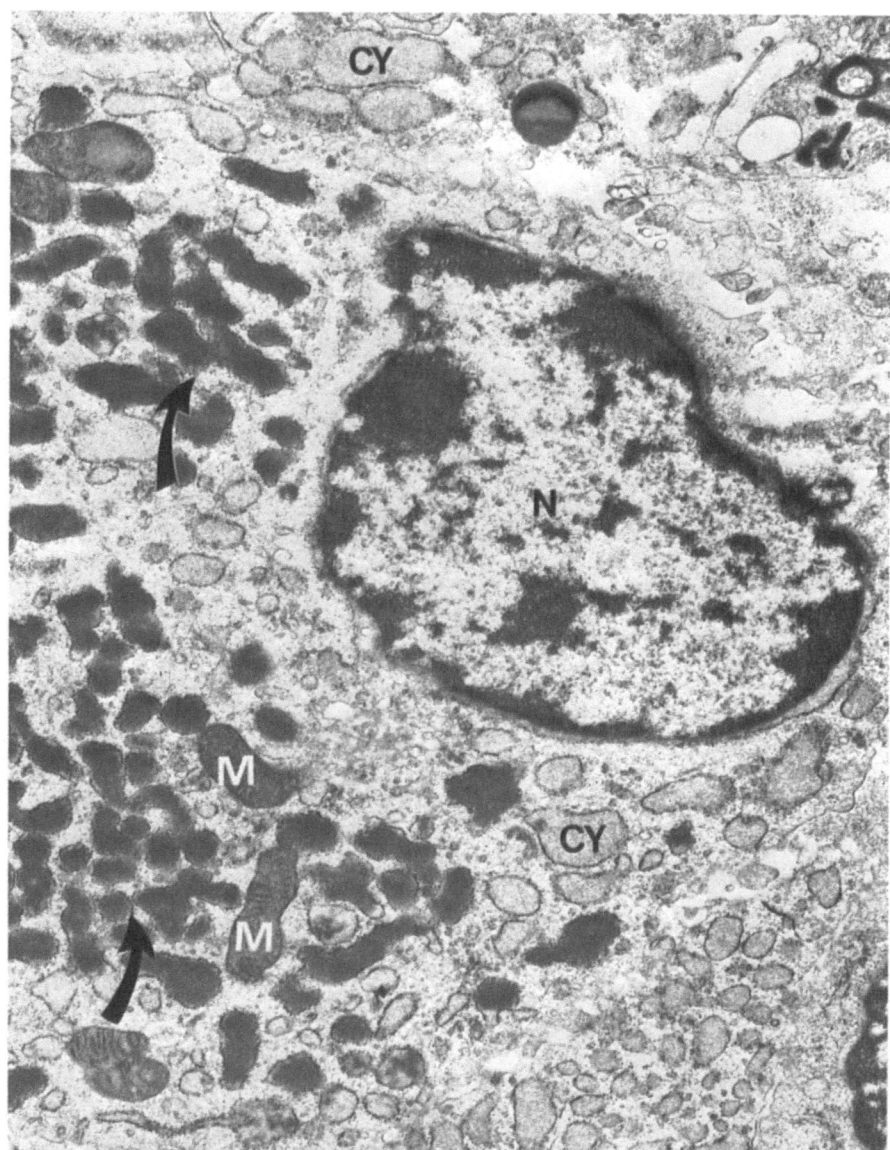

Fig. 5.8. Part of a plasma cell showing a nucleus (*N*) with irregular contours. The cytoplasmic cisternae (*CY*) are arranged in irregular fashion and some (*arrows*) contain material of greater than normal electron density. *M*, mitochondria. Alpha-chain disease. (×11 340)

◁ **Fig. 5.6.** Histology of the mucosa in a patient with alpha-chain disease showing absence of villi, normal enterocytes (*EN*) and dense cellular infiltration of the lamina propria with plasma cells (*arrows*). Part of a crypt of Lieberkühn is present (*thick arrow*). (×600)

◁ **Fig. 5.7.** Part of an abnormal plasma cell from the same patient's mucosa showing the following features: two nuclei (*N*), dilated and irregularly arranged cytoplasmic cisternae (*CY*) and large autophagic vacuoles (*Va*) containing lysosomes (*L*), mitochondria (*M*), RER and ribosomes. (×12 090)

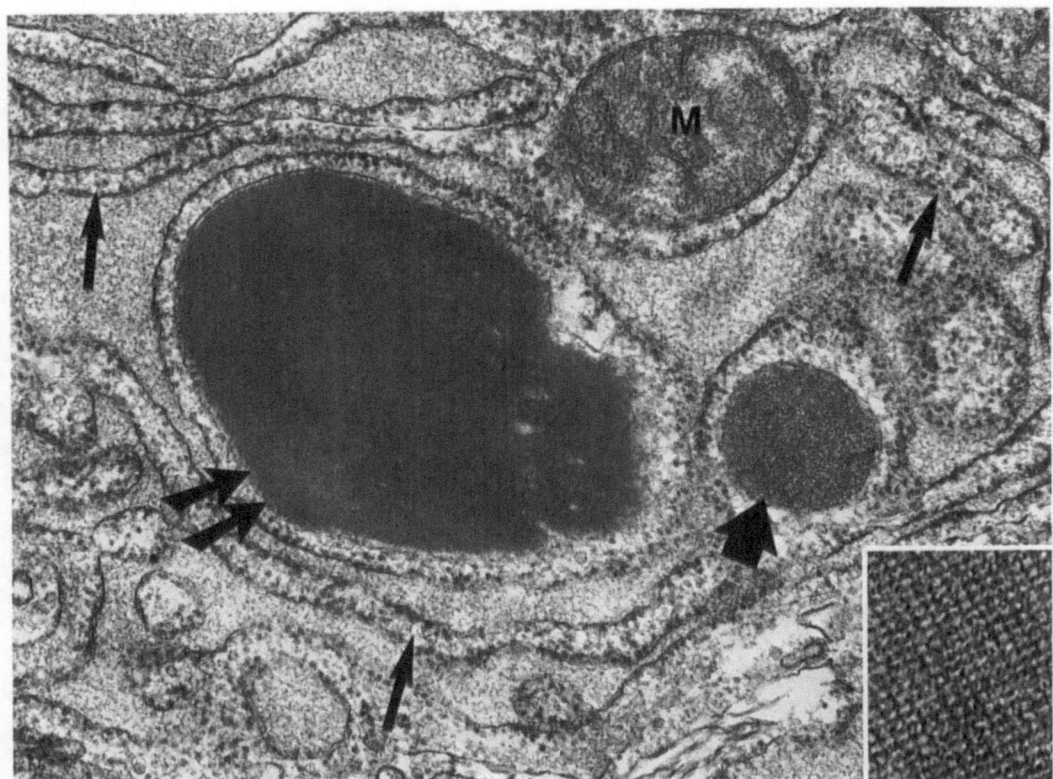

Fig. 5.9. △   **Fig. 5.10.** ▽

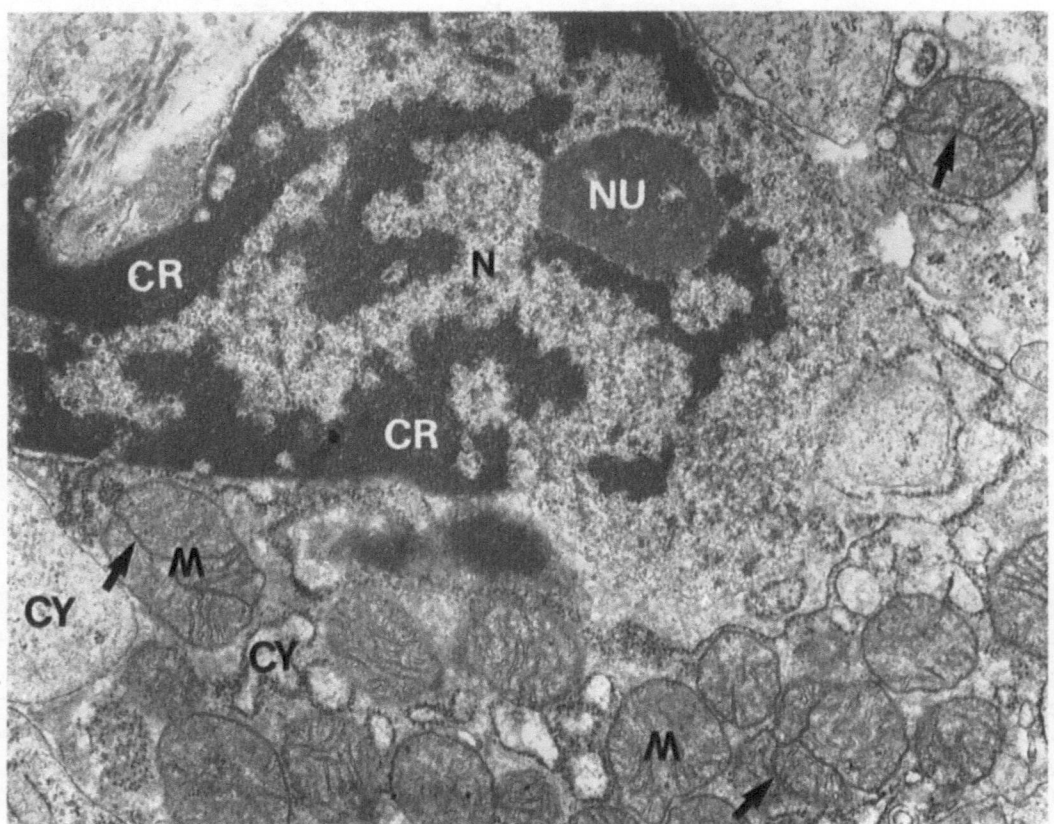

Fine structure of uninvolved mucosa in lymphoma

All patients had long-standing malabsorption (eventually fatal). Two patients had ileal lymphomas, and in the other two only the mesenteric glands were infiltrated with lymphoma cells. Serial jejunal biopsies of these four patients were available and were reported as histologically normal. Fine-structural examination of the plasma cells, lymphocytes and histiocytes revealed some cells which resembled those described in the previous patients with IPSID and alpha-chain disease and were therefore regarded as abnormal (Figs. 5.10–5.13). These cells were often so bizarre in nuclear and cytoplasmic appearance that it was difficult to recognise their cell type.

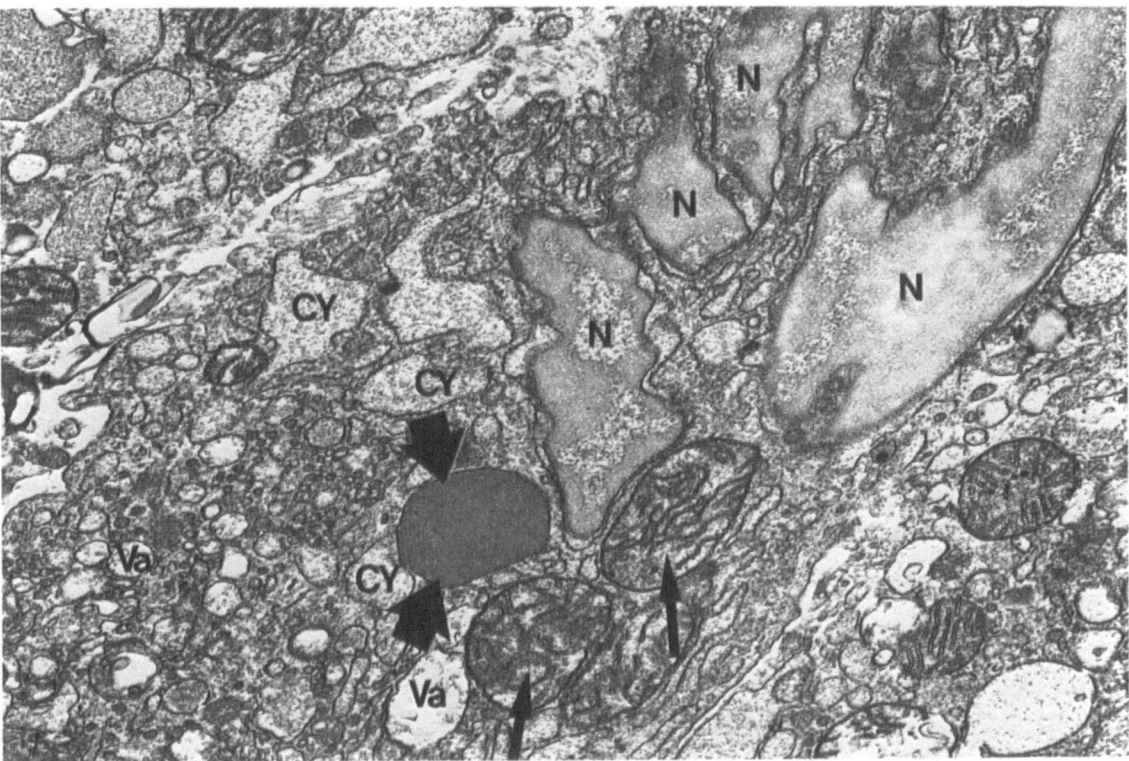

Fig. 5.11. Multinucleated (*N*) plasma cell from the uninvolved mucosa of another patient with lymphoma, showing gross cytoplasmic abnormalities such as increase in small and large vacuoles (*Va*), bizarre shaped cristae mitochondrales (*arrows*), and irregular cisternae (*CY*), one of which contains crystalline material (*thick arrow*). (× 23 480)

◁ **Fig. 5.9.** Higher magnification of plasma cell cisternae containing floccular material of normal electron density (*arrows*), of increased density (*thick arrow*) and of crystalline consistency (*double arrows*) (*see also inset*). *M*, mitochondria. Alpha-chain disease. (× 42 350; inset × 256 000)

◁ **Fig. 5.10.** Plasma cell from the uninvolved mucosa of a patient with lymphoma of the small intestine. A single nucleus (*N*) is present which is bizarre shaped, has an abnormal yet still characteristic chromatin pattern (*CR*) and a large nucleolus (*NU*). The mitochondria (*M*) appear rounder than normal but show no damage. The mitochondrial cristae show alteration of their normal pattern (*arrows*). *CY*, cisternae. (× 25 500)

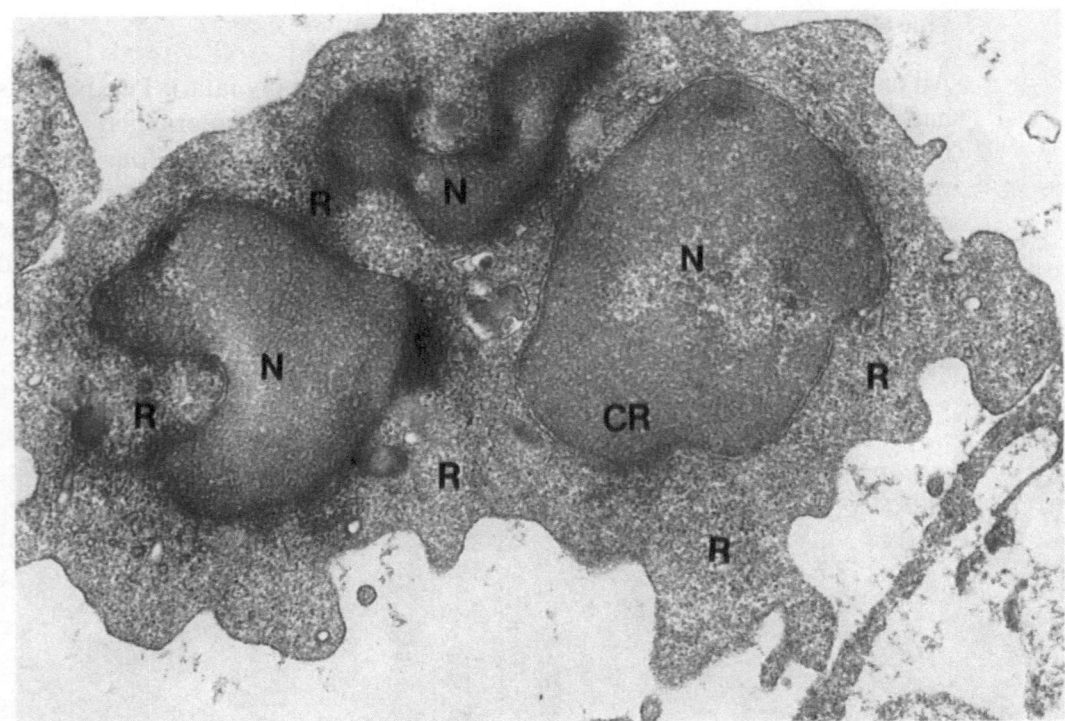

Fig. 5.12. △   **Fig. 5.13.** ▽

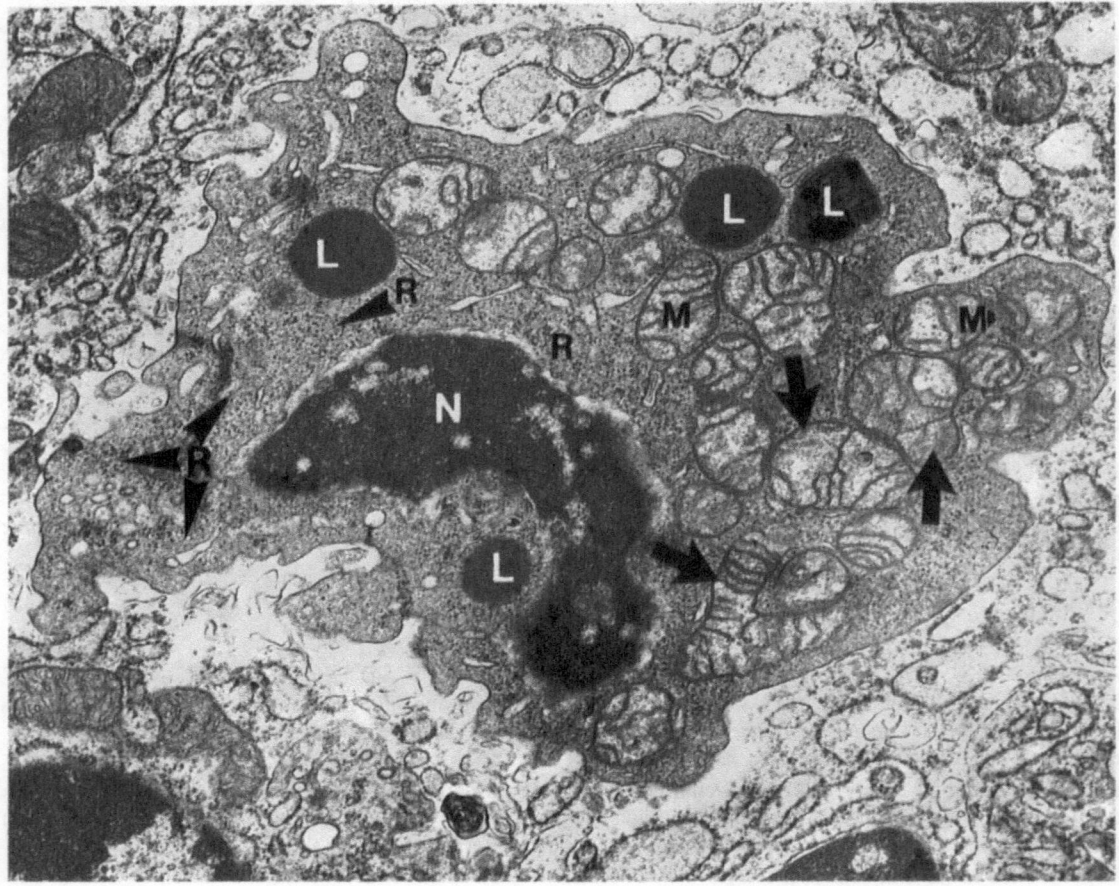

Ultrastructural recognition of abnormal inflammatory cells

The search for isolated cells with abnormal structure in uninvolved mucosa in patients with suspected lymphomatous infiltration of the small bowel is usually unrewarding with light microscopic examination but could be well worth while at the ultrastructural level. This has been pointed out in the case of abnormal plasma cells [19] and of histiocytes [22, 23]. In our study of the eight patients with lymphoma [8] we have shown fine-structural abnormalities affecting plasma cells, histiocytes or lymphocytes. These cells may be so bizarre that the original cell type is in doubt, or the cells may show features resembling more than one cell type. Although it has been possible to identify plasma cells, histiocytes or lymphocytes as ultrastructurally abnormal, the problem of interpretation remains: what is the significance of a few cells with abnormal features amongst others that appear normal? Are the abnormal cells reactive, hyperplastic, premalignant or malignant? It is too early to answer these questions but the electron microscopist should be on the lookout for fine structural changes in isolated plasma cells, histiocytes or lymphocytes, even if these are few in numbers, because of their eventual significance in diagnosis.

Giardia lamblia

These protozoa are a common cause of infection in tropical and non-tropical areas and are more likely to cause symptoms in temperate regions. They are found in large numbers in the small intestinal lumen and are easily identified by light and electron microscopy (Fig. 4.6), lying immediately above the luminal end of the microvilli close to the glycocalyx (Fig. 4.5). The area to be looked for is the brush border of the villous enterocytes and more rarely the crypt epithelium. The parasite may or may not make contact with the microvilli, but even where contact is made there may not be any significant fine-structural damage to the microvilli or the epithelial cytoplasm. Intracytoplasmic lysosomes may be increased [3] and show active phagocytosis but this is variable. It is therefore possible that a symbiotic existence between parasite and host mucosa exists. Are *Giardia* invasive under certain circumstances? They have been shown to cause mucosal injury [3, 41] and were seen in recognisable form within mucosal epithelial cells and below the epithelium in the lamina propria [6]. It is possible that they only invade epithelial cells in which lysis is imminent and thus gain access to the lamina propria [6] or that they are invasive in the immune compromised patient. Enzyme deficiencies of the absorptive cells, presumably caused by the parasite, have been reported [3]. The detailed structure of this protozoa has been well described [6,7,29].

◁ **Fig. 5.12.** Multinucleated cell, probably a lymphocyte, from the uninvolved mucosa of a patient with lymphoma. There are three nuclei (*N*) with a somewhat indistinct thick chromatin pattern (*CR*). The cytoplasm contains few organelles apart from numerous ribosomes (*R*). (× 15 192)

◁ **Fig. 5.13.** Lamina propria cell with single irregularly shaped nucleus (*N*) from the same mucosa as Fig. 5.12. The cytoplasm contains grossly abnormal mitochondriae (*M*) and cristae mitochondrales (*arrows*). There are numerous ribosomes (*R*) and four dense bodies, probably lysosomes (*L*). (× 21 940)

Cysts

Some encysted parasites appear to undergo lysis as they come in contact with epithelial enzymes as part of a protective barrier against the physical entry of the live organism into the mucosa. An example of this mechanism whereby cysts are destroyed is illustrated in the series of photographs (Figs. 4.7, 4.8, 5.14, 5.15) from a single biopsy. This shows unidentified encapsulated cysts approaching the microvilli of enterocytes in an intact state. On contact with the microvilli partial lysis of the cyst membranes occurs. The microvilli appear to engulf the cyst further and contact is made with the upper part of the enterocyte

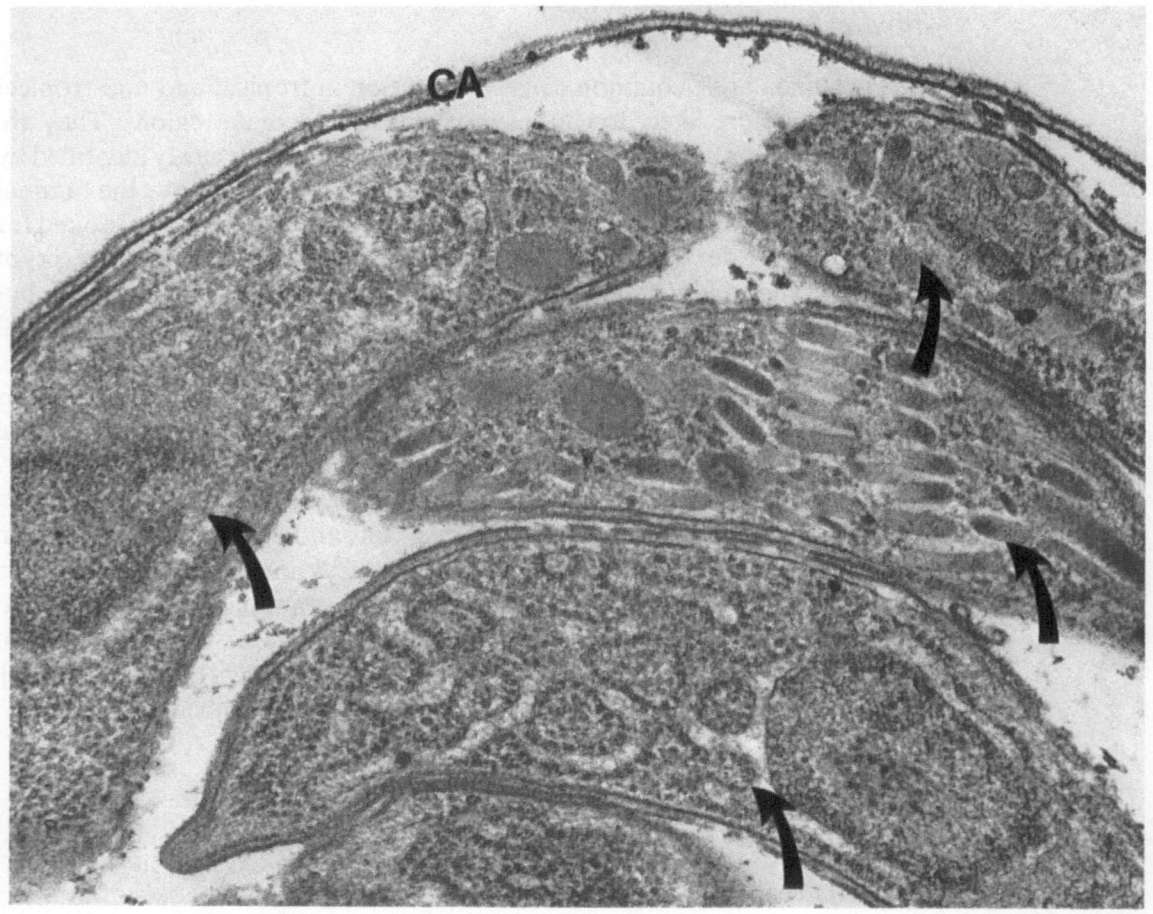

Fig. 5.14. Encapsulated trophozoites (*arrows*). *?Giardia lamblia* seen in the lumen of the jejunum close to the mucosal brush border. From a patient with malnutrition. *CA*, capsule. (× 65 600)

itself. At this point lysis progresses to the organelles of the cyst. Eventually the cyst is wholly engulfed within the enterocyte cytoplasm, walled off by membrane of the smooth endoplasmic reticulum. The end product of the lysed cyst appears as a mass of whorl-like fibrils and homogeneous material enclosed in single membrane. It is noteworthy that no apparent damage to the enterocyte and its organelles is visible and the cell apparently remains viable.

The cysts of certain *Coccidia* (Figs. 5.16–5.20) on the other hand appear to be more invasive [40, 42, 43] in that they can be seen not only on the surface of the microvilli but also in more recognisable form within the epithelial cells and possibly beyond.

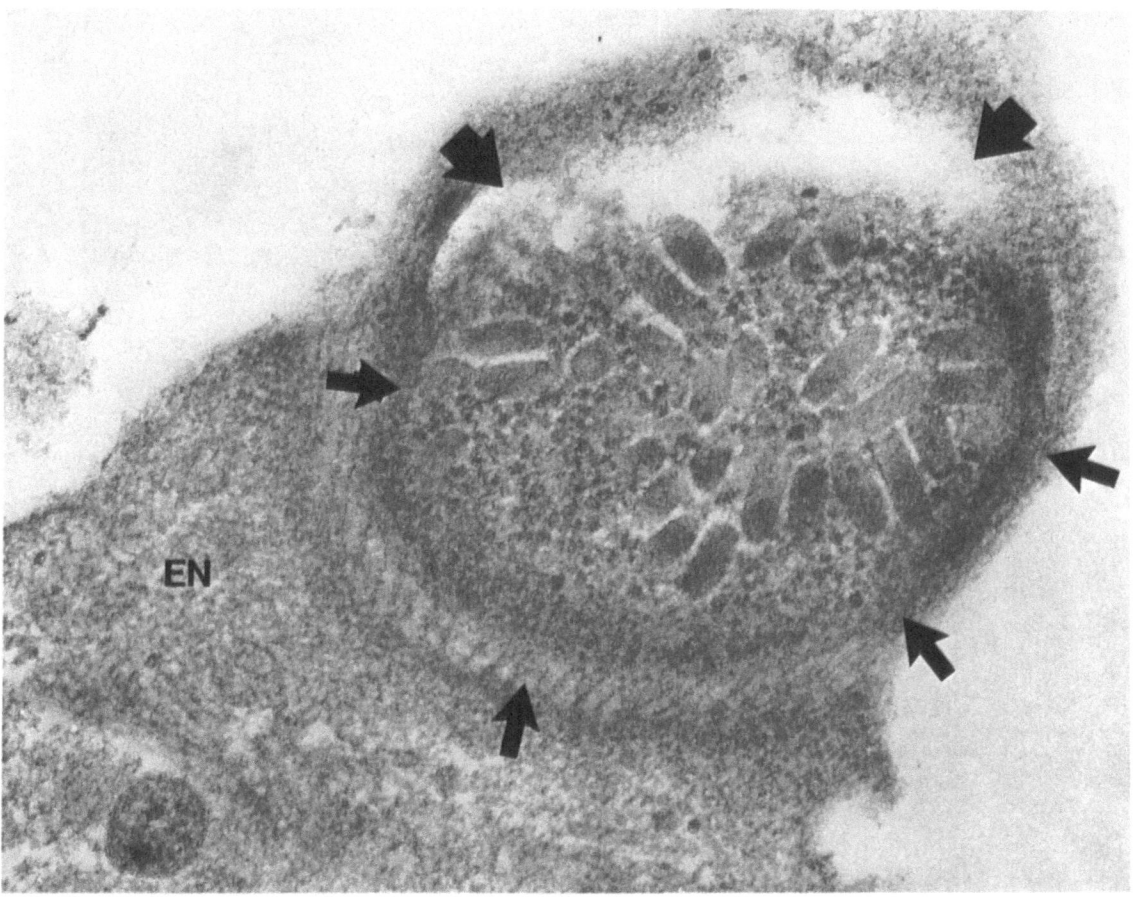

Fig. 5.15. Transverse section of the individual trophozoite (*arrows*) as in Fig. 5.14 in intimate contact with an enterocyte (*EN*). Note that the invading protozoon has lost its capsule and is undergoing partial lysis (*thick arrows*). (× 98 400)

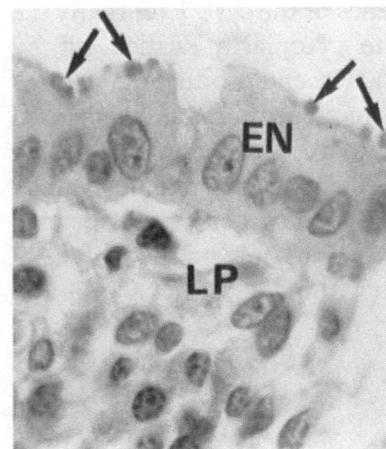

Fig. 5.16.

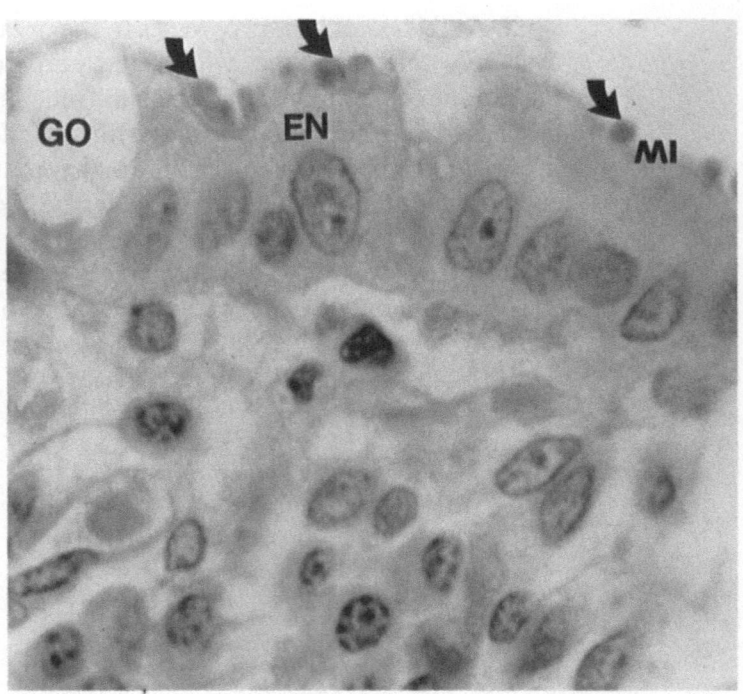

Fig. 5.17.

Fig. 5.18.

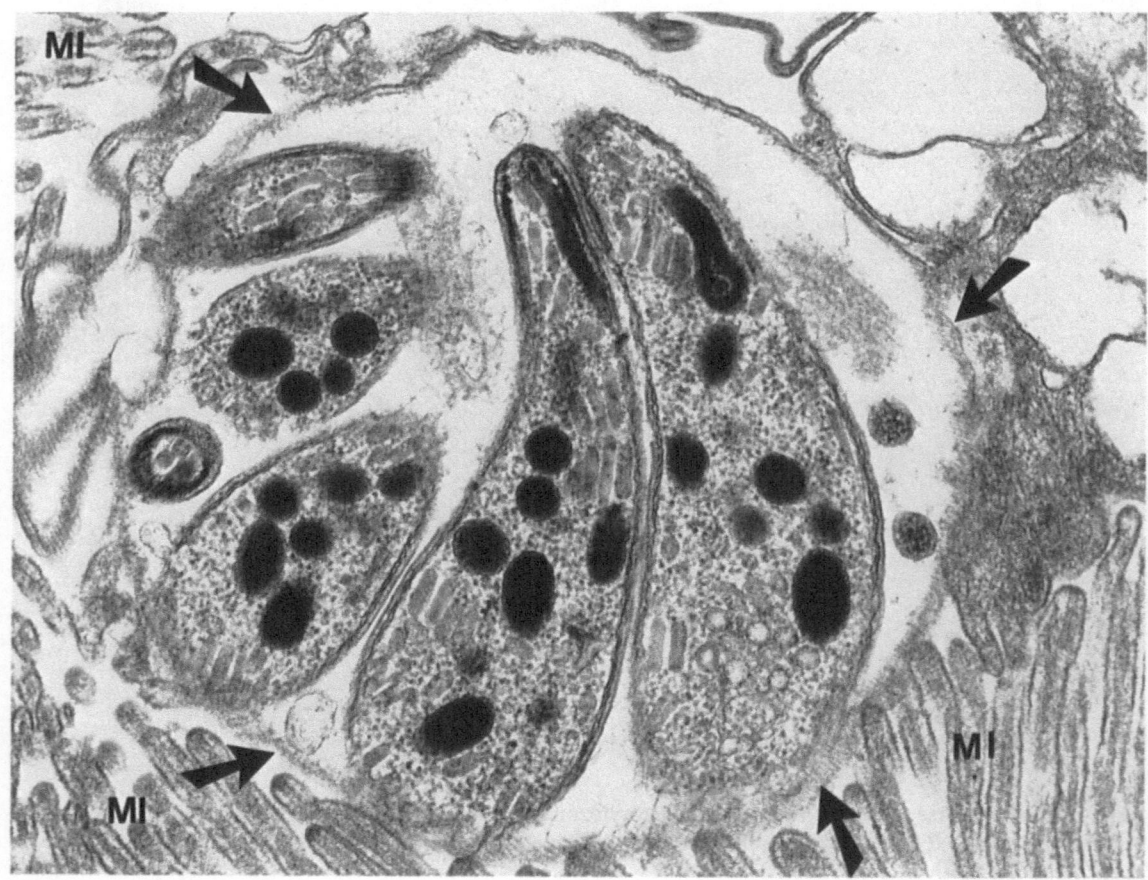

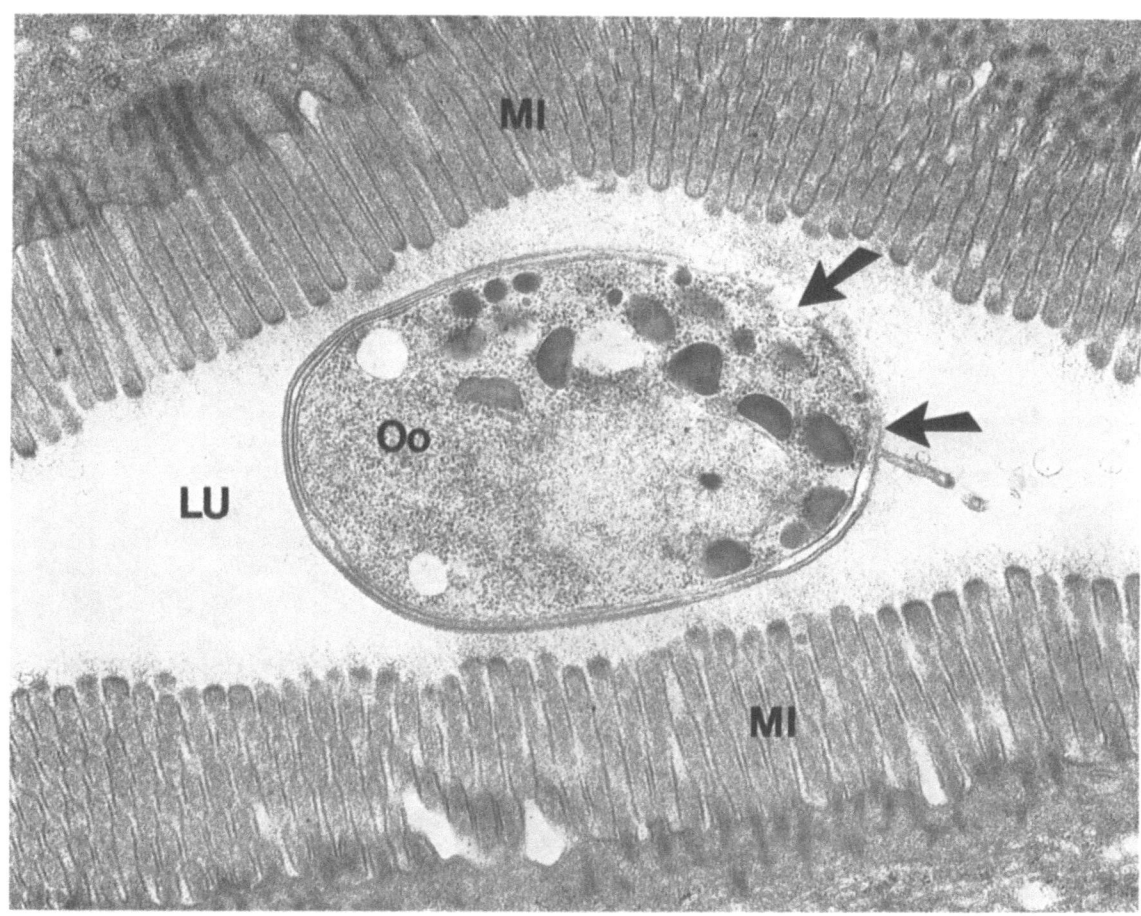

Fig. 5.19. Oocyst (*Oo*) of *Cryptosporidium wrairi* in the lumen (*LU*) near the mouth of a crypt. Note that the microvilli (*MI*) of enterocytes on either side are intact but that lysis of the oocyst capsule has occurred (*arrows*). (× 23 730)
Courtesy of Dr. R. Dourmashkin.

◁ **Fig. 5.16.** Light microscopy of the jejunal mucosa of a child with coccidial infection showing small cyst-like bodies in contact with the brush border (*arrows*). *EN*, enterocytes; *LP*, lamina propria. (H & E × 480)

◁ **Fig. 5.17.** Phase contrast micrograph of Epon-embedded tissue of same mucosa at higher magnification. The round, dense bodies (*arrows*) appear in intimate contact wth the microvilli (*MI*) but invasion of the enterocytes (*EN*) is not clearly visible. *GO*, goblet cell. (× 1320)

◁ **Fig. 5.18.** Ultrastructure of a trophozoite, probably *Cryptosporidium wrairi*, overlying the luminal end of microvilli (*MI*). Note lysis of the capsule surrounding the trophozoites (*arrows*). From the same patient as Figs. 5.16 and 5.17. (× 43 420)
Courtesy of Dr. R. Dourmashkin.

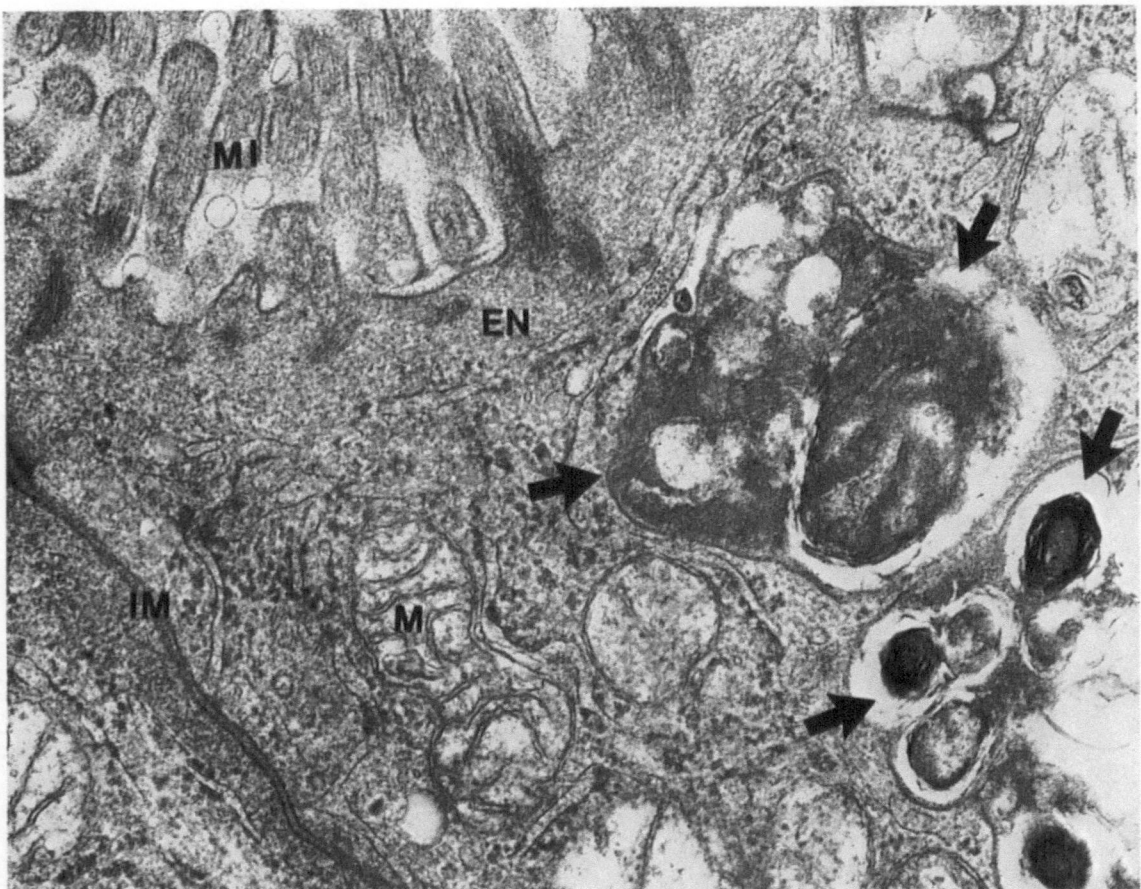

Fig. 5.20. Upper part of an enterocyte (*EN*) from the same mucosa showing apparent invasion and destruction of the trophozoite (*arrows*) within the cell cytoplasm. Lysis of the parasite by the enterocyte may be associated with minimal damage to the epithelial cell itself. *MI*, microvilli; *M*, mitochondria; *IM*, intercellular membrane. (× 55 400)

Whipple's Disease (Fig. 5.21)

The contribution of electron microscopy in Whipple's disease is an important one. Numerous reports [2, 15, 17, 26, 30, 33, 36] have described the presence of intact bacteria in close proximity to the enterocyte brush border, and probably also within the crypt lumen, and their ability to invade the mucosa in an intact state. Once the lamina propria is invaded (Fig. 5.22) the bacteria are taken up into the macrophages (Fig. 5.23) and mast cells [10] which, although they appear to be the primary defence mechanism, cannot readily destroy them. Although bacteria can be recognised within macrophages in free form, large vacuoles (?phagolysosomes) are also evident within these cells and are probably intimately related to the presence of the bacteria (Fig. 5.23). After treatment (antibiotics or steroids) the bacteria cannot be seen any longer within the lamina propria and the macrophages show an accumulation of granular, fibrillar or crystalline bodies, enclosed in smooth-membraned vesicles, in their cytoplasm (Figs. 5.24, 5.25). The crystalline material appears to persist long after treatment has begun and is probably responsible for the positive staining of the macrophages with periodic acid (Fig. 5.21).

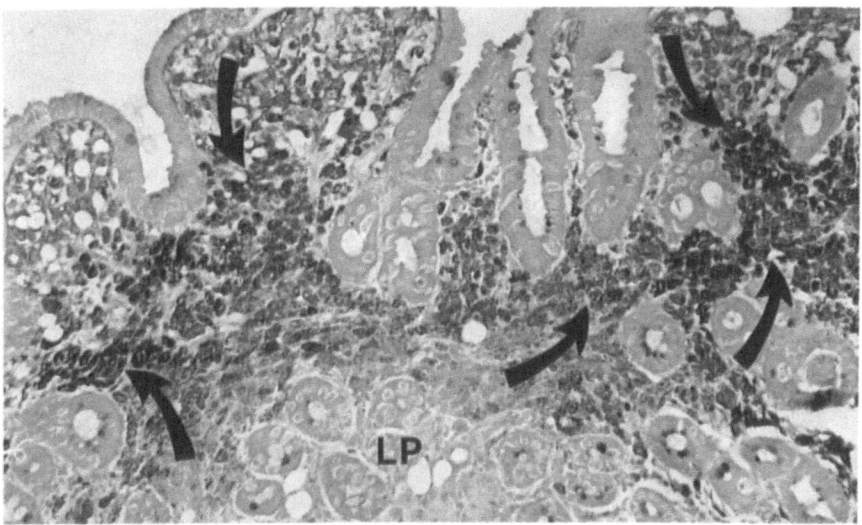

Fig. 5.21. Light micrograph of the jejunal mucosa from a patient with untreated Whipple's disease. Numerous macrophages (*arrows*) are seen in the lamina propria (*LP*). Periodic acid-Schiff stain. (× 200)

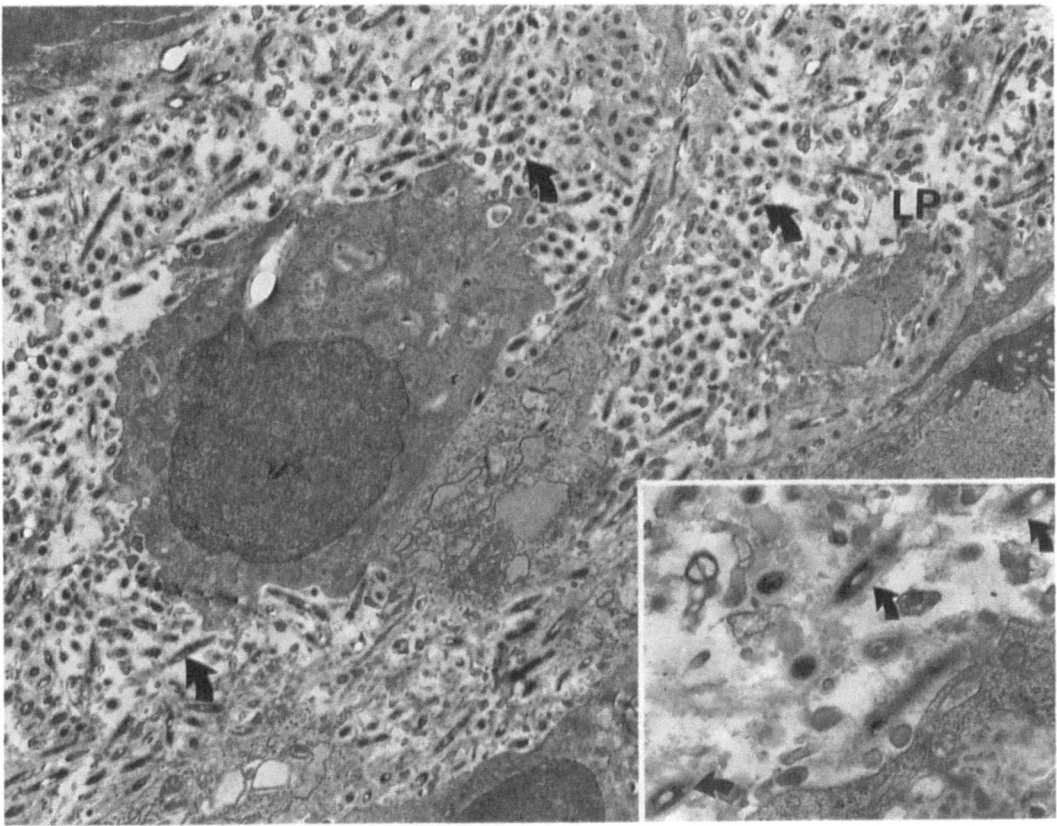

Fig. 5.22. Electron micrograph of lamina propria (*LP*) from a patient with Whipple's disease showing invasion of the connective tissue spaces by numerous bacteria (*arrows*), both rod shaped and coccal (*inset*). The bacteria do not show lysis. (× 2770)
Courtesy of Dr. F. Tavarela Veloso.

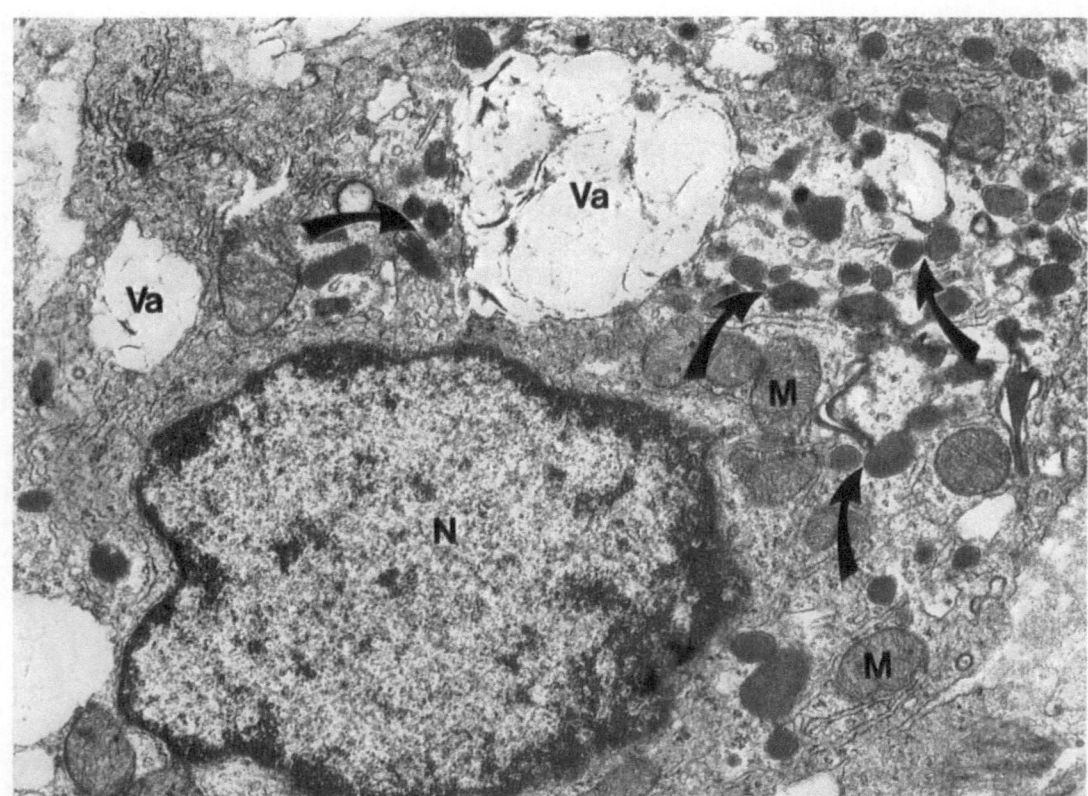

Fig. 5.23. △   **Fig. 5.24.** ▽

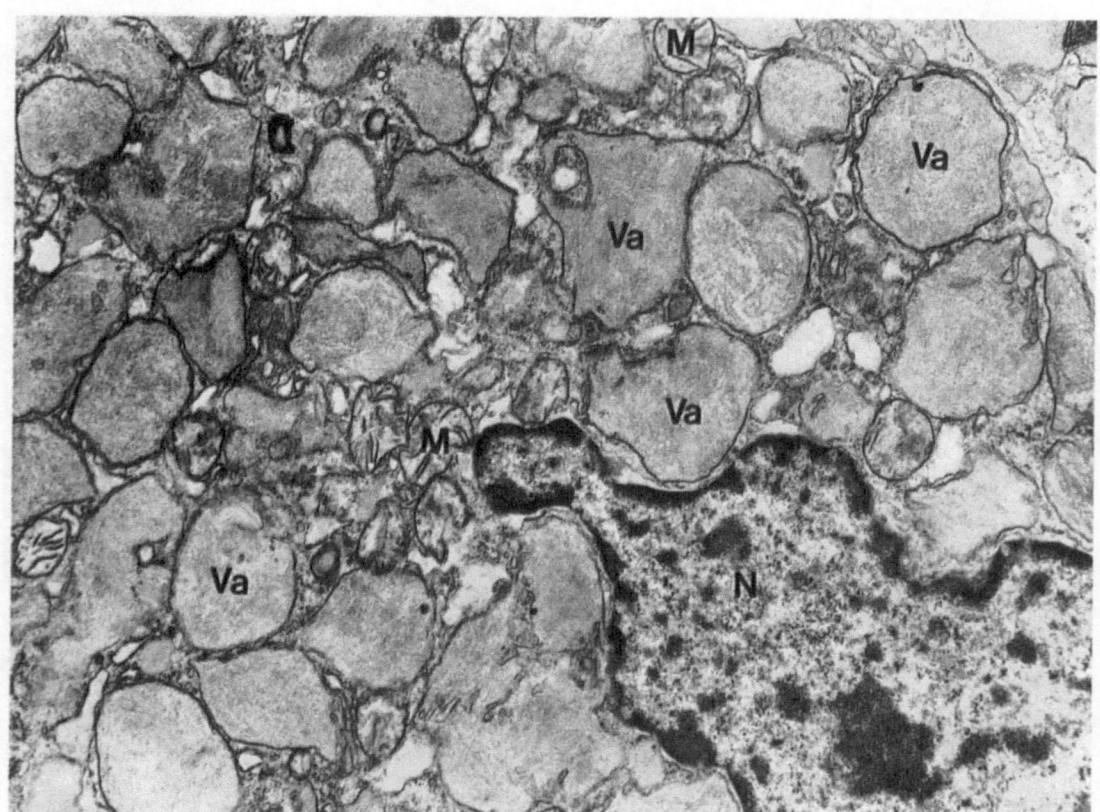

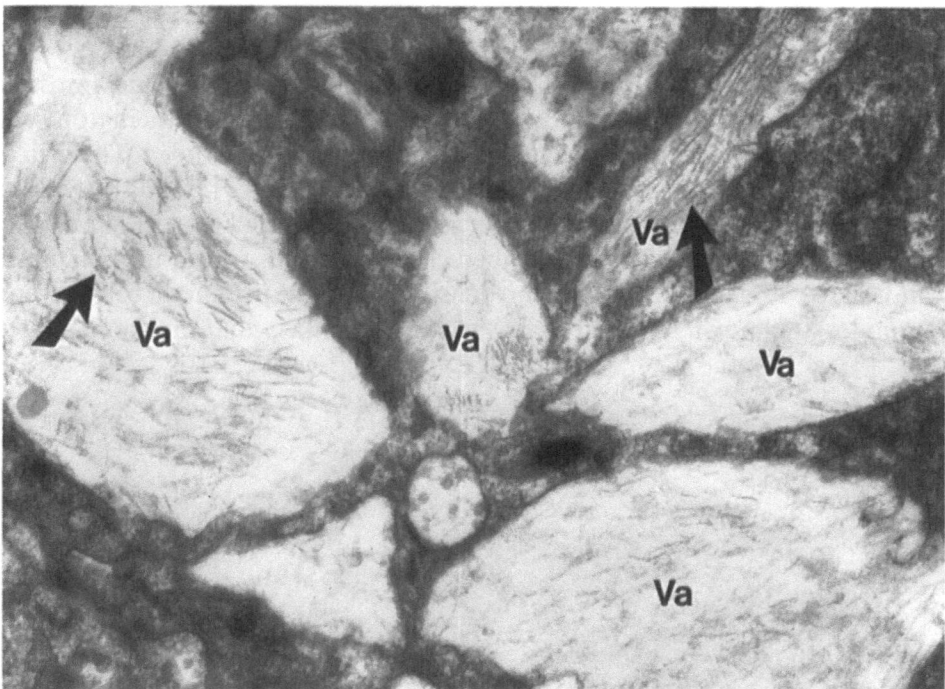

Fig. 5.25. Higher magnification of the cytoplasmic vacuoles (*Va*) of macrophages from the mucosa of a patient with Whipple's disease in remission. The vacuoles may be large and confluent and may contain fibrillar and crystalline material (*arrows*). (× 29 290)

Despite an extensive search into the type of bacteria which invade the mucosa in Whipple's disease, it is still not clear which of the invading organisms are responsible for the mucosal reaction. It seems certain that pathogens are not involved. The bacteria have been reported by some authors as gram positive, by others as gram negative rods or cocci. Since Whipple's disease is, in its late stages, a generalised disease which may affect other organs, it is likely that the pathogenetic defect lies in an abnormal response of the body to certain bacteria, possibly due to a lack of the normal immune defence mechanisms. The gut lumen, normally containing a bacterial flora, appears to be the primary route of invasion.

◁ **Fig. 5.23.** A macrophage from a patient with untreated Whipple's disease showing recognisable bacterial bodies (*arrows*) and large vacuoles (*Va*) in the cytoplasm. The presence of the vacuoles may indicate active phagolysis. *N*, nucleus of macrophage; *M*, mitochondria. (× 20 600)

◁ **Fig. 5.24.** A macrophage from the mucosa of a patient with Whipple's disease after treatment. The cytoplasm contains numerous large vacuoles (*Va*) enclosing fine granular or fibrillar material. No bacterial shapes can be recognised. *N*, nucleus; *M*, mitochondria. (× 15 350)
Courtesy of Dr. F. Taverela Veloso.

Acrodermatitis enteropathica

This congenital disorder of children, probably inherited as an autosomal recessive gene, shows the clinical features of an extensive erythematous rash, particularly around the orifices, associated with severe diarrhoea. The primary aetiological factor is a deficiency of zinc. Recently [5,18,31,34] ultrastructural abnormalities within the jejunal mucosa and particularly of the Paneth cell secretory granules have been described. These granules appear irregular in size and shape and heterogeneous in density (Fig. 5.26). Paneth cell secretory granules are known to incorporate zinc and it is likely that the comparatively

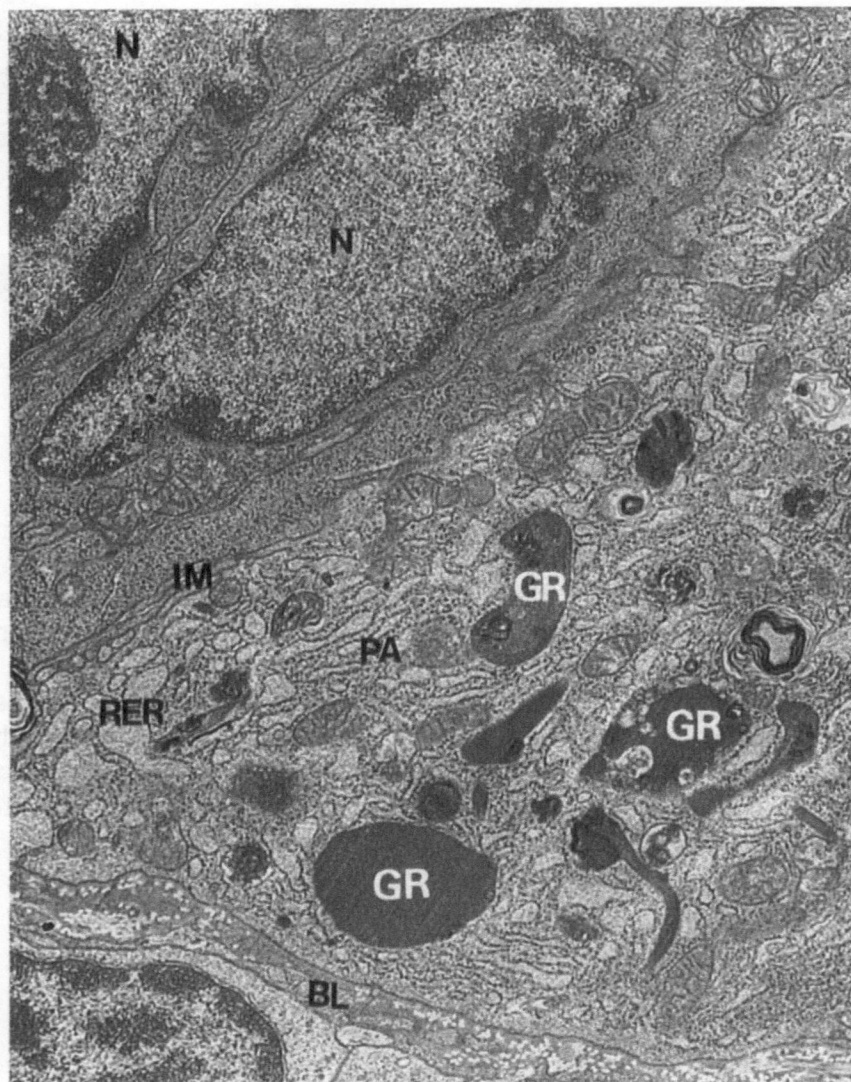

Fig. 5.26. Crypt epithelium from the jejunal mucosa of a child with acrodermatitis enteropathica. The Paneth cell (*PA*) shows several densely staining granules (*GR*) but these are abnormal in shape and lack uniformity in consistency (compare with Fig. 1.31), thus resembling lysosomes. The cell is rich in *RER*. The nuclei (*N*) of two adjacent crypt cells are seen resembling immature cell types. *BL*, basal lamina; *IM*, intercellular membranes. (× 12 560)

sparse and irregular granules seen in this disease owe their structural abnormality to a general deficiency of zinc. The clinical features of acrodermatitis enteropathica disappear when zinc sulphate is given orally.

Multiple sclerosis

The interest in the gut in this patchy demyelinating disease of the CNS is twofold: 1) Is the gut the mode of entry of agents which select their site of action in different organs (the central nervous tissue), for example a virus

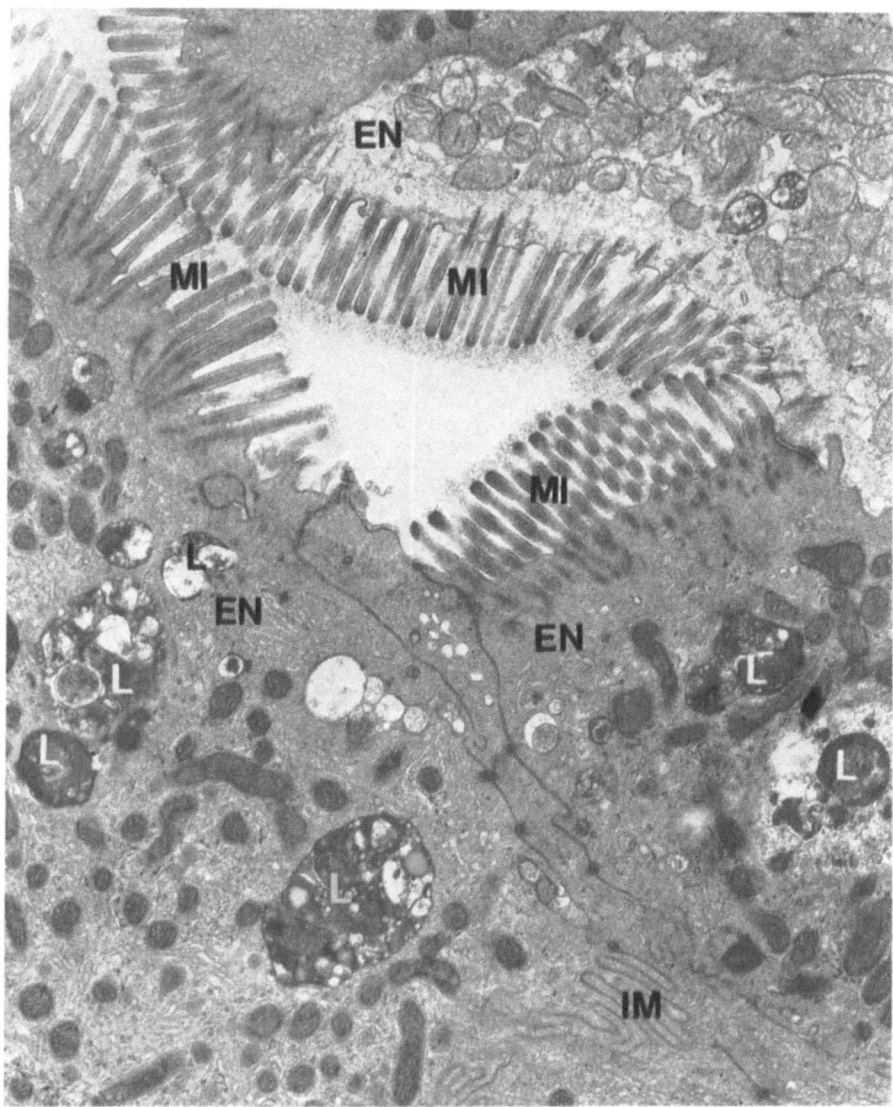

Fig. 5.27. Several enterocytes (*EN*) with normal microvilli (*MI*) from the villous region of the jejunal mucosa in multiple sclerosis. The cells appear essentially normal but lysosomes (*L*) are increased. *IM*, intercellular membranes. (× 10 654)

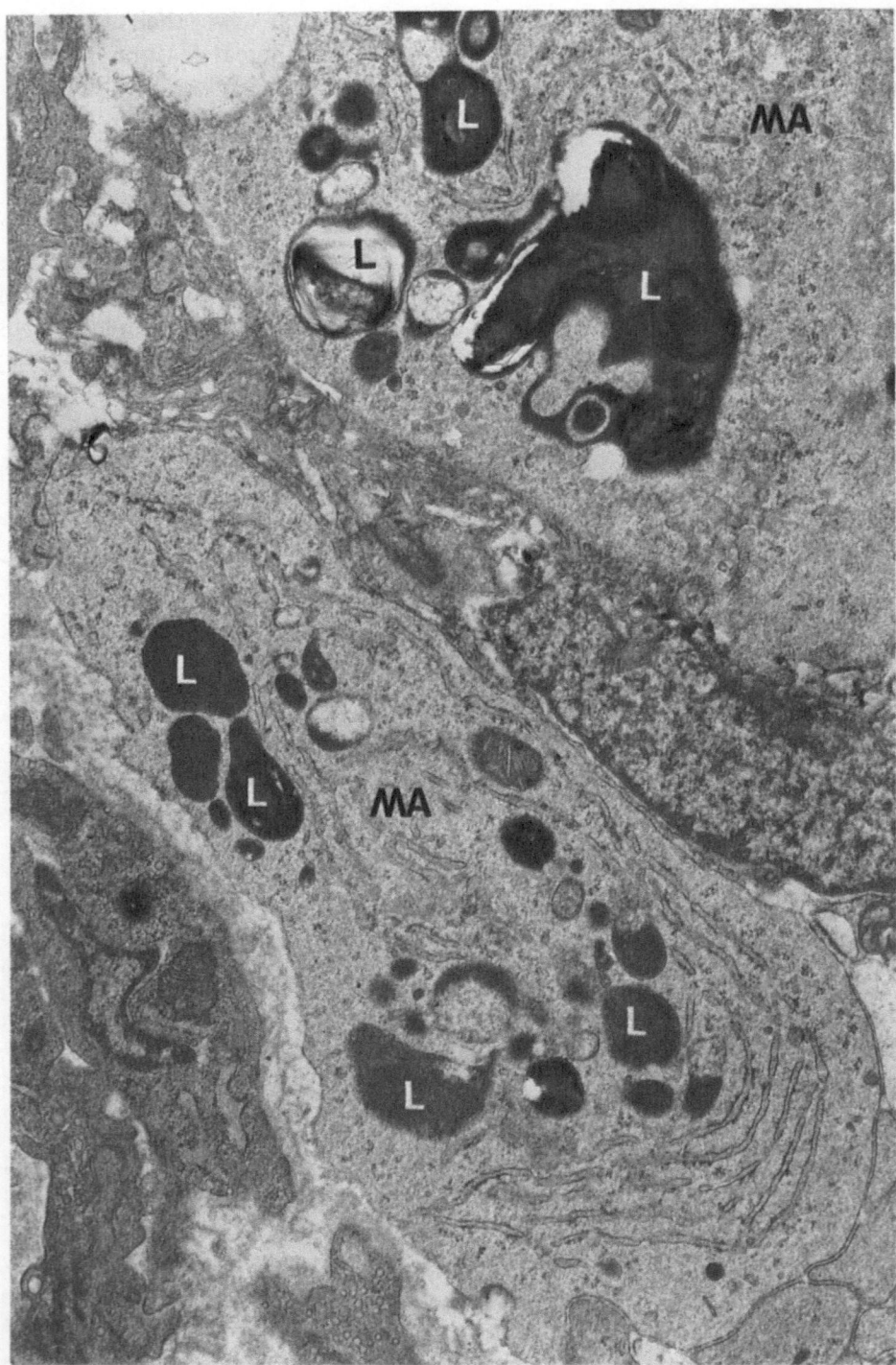

Fig. 5.28. Part of the cytoplasm of two macrophages (*MA*) in the lamina propria of the jejunal mucosa in multiple sclerosis showing large, densely staining lysosomes (*L*) which contain heterogeneous material. (×7210)

harboured in the gut which becomes activated at intervals? 2) Is the gut absorbing an abnormal substance (e.g. essential fatty acids) or polypeptides such as gluten which could be toxic to the neurons of the brain? In either case an abnormal immune response, caused by viral or protein antigens or a deficiency of the lipid components of the lymphocyte membranes[28], might be involved in the inflammatory response in the brain tissue, ultimately leading to a patchy necrosis.

Bearing in mind all the above-mentioned aetiological factors which might affect the jejunal mucosa in multiple sclerosis, it is easier to describe those which can be excluded than those actually found abnormal. The jejunal mucosal appearances do not show villous atrophy suggestive of coeliac disease, although in our study [27] 1 of 11 patients had a subtotal villous atrophy. The inflammatory cells within the lamina propria show some increase but this could be considered non-specific. Ultrastructurally the plasma cells, lymphocytes and eosinophils appear normal but lysosomes may be increased in the enterocytes (Fig. 5.27). Macrophages are numerous and their cytoplasm is filled with large phagolysosomes containing dense homogeneous or hetero-geneous material (Fig. 5.28). This substance does not appear to be lipid because oral feeding with linolenic acid, a lipid thought to be deficient in

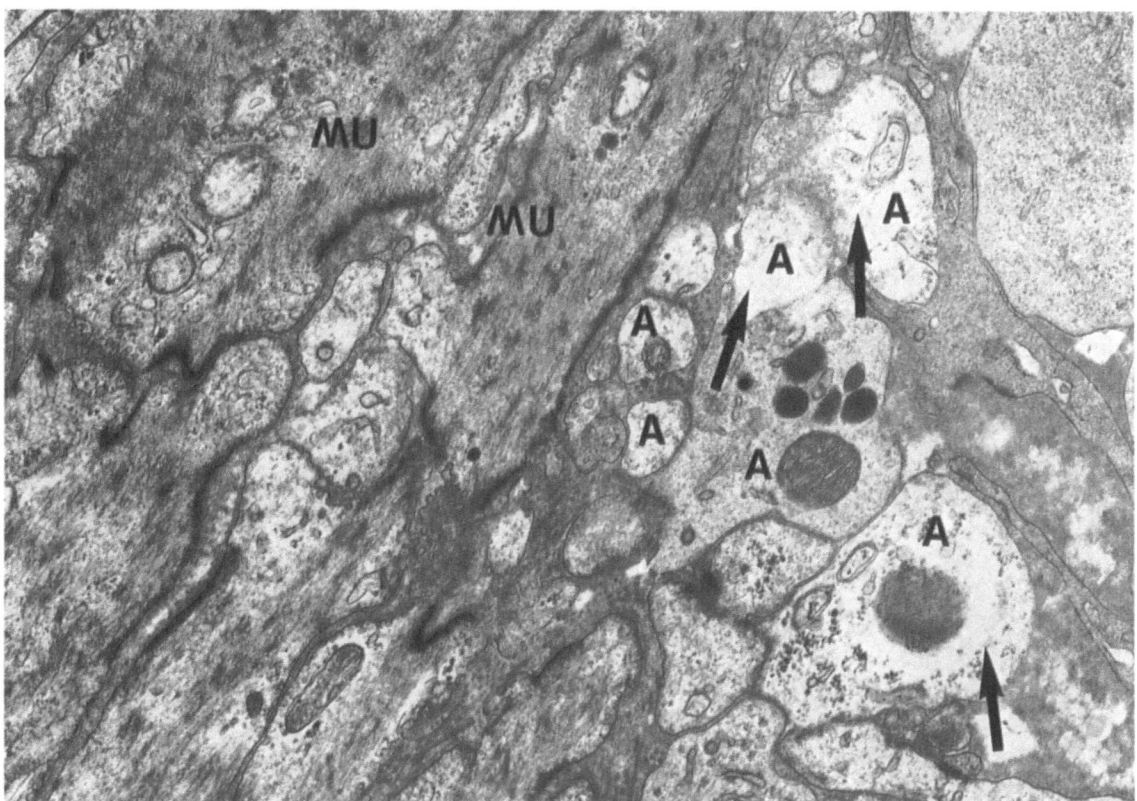

Fig. 5.29. Several axons (*A*) in close association with smooth muscle fibres (*MU*) of the muscularis mucosae in multiple sclerosis. There is swelling of some of the axons (*arrows*) with loss of electron density of their axoplasm. (×18 130)

multiple sclerosis [1], shows that the fat is taken up normally by the villous epithelium and that it is not retained abnormally in macrophages (personal observation). The nature of the lysosomal bodies within the jejunal macrophages remains obscure. It could signify active phagocytosis of a toxic or infective agent which has been absorbed or it could be part of an abnormal local immune response. We also observed an increase in fibrocytes and collagen in close association with swollen nerve cell axons (Figs. 5.29, 5.30). On the other hand a more recent study [4] failed to demonstrate any histological or ultrastructural abnormalities in multiple sclerosis resembling coeliac disease. A search for virus antigens in the jejunal mucosa has been unsuccessful [25], but some investigators [32] have claimed the recovery of paramyxovirus from the jejunal mucosa of patients with multiple sclerosis.

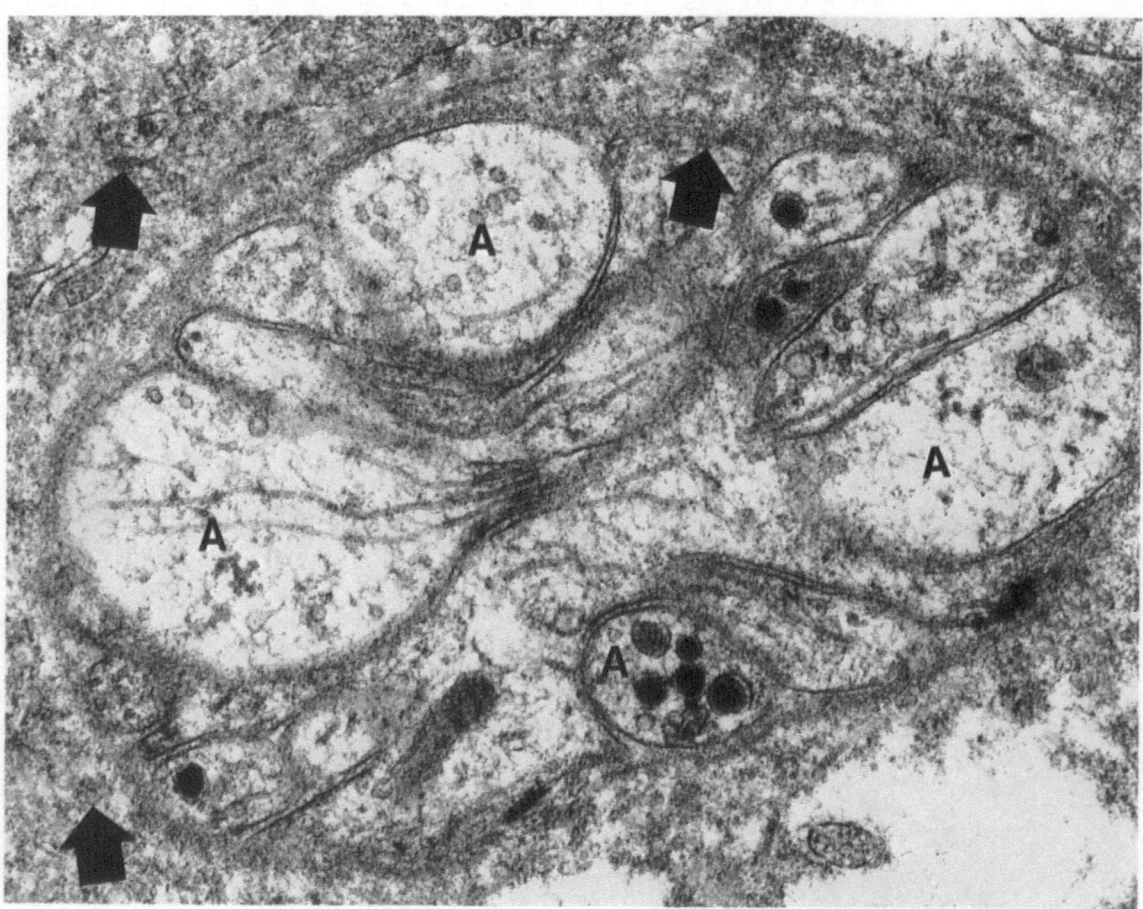

Fig. 5.30. A bundle of several axons (*A*) in the lamina propria in multiple sclerosis, surrounded by dense fibrous tissue (*arrows*). The axoplasm appears less electron dense than normal (compare with Fig. 1.50). (× 34 710)

Crohn's disease

The aetiology of this inflammatory bowel disease is as obscure as that of multiple sclerosis, but the site of pathological involvement and the major cell types involved are very different. The ultrastructure of the mucosa and submucosa at the site of the lesion has been described in detail [8, 12, 13, 14] and in particular, fine structural proof of viral particles has been sought [16, 35]. It is known that functional changes can occur in the small bowel which is not pathologically involved. We have therefore studied the 'uninvolved' mucosa, which appeared histologically normal or showed a mild partial villous atrophy, often with excessive vacuolation of the enterocyte of the jejunal villi (Fig. 5.31).

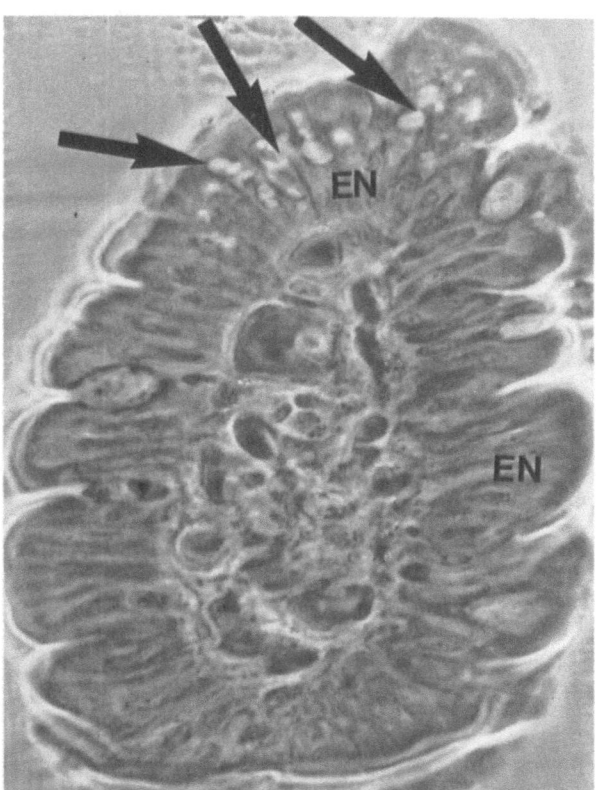

Fig. 5.31. Phase contrast micrograph showing a cross-section of a villus from the 'uninvolved' jejunal mucosa in Crohn's disease. There is vacuolation (*arrows*) in the enterocytes (*EN*). (× 1100)

Ultrastructurally the microvilli appear somewhat shorter than normal (Fig. 5.32) and sometimes they are unusually irregular. There is excessive extrusion of enterocytes (Fig. 5.33) and when this affects several cells it could lead to the formation of shallow micro-ulcers. The cytoplasm of the enterocyte often shows an excess of vacuoles (Fig. 5.34) lined by smooth endoplasmic reticulum. These vacuoles do not appear to contain any recognisable material and may be regarded as dilated ER, perhaps secondary to cytoplasmic damage.

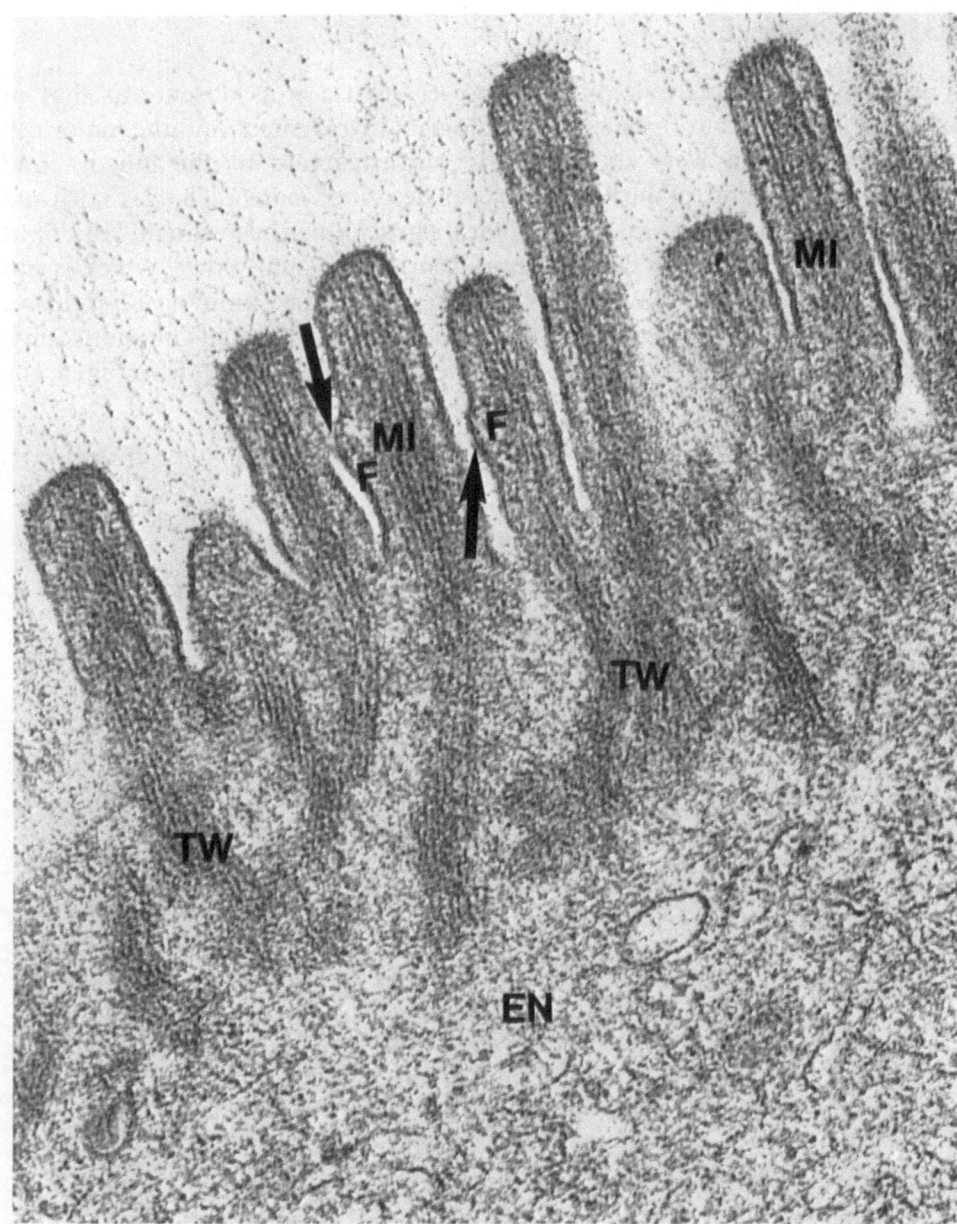

Fig. 5.32. Upper part of an enterocyte (*EN*) from the villous region of the uninvolved jejunal mucosa in a patient with Crohn's disease showing short irregular microvilli (*MI*). Some of these have bulbous outgrowths (*arrows*) and at these sites the microvillous membranes and the microvillous filaments (*F*) may appear damaged. *TW*, terminal web. (×81 760)

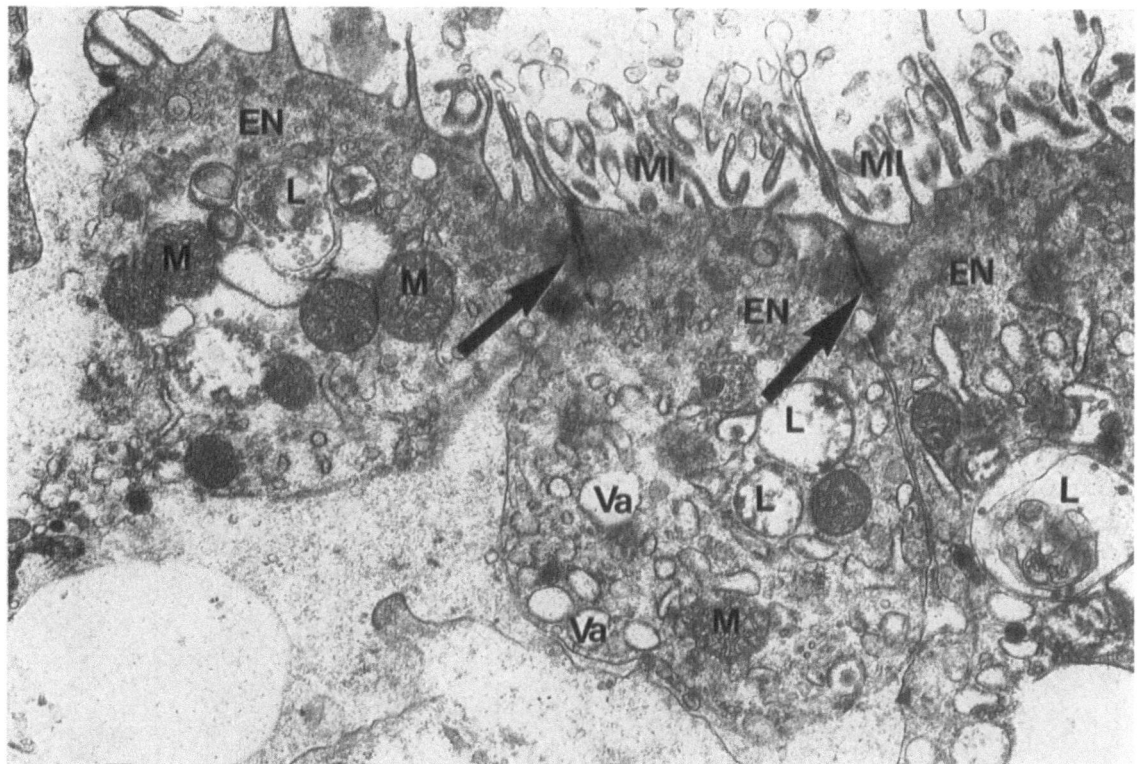

Fig. 5.33. Three enterocytes (*EN*), near the tips of villi in Crohn's disease, in the process of extrusion. The cells appear obviously damaged though they are still joined by intercellular junctions (*arrows*). The microvilli (*MI*) are bulbous and irregular. The intracellular organelles show an increase in lysosomes (*L*) and vacuoles (*Va*), though the mitochondria (*M*) appear normal. (× 8890)

The mitochondria may be normal or may show swelling and disruption of their cristae (Fig. 5.34). The enterocyte nucleus appears normal. Other fine-structural changes such as thickening of the basal laminae of enterocytes and endothelium (Fig. 5.35), increase in the fibrous tissue of the lamina propria, and degranulation of mast cells (Fig. 5.36) have been observed. There appears to be no increase in the number or activity of the macrophages but histiocytes are numerous in the lamina propria (Fig. 5.35). Viruses or viral particles have not been identified in the uninvolved mucosa. It is uncertain whether the changes described in the enterocytes have any significance but they may explain some of the defects in the absorptive capacity of the small bowel described. If this is so, the fine structural appearances of the enterocyte may offer one more proof that Crohn's disease affects the bowel to a much larger extent than can be attributed to observed macroscopic or microscopic involvement.

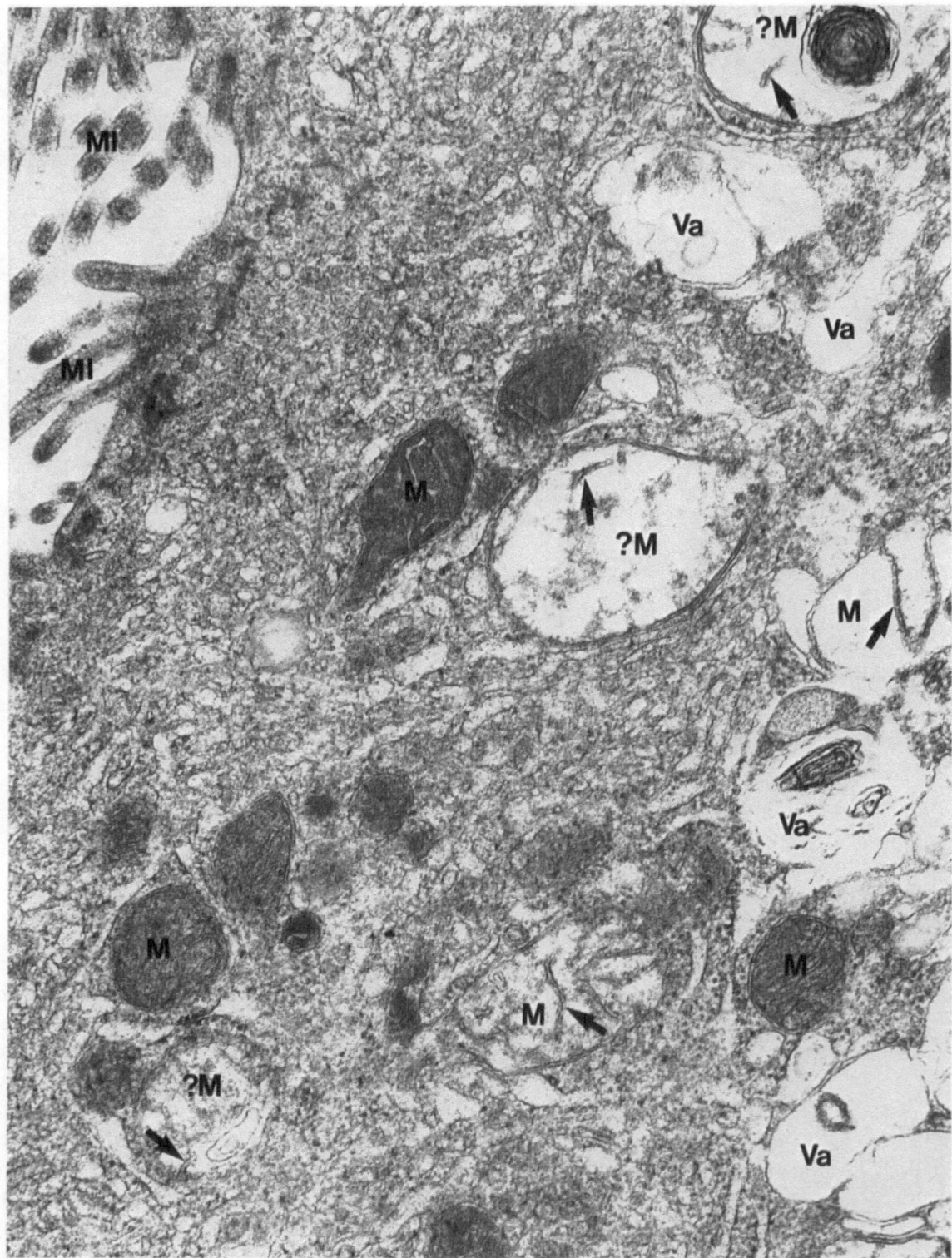

Fig. 5.34. Upper half of an enterocyte from the mid-villous region in Crohn's disease showing large cytoplasmic vacuoles (*Va*) lined by smooth membrane. Other vacuoles appear to be surrounded by double membranes and may represent swollen mitochondria because a few disrupted cristae are still visible (*arrows*). Some mitochondria (*M*) appear normal. *MI*, microvilli. (× 14 360)

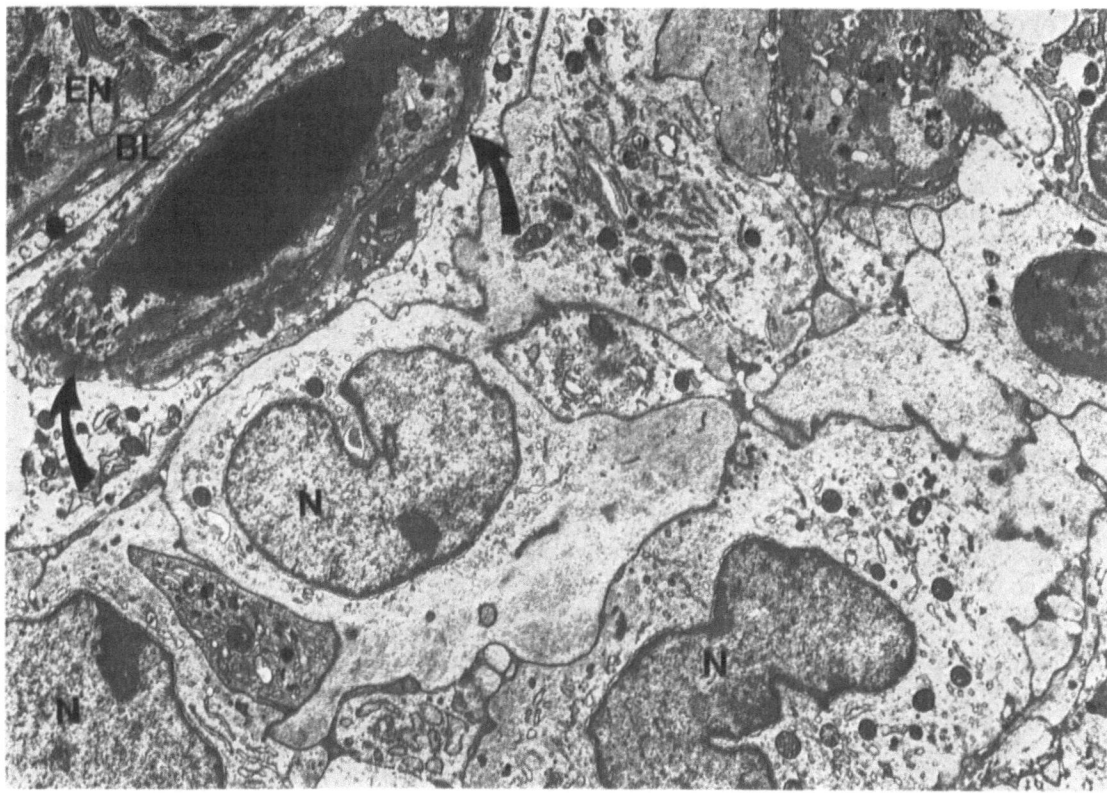

Fig. 5.35. Lamina propria in Crohn's disease immediately below the enterocytes (*EN*), showing thickening of the basal laminae (*BL*) of enterocytes and small blood vessel endothelium (*arrows*). Below the blood vessel the nuclei (*N*) of three histiocytes can be identified. (× 5790)

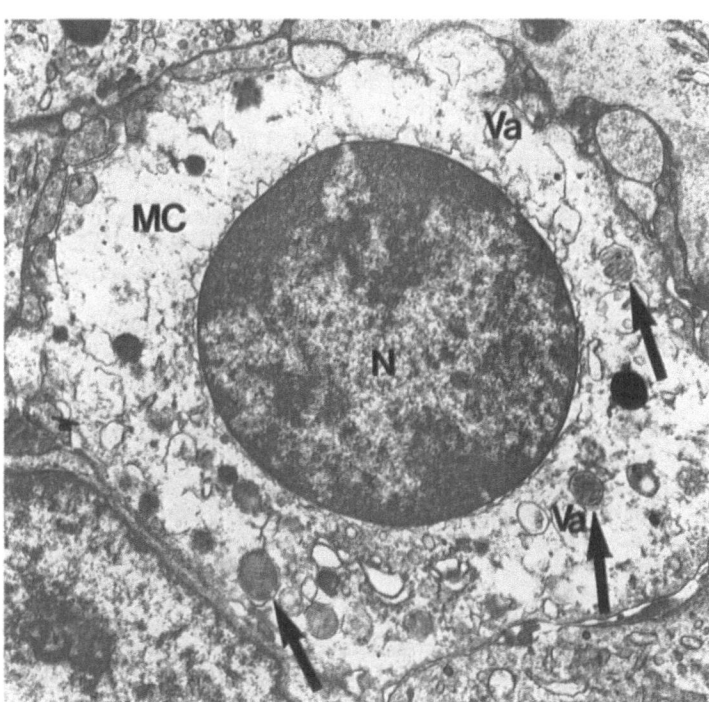

Fig. 5.36. An almost totally degranulated mast cell (*MC*) with its central nucleus (*N*) in the lamina propria in Crohn's disease. The cytoplasm contains a few small dense and heterogeneous granules (*arrows*) and some empty vacuoles (*Va*). (× 8750)

References

1. Baker RWR, Thompson RHS, Zilkha KJ (1964) Serum fatty acids in multiple sclerosis. J Neurol Neurosurg Psychiatry 27:408–414
2. Ballazs M (1979) Repeated light- and electron-microscopic studies of the small-bowel mucosa in Whipple's disease. Exp Pathol (Jena) 17:249–263
3. Barbieri D, DeBrito T, Hoshino S et al. (1970) Giardiasis in childhood. Absorption tests and biochemistry, histochemistry, light and electron microscopy of jejunal mucosa. Arch Dis Child 454:466–472
4. Bateson MC, Hopwood D, McGillivray JB (1979) Jejunal morphology in multiple sclerosis. Lancet i:1108–1110
5. Baudon JJ, Fontaine JL, Larrègue M, Feldmann G, Laplane R (1978) Acrodermatitis enteropathica. Anatomo-clinical study of 2 familial cases treated with zinc sulfate. Arch Fr Pediatr 35:63–73
6. Brandborg LL, Tankersley CB, Gottlieb S, Barancik M, Sartor VE (1967) Histological demonstration of mucosal invasion by giardia lamblia in man. Gastroenterology 52:143–150
7. Brooks SE, Audretsch J, Miller CG, Sparke B (1970) Electron microscopy of giardia lamblia in human jejunal biopsies. J Med Microbiol 3:196–199
8. Cook MG, Turnbull GJ (1975) A hypothesis for the pathogenesis of Crohn's disease based on an ultrastructural study. Virchows Arch (Pathol Anat) 365:327–336
9. Djaldetti M (1976) Crystalline inclusions in multiple myeloma. Case histories in human medicine, No 10. Philips, Holland
10. Dobbins WO III, Kawanishi H (1981) Bacillary characteristics in Whipple's disease: an electron microscopic study. Gastroenterology 80:1468–1475
11. Doe WF, Henry K, Hobbs JR et al. (1972) Five cases of alpha chain disease. Gut 13:947–957
12. Dvorak AM (1980) Ultrastructural evidence for release of major basic protein-containing crystalline cores of eosinophil granules in vivo: cytotoxic potential in Crohn's disease. J Immunol 125:460–462
13. Dvorak AM, Dickersin GR (1979) Crohn's disease: electron microscopic studies. Pathol Annu 14: 259–306
14. Dvorak AM, Dickersin GR (1980) Crohn's disease: transmission electron microscopic studies. I. Barrier function. Possible changes related to alterations of cell coat, mucous coat, epithelial cells, and Paneth cells. Hum Pathol 11:561–571
15. Dybker R, Kok N (1965) Bacteria in Whipple's disease. 3. Studies in two patients of antibodies in serum and cutaneous hypersensitivity against some bacterial antigens. Acta Pathol Microbiol Scand 64:373–380
16. Gitnick GL, Rosen VJ (1976) Electron microscopic studies of viral agents in Crohn's disease. Lancet ii:217–219
17. Greenberger NJ, DeLor CJ, Fisher J et al. (1971) Whipple's disease. Characterization of anaerobic corynebacteria and demonstration of bacilli in vascular endothelium. Am J Dig Dis 16:1127–1136
18. Heilmann K, Rossner JA, Braun O (1973) Light and electron microscopy studies on biopsies of the small intestine in acrodermatitis enteropathica. Verh Dtsch Ges Pathol 57:450
19. Henry K (1975) Electron microscopy in the non-Hodgkin's lymphomata. Br J Cancer 31 [Suppl II]: 73–93
20. Henry K, Farrer-Brown G (1977) Primary lymphomas of the gastrointestinal tract. I. Plasma cell tumours. Histopathol 1:53–76
21. Horowitz A, Shiner M (1981) The recognition of premalignant change in jejunal mucosal biopsies of patients with malabsorption. J Submicrosc Cytol 13:423–443
22. Isaacson P, Wright DH (1978) Intestinal lymphoma associated with malabsorption. Lancet i:67–70
23. Isaacson P, Wright DH (1978) Malignant histiocytes of the intestine. Its relationship to malabsorption and ulcerative jejunitis. Hum Pathol 9:661–667
24. Isaacson P, Wright DH (1980) Malabsorption and intestinal lymphomas. In: Wright R (ed) Recent advances in gastrointestinal pathology. Saunders, London-Philadelphia-Toronto, pp 193–212
25. Kingston D, Shiner M, Lange LS, Mertin J, Meade C (1977) Measles antigen in jejunal mucosa in multiple sclerosis. Lancet i:1313
26. Lamberty J, Varela PY, Font RG, Jarvis BW, Coover J (1974) Whipple's disease: light and electron microscopy study. Arch Pathol 98:325–330

27. Lange LS, Shiner M (1976) Small bowel abnormalities in multiple sclerosis. Lancet ii:1319–1322

28. Mertin J, Hughes D, Stewart-Wynne E (1974) P.H.A. transformation in multiple sclerosis. Inhibition by linoleic acid. Lancet i:1005–1006

29. Morecki R, Parker JG (1967) Ultrastructural studies of the human giardia lamblia and subjacent jejunal mucosa in a subject with steatorrhoea. Gastroenterology 52:151–164

30. Morningstar WA (1975) Whipple's disease. An example of the value of the electron microscope in diagnosis, follow-up, and correlation of a pathologic process. Hum Pathol 6:443–454

31. Polanco I, Nistal M, Guerrero J, Vázquez C (1976) Acrodermatitis enteropathica, zinc, and ultrastructural lesions in Paneth cells. Lancet i:430

32. Prasad I, Broome JD, Pertschuk LP, Gupta J, Cook AW (1977) Recovery of paramyxovirus from the jejunum of patients with multiple sclerosis. Lancet i:1117–1119

33. Puppala AR, Singh S, Munaswamy M (1978) Whipple's disease. Endoscopic documentation, light and electron microscopic features in an 80-year-old man. Am J Gastroenterol 70:407–411

34. Rayhanzadeh S, Dantzig P (1974) Acrodermatitis enteropathica, with pathologic findings in jejunum and skin. Pediatrics 54:77–80

35. Riemann JF (1977) Further electron microscopic evidence of virus-like particles in Crohn's disease. Acta Hepatogastroenterol (Stuttg) 24:116–118

36. Roberts DM, Themann H, Knust FJ, Preston FE, Donaldson JR (1970) An electron-microscope study of bacteria in two cases of Whipple's disease. J Pathol 100:249–255

37. Sanel FT, Lepore MJ (1968) Granular and crystalline deposits in perinuclear and ergastoplasmic cisternae of human lamina propria cells. Exp Mol Pathol 9:110–124

38. Scotto J, Stralin H, Caroli J (1970) Ultrastructural study of two cases of alpha-chain disease. Gut 11:782–788

39. Shiner M (1979) Malignant potential of intestinal plasma cells in alpha-chain disease. Lancet i:156–157

40. Stemmermann GN, Hayashi T, Glober GA (1980) Cryptosporidiosis. Report of a fatal case complicated by disseminated toxoplasmosis. Am J Med 69:637–642

41. Tandon BW, Puri BK, Ghandi PC, Tewari SG (1974) Mucosal surface injury of jejunal mucosa in patients with giardiasis: an electron microscopic study. Indian J Med Res 62:1838–1842

42. Trier JS, Moxey PC, Schimmel EM, Robles E (1974) Chronic intestinal coccidiosis in man: intestinal morphology and response to treatment. Gastroenterology 66:923–935

43. Weinstein L, Edelstein SM, Madara JL et al. (1981) Intestinal cryptosporidiosis complicated by disseminated cytomegalovirus infection. Gastroenterology 81:584–591

Subject Index